Serenades for A Tango with Cancer

"This is one of those stories none of us envision ourselves being the heroine (or the hero), but the sad reality of our times is that we most likely we will be. Apryl Allen's well-written and riveting memoir of her battle, not just with a dreaded and frightening disease, but with our insensitive, uncaring, and inhumane healthcare system, is compelling, engrossing and alarmingly accurate. *A Tango with Cancer* is one of those vital books that should sit on every American's nightstand, because even if you escape cancer yourself, it's a good bet one of your family members or a close friend won't. As a cancer survivor myself and, as of six months ago, having endured sarcasm, duplicitousness and disdain during the care of my husband who died of leukemia, I know of wherefore I speak. The torture of this painful disease was ungodly, but because he was an "unhealthy" patient, translate that to "terminal", he was only valuable to the hospital as long as his insurance held out. Shockingly, we have devolved in our efforts to help our fellow human beings. This spot light that Apryl Allen illuminates, is not centered on herself. This selfless, passionate and courageous woman has spent two years of her life bringing this book to the public domain—her only wish is to help others through this maze of insanity."

— *Catherine Lanigan*
Cancer Survivor
Caregiver to Spouse with Cancer
Author of: Romancing the Stone
　　　　　The Jewel of the Nile
　　　　　Angel Watch Series
　　　　　and forty novels

"A very interesting read for me, a cancer survivor. Apryl shares her story in an educational and emotional way that made me think about how different yet the same we all are. She is a true story teller deep from her heart. *A Tango with Cancer* is full of enlightenment, spirit and passion."

— *Billie Jo Herberger*
Cancer Survivor
Author & Philanthropist

Serenades Continued...

"This heartfelt compelling guide, a lifesaver for any patient, caregiver, or loved one is a must read for anyone confronted with cancer. Apryl Allen shares her compassion, experience, and wit. Read Apryl's book and you have a new caring friend."

— *Pat (Patricia) Brilliant*
Loyal Friend & Supporter

"I first met Apryl at the Gym we both work out at. I noticed one day she seemed very quiet not the Apryl we all know! It is then she shared with me her diagnosis of Cancer. She wanted to reach out to me because I was a friend but also I lost my wife to Cancer after a 22-year battle. When I first met with Apryl and Ken to discuss my experiences with Cancer we discussed many things associated with it but also I tried to prepare them both for some of what was to come.

Cancer is a team event you have many Doctors and professionals on the medical side of things as you can imagine. But you also better prepare and set up your own team for support and help as you fight your battle. Cancer is all consuming to the one inflicted and it also creates collateral damage to those around you. Your caregivers and family need to know what is ahead of them and be prepared.

Apryl and I discussed this at length but I don't think it really sunk in until she was in the middle of the battle. Cancer can be defeated with all the new treatments available but if you as a patient or caregiver are not leading that charge and have the mind set to do that it will be a long battle. I unfortunately had to learn that from 22 years watching the strongest woman I have ever known deal with cancer head on and with Grace.

This book is a great look into just what to expect when confronting Cancer. I wish a book like this was available to me 22 years ago, we might have prepared differently for my families battle with the disease. Thank you Apryl for sharing your experience."

— *Scott McPherson*
Husband
Caregiver to Spouse with Cancer

A Tango with Cancer
My Perilous Dance with Healthcare & Healing

Apryl Allen

Genuine gratitude is expressed for permission to use lyrics from
"Keep It Loose, Keep It Tight" and "All My Friends" by Amos Lee
Copyright ℗ © 2005 Blue Note Records
a trademark of Capitol Records, Inc. All rights reserved.

Oray Publishing, [2016]

This publication contains the opinions and ideas of its author. It is intended to provide helpful and informative material on the subjects addressed in the publication. It is sold with the understanding that the author and publisher are not engaged in rendering medical, health, or any other kind of personal professional services in the book. The reader should consult his or her medical, health, or other competent professional before adopting any of the suggestions in this book or drawing inferences from it. The author and publisher specifically disclaim all responsibility for any liability, loss, or risk, personal or otherwise, which is incurred as a consequence, directly or indirectly, of the use and application of any of the contents in this book.

Copyright © 2016 by Apryl D. Allen

All Rights Reserved

No part of this book may be reproduced, stored in a retrieval system, or transmitted by any means, electronic, mechanical, photocopying, recording, or otherwise, without written permission from the author.

ISBN: 978-1-943767-75-5 (hardback)
ISBN: 978-1-943767-74-8 (paperback)
ISBN: 978-1-943767-76-2 (eBook)
LCCN: 2016914234

Jacket & Interior Book Design by Apryl Allen
Jacket Artwork by Jacques Barbey

LCSH: Allen, Apryl. | Breast–Cancer–Patients–United States–Personal narratives. | Cancer–Patients–United States–Personal narratives. | Breast cancer patients' writings, American. | Breast–Cancer–United States–Economic aspects. | Cancer–United States–Economic aspects. | Breast–Cancer–Patients–Care. | Medical care–United States–Economic aspects. | Medical care, Cost of. | Medical personnel–United States–Psychological aspects. | Medical personnel–United States–Social aspects. | Altruism–United States. | BISAC: HEALTH & FITNESS / Diseases / Cancer. | HEALTH & FITNESS / Women's Health. | BIOGRAPHY & AUTOBIOGRAPHY / Medical.

LCC: RC280.B8 A45 2016 | DDC: 362.19699/4490092–dc23

for:

My husband
Kenneth Lewis Allen
You are my every breath

My mother
Ada Riddles Hettich
1922 - 2002
You taught me courage
You give me strength
I miss you dearly

My friend
Katherine Amalie Koppel
1966 – 2016
The circle of a bracelet is forever

Soundtrack

	Prelude	1
	Introduction	
	1. In The Air Tonight	5
	Phil Collins	
	2. Wildfire	13
	Michael Martin Murphy	
	3. Rumor Has It	25
	Adele	
	4. Keep It Loose, Keep It Tight	31
	Amos Lee	
	5. My Way	40
	Los Lonely Boys	
	6. Face the World	54
	Apryl Allen	
	7. Freedom	69
	Anthony Hamilton & Elayna Boynton	
	8. Qué Sera Sera	80
	Pink Martini	
	9. Time in a Bottle	97
	Jim Croce	
	10. Morningstar	111
	Apryl Allen	
	11. I'll Wait	119
	Taylor Dane	
	12. Silent Strength	128
	Apryl Allen	
	13. I Believe	142
	Apryl Allen	

Soundtrack Continued...

14. **It's Too Late**		153
Sabrina Malheiros		
15. **Erased**		169
Annie Lennox		
16. **El Tango** *(de Roxanne)*		187
Jose Feliciano, Ewan McGregor & Jacek Koman		
17. **Black & White**		198
Apryl Allen		
18. **Nowhere to Run**		207
Michael McDonald		
19. **A Million Miles Away**		224
Lenny Kravitz		
20. **Tangled**		236
Maroon 5		
21. **Tightrope**		251
Stevie Ray Vaughan		
22. **Money**		258
Pink Floyd		
23. **Windmills of Your Mind**		267
Sting		
24. **Velvet Voice**		286
Apryl Allen, Julio Fernandez & Richie Cannata		
25. **Million Years Ago**		297
Adele		
A Final Note		312
Conclusion		
Acknowledgements		314
About the Author		315

Prelude

A mirror doesn't lie. The hard cold truth in its reflection is *fear* when you hear the word *Cancer*. What follows is a terrifying reality that completely strips you of the life you currently know. Throughout this insidious period, you learn that fighting *Cancer* isn't necessarily limited to eradicating it from your body. Too often it continues with the healthcare system that's supposed to heal us.

The mere mention of *Breast Cancer* conjured what I had seen in the media and have experienced within our society: Bald women, scarves, pink, a "Spiritual Journey," the Susan G. Komen Foundation, Race for the Cure, pink ribbons, emotional women with their daughters at a finish line, and well *(big breath)* . . . PINK again!

Tragically, my mother passed away from breast cancer at the age of 79. However, I remained optimistic about my own health, primarily because my family does not have a history of *Cancer*. My mother began taking estrogen at age 76 to alleviate a throbbing pain in her shoulder—which it did. But shortly thereafter all sorts of health issues ensued, eventually leading to breast cancer. She was initially diagnosed in 1999, and after her surgery, was in remission until 2001. In September of that year, the cancer came back with a vengeance, this time throughout her entire body. Her doctor gave her six months to live. She passed away on April 20, 2002. My last conversation with her was on my 35th birthday.

April 20th was a Saturday in 2002. The following Monday I was diagnosed with melanoma. A year later I found myself in need of a hysterectomy, and a couple of weeks prior to that surgery had another melanoma removed. I remember thinking, *Okay, if this is the cancer I am to be labeled with I can deal with it.* Of course, we never know what our future holds . . .

My former self: Miss Arizona USA 1993, an actress, musician, singer, songwriter, Comanche storyteller and author, who has written and recorded two award-winning albums, currently authoring a Native American trilogy while simultaneously composing its musical. (Breath.) Falling madly in love, I married a high-profile architect and became not only his wife, but his firm's CFO overseeing administrative, legal, financial and human resource issues (including negotiating our company health insurance).

That's who I was until my life came to a screeching halt in 2013 — *Breast Cancer*. Now I consider myself well equipped to battle this disease: I'm in good health, my husband and I (to some extent) are well-connected with friends who are doctors, we know individuals who are highly respected within our medical community, we have good insurance and are financially sound.

Speaking of sound, I have named each chapter after various songs. I've indicated which version by the vocalists' rendition (in some instances I've included the names of instrumentalists that are showcased too). The reasons why I chose these songs vary: a couple played a role in my healing, some I sang to the cancerous nodule as if it were a person or illicit lover, others reflect how I felt at the time — the constant baring of my breasts and having them fondled by strangers left me feeling exposed and vulnerable.

As I refuse to give into this disease completely, I changed the titles of my doctors that had anything to do with, *ahem* . . . *Cancer*. I chose names I felt were more befitting due to the doctors' physical and personality traits, or what they represented to me. Okay, and yes, I renamed a few others who played a not so endearing role during this period of my life. Eventually the cancerous nodule and lymph node were renamed too. Throughout this book you will come to know them as the following:

Breast Cancer Nodule	Jorge
1 Cancerous Lymph Node	Lymph-Along-Kid
Family Physician	Dr. KnowItAll
Radiologist	Breast Investigator
Breast Surgeon	Medicine Woman
Oncologist #1	Mad Scientist
Nurse Navigator #2	Nightmare Navigator
Radiation Oncologist	Radiation Man
Reconstructive Surgeon	Shape Shifter
Life Coach & Therapist	High Priestess
Oncologist #2	The King
Oncologist #3	Dr. Cool
Health Insurance	ACME Insurance

Besides the renaming of my doctors, there are a few very special individuals I had to choose unique names for in the retelling of my *Tango*. They simply had to have meanings that would reflect the loving qualities they brought to me during this period of my life. Below are their names, meanings and pronunciations:

Adelaide – (A-də-layd)
In French the meaning of the name Adelaide is Nobility. French form of the Old German is a compound of 'athal' (noble) and 'haida' (hood).

Clíona – (KLEE-a-na)
According to Old Irish legends, Clíona is the name of one of the three beautiful daughters of the poet Manannán mac Lir. In other myths, she is a goddess of love and beauty. Yet others depict her as a fairy and the guardian spirit of the MacCarthy's. Clíona is said to have three brightly colored magical birds who eat apples from an otherworldly tree and whose sweet song heals the sick.

Malaika – (muh-lī-kuh)
In Swahili the meaning of the name Malaika is Angel. As is the case with many Swahili words, it is ultimately derived from Arabic.

Pedro
The name Pedro is of Spanish and Portuguese origin and derived from the Latin word "Petra" meaning "rock" or "stone".

Aliza
Means joy. In Kabbalah it signifies the joyful ability to rise above nature.

Lastly, as they say . . . all names in this book have been changed to protect the innocent, the not so innocent, and the downright mean and guilty!

1

In The Air Tonight
Phil Collins

In the back of my mind I knew I was past due for a couple of annual exams. The two I dread most are my mammograms and skin check-ups. Most women can relate to my fear of mammograms, but mine was a little more personal. First, I always think of my mother and find myself holding back tears and other emotions. Second, a couple of these appointments turned into biopsies—who needs that added stress! And third, a mishap caused by the Imaging Center itself.

Annually I check my credit reports and noticed a blemish on my otherwise perfect score. It reflected a medical bill for $60 that had been sent to collections. To make a weeklong saga to correct this mistake short, the Imaging Center had entered the wrong mailing address—ergo I never received the invoice. No other attempts were made to contact me and the unpaid bill was sent to collections. As I pointed out to the collections agent, "You don't get perfect credit by ignoring $60 bills." This only fueled my procrastination over scheduling my mammogram.

As for the skin check-ups, I attribute its postponement to travel and busy schedules. It seemed every time I made appointments for my husband and myself, they inevitably would be cancelled. Either our dermatologist would be out of town, or vice versa. Then we were told she decided to focus her practice in other areas and turned all of her patients over to a *younger* woman. It had taken me several years to find someone with whom I felt comfortable. Trust in healthcare is something rare and I really liked our dermatologist.

Postponing these appointments became easier as my sole focus was placed on my husband's business. Small business and the economy took all of our attention, and while I kept up with other health appointments, I let the two aforementioned slide. Stress took center stage as our business began treading water. Our main focus became keeping our business alive and employees employed. This was how 2010 ended for us.

Fast forward to mid-May 2013 . . . my friend Adelaide and I booked ourselves a four-day spa retreat in Sedona, Arizona. From Thursday, June 27th through Sunday, June 30th we would be pampered nonstop with various spa treatments and elixirs. Throughout this glorious weekend we'd be oiled, rubbed, exfoliated, wrapped in hot linens, hot stoned and hot tubbed. We'd also embark upon various activities and adventures meant to stimulate our mind, body and soul—hiking, walks, workouts, water aerobics and yes . . . meditation.

During this same period, I ran into a friend at the gym, and for whatever reason we began discussing dermatologists. It ends up he goes to the same dermatologist we do. "I really like who she chose to take over her practice," he informed me.

"Okay, I've got to schedule an appointment." And for the next couple weeks every time I ran into our friend Seth, I was embarrassed to report, "No, I haven't scheduled the appointment."

Eventually I succumbed and scheduled appointments with *all* of our doctors—our annual physicals, eye exams, dermatologist, you name it, I scheduled it. Earlier that year I had appointments with both my dentist and gynecologist, wherein Dr. Gyno reminded me I needed to go in for my annual mammogram. Promises were made, but quickly placed on the back burner.

During my routine physical with our internist Dr. KnowItAll, he too inquired, "Have you gone in for a mammogram lately?"

"*Argh*—no, but I'll get it scheduled soon."

"I'm showing the last time you were in was June of 2010—two years ago."

"Wow . . . has it been that long?" *Well, no worries, I'm healthy and am confident nothing will come of it.* "Okay, I'll get it scheduled," thinking in the back of my mind I'd push it off until the fall—*who has time?*

My husband and I attempt to schedule our doctors' appointments together late in the afternoon. This way we can end our day with a martini. It's just something nice to look forward to—more so to take the edge off—allowing us to revel in our health and life!

In most cases we have the same doctors and I take the first appointment. Such was the case on June 21, 2013, with Dr. KnowItAll. Concluding my annual physical he invites me to join him in his office after

I realign my ensemble. Entering the small room, I take a seat across from him at his desk and we catch up on the various trips we've each taken over the past year. In the meantime, Ken enters the recently vacated exam room and readies himself for his physical. Concluding the details of his latest trip, Dr. KnowItAll excuses himself and disappears to greet Ken at his best. Looking around the room I spot a gossip magazine sitting on the chair next to me and start flipping through its pages to amuse myself. The hot topic with its scorching headline: *"Angelina Jolie opted for a double mastectomy."* Yikes . . . poor girl!!!

Dr. KnowItAll finished with Ken and joined me in his office again. Soon Ken followed. "Ken I'm a bit concerned with the rhythm of your heart — notice here how this beat is different from the others? I'd like to get you back on the EKG. It could just be the anxiety of being here. Ruford, please get Ken back on the EKG and let's get another reading of his heart."

Again the same strange rhythm was seen on the tape. "You should make an appointment with your cardiologist. I don't think it's anything we should be too concerned about, but just to be on the safe side, get the appointment scheduled. Also, I'd like you to have a chest X-ray. They'll do that for you downstairs."

Over the years, Ken and I have had X-rays completed downstairs. If Dr.KnowItAll's office was open, they were too. However, on this day fate played its role — they were closed. Ken and I were a bit in disbelief and simultaneously looked at our watches. He soon uttered exactly what I was thinking, "*Humph* . . . that's odd they're closed. In all the years we've been coming here I've never known them to be closed."

"Well, I guess it's for the best," I replied. "I need a mammogram and rather than putting it off until October I might as well get it over with. I'll call and schedule a chest X-ray for you and a mammogram for me." The next day we were set; I scheduled them both for Tuesday, June 25th. Unbeknownst to me my entire world was about to turn upside down!

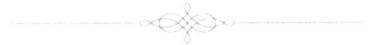

It's going to be a typical mammogram, I keep telling myself, *it has to be, Ken's here and nothing ever goes wrong at a doctor's appointment when he's with me — he's my lucky charm!* And then my name's called.

I follow the technician through a maze of hallways to the changing room. I know the drill, change into the gown with the opening in the front. She'll be back shortly to get me. Piece of cake—this is definitely *not* going to end with a biopsy like the last one did in 2010. Deep inside I wish Ken could be by my side for this entire process—primarily because I can't seem to shake a looming feeling that a storm is coming.

After donning the lovely gown, I take a seat in the waiting room. *Hmmm ... what to read—Angelina Jolie seems to be everywhere.* Well it doesn't matter, the tech's returned asking me to follow her to the infamous "Mammo Room." And here I stand, with my left breast in the machine all twisted and pressed, with one arm up and the other down.

"Okay, take a deep breath and hold it," the tech instructs. The soft whirring of the machine begins and I'm asked to do a couple more poses, then, "Okay, let's do the right side." And we repeat the same acrobatics on my right breast. "I love your skirt! Such beautiful tranquil blue colors. Where did you get it, in the Caribbean?" she asked while taking the last image.

"No, believe it or not, I found it at the mall."

"I wish I could find something like that," she mused. "We're finished here; I'll take you back to the waiting room while the Breast Investigator takes a look at your mammograms." *Okay and I'll get back to something other than Angelina Jolie and her "Double M."*

And there I sat, rummaging through the much handled magazines when the tech reappeared. "The Breast Investigator noticed a little something she'd like to get a better look at. Can you come back tomorrow for an ultrasound?"

Rats! "Yeah, sure."

"Okay, let's get you back up to the front to get it scheduled." Walking back seemed more confusing than the initial walk for the mammogram. Once at the front desk I scheduled my ultrasound for the next day, Wednesday, June 26th, at 1:30. Returning to the waiting area, I locked eyes with my husband's baby blues, now filled with trepidation. Without saying a word he asked, *"Another appointment?"*

"The doctor saw something she wants to get a better look at. I'm sure it's nothing, but they'd like me back tomorrow for an ultrasound." A bit disheartened, I left with high spirits. Surely it was nothing, just a little blip on the big screen of life.

In the meantime, the results for Ken's chest X-ray were sent to his cardiologist and Dr. KnowItAll. His cardiologist told him he'd like to monitor his heart for a few days and equipped Ken with a heart monitor. It would be removed on Tuesday, *after* my return from Sedona.

In my heart I knew Ken was fine—his chest X-ray played its role as the instigator for me to get a mammogram. Now we were just following the needed steps to assure this indeed was the case.

"Honey, maybe I should cancel the Sedona trip and stay home with you," I offered, feeling a bit concerned. I don't know, there just seemed to be something in the air tonight . . . a feeling . . . a warning possibly . . . but I couldn't quite place it.

"Absolutely not! If you do we'll just sit here staring at each other, wringing our hands waiting for its removal. I'd rather you go and enjoy a wonderful weekend with Adelaide. Besides, you've always wanted to go away with a girlfriend for a spa retreat." And that's my husband, always looking out for others first.

Since an ultrasound is relatively simple, I insisted Ken spend his day at the office. Once again I find myself waiting for my name to be called. Although, I didn't have to worry about idle time—it appears the office lost the paperwork I completed yesterday—because I was asked to complete the forms again. Once finished I turned my attention to a movie that was playing on a flat screen.

Eventually, "Apryl Allen?" rang through the waiting area. This time Penelope greeted me. Escorting me through the maze of halls, she took me to another changing room and handed me a folded sanitized gown with ties.

After changing I follow her into a 10 x 14-foot room where she instructs, "Please lay face-up on the bed. Are you warm enough? If not, I can get you a warm blanket?"

"No, I'm good. Thanks."

Feeling a bit apprehensive, we discussed how long she'd been doing this type of work while I watched her place clear gel on top of a magical wand. She then started the procedure. Thankfully, the gel was warm and I was saved from the shock of it being ice cold. We then scrutinized the monitor. "There's the little guy!" she exclaimed as she repeatedly moved the sensor over the lower left portion of my underarm. "*Hmmm*, he does look a little angry," she noted.

"Where exactly is he at?" I asked. After pointing him out to me on the black and white monitor I thought, *Yeah, he does look a little dark, and my underarm in that area has been feeling a bit sore. But that's just due to the time of month—I think. I mean, didn't he always get a little grumpy during this time?* Although I had a hysterectomy, they did leave my ovaries intact, as in I still have the monthly symptoms, just not my . . . *ahem, well, you know!*

"Let me get the Breast Investigator to take a look at him. She may want me to take a few more pictures."

"Okay, I have nowhere else to go," I said with an anxious smile.

When she returned, she relayed, "Yeah, she does want a few more."

I watched as Penelope worked the red ball on her mouse—clicking on various sides of the angry little guy, attempting to capture his best attributes. "Okay, you can sit up now. We're finished." She grabbed a handful of tissues for me to wipe off the gel. "The Breast Investigator wants to take a look at these and may want to speak with you. Please wait here," and she disappeared behind the door for the private screening.

Sitting on the table I looked around the room. *This is not my reality. This is not going to be my reality*, I silently assured myself. I then stood and walked to the end of the table and leaned with my back against the counter. *This is not what my future holds—I'm healthy!* I looked down at the bed I was just on and then around the room. I closed my eyes, taking a deep breath, and began releasing the air slowly between my lips.

That's when the door opened. Penelope had returned with the Breast Investigator. "Hi, Apryl, I'd like to have you come back for a biopsy. This little guy doesn't look too happy and I want to make sure everything's okay," were the first words the Breast Investigator uttered to me.

Double Rats! I felt my heart sink deep inside and my eyes immediately filled with tears. *Don't lose it, Apryl, be strong like Mom—find her strength. This is nothing. I know it is, just like before—nothing. Oh why didn't I have Ken, my lucky charm, come to this appointment?* "Do you think it's anything serious?" My voice was barely audible.

"We don't think so. We just want to rule out *any* possibilities."

"Okay, when would you like me back?"

"How about Friday morning?" Penelope inquired.

"Sure. Oh wait . . . what am I thinking? My girlfriend and I are going to Sedona for a spa retreat. We return Sunday night. Can it wait until Monday morning?"

"Penelope, introduce Apryl to Iris and see what times we have available on Monday morning. Apryl, besides having a wonderful time in Sedona, we'll need you to fast the morning of the biopsy. The procedure will take about two hours." The Breast Investigator then excused herself to return to, well . . . more investigating.

"All right, let's go see what we have available." I quickly changed and followed Penelope back through the maze of halls to meet Iris.

After cordialities, "What time would you like the appointment?" Iris inquired.

"What's the earliest you have?"

"Does 7:30 work?"

"Perfect! I'll see you bright and early Monday morning."

"Have a wonderful weekend in Sedona! And don't worry . . . we just want to rule out any *uncertainties*," Iris added.

Walking out the front door of the Imaging Center, I took a deep breath and let it out. Once in the car I slid my phone from my purse and dialed Ken's private line.

"Hey, Baby, how did it go?"

Big breath. "Well, they want me to come back for a biopsy."

"No! Oh, Apryl."

"Ken, I'm sure it's *nothing*, just like before. Besides, I really like the Breast Investigator. She makes me feel comfortable, and I know I'm in good hands. Plus, I remember my last biopsy being relatively easy—other than when she numbed me, but even that was reasonably painless. We're doing it when I return from Sedona on Monday morning first thing."

"Are you sure you're okay?"

"A little shaken, but fine."

"Okay, I'll see you at home shortly."

After I hung up, I sat there thinking, *it really is nothing*. I felt a calmness come over me and the strength of my beautiful mother enveloped me. I then picked up the phone and called my friend Adelaide.

"Hey, how'd it go?" she asked, skipping cordialities.

"Well . . . they want me back for a biopsy."

"No!"

"Yeah, but it's going to be fine. I really like this doctor. They just want to make sure it's nothing. She's done a biopsy on me before and it wasn't bad at all."

"When are you having it done?"

"At 7:30 Monday morning after we return from Sedona."

"Are you sure you still want to go?"

"Yes! It'll help keep my mind off of it."

"Okay then, we're on!"

"I'm headed home now—I'll talk to you later. Big hug and kiss!"

"You, too—bye."

Driving home I felt a bit uneasy. But my mind was already fast at work consoling me. *Apryl, you've been here before—you're going to be just fine! It really will be nothing!*

2
Wildfire
Michael Martin Murphy

Whether you believe in it or not, at some point *fate* will play a role in your life. Its guises are endless—mostly portraying the misconception that you're in control. In some instances, its mystical spinning threads lure its prey with a subtle intoxicating proposition; other times it's a euphoric feat or accomplishment. Of course there are those times when the deck's stacked against you—with no warning at all it slams you up against a wall, knocking the very breath from you. That's when you realize you're but a puppet in its mindless game. The truth is *fate* has the ability to catapult you into another world, another realm, and sometimes a completely different life.

If you ever find yourself in need of a biopsy, I *highly* recommend a spa retreat prior to having it. It relaxes you completely, allowing you to revel in life and your health. And that's exactly what Adelaide and I experienced—blissful, calming and tranquil. Honestly, it seemed there were no spare moments; there was always a treatment or activity we were scheduled for. Whenever the thought of my biopsy came to mind, I dismissed it knowing it would end as it did in June 2010 as *a non-event*. At the end of the weekend I actually forgot about my imminent appointment.

When I arrived home, after being greeted by our two sweet dogs, Princess Maddy and Loco Hugo, my loving and thoughtful husband reminded me of my notorious appointment. "Wow, I completely forgot about it!" and I really had!

That evening we went out for a quick dinner and then retired to bed early, to assure I had ample rest for my appointment. Thankfully, I felt refreshed and relaxed when I awoke the next morning. Although, what I didn't fully comprehend is this biopsy was on a lymph node, not the breast.

Regardless, I was feeling confident because I had brought my lucky charm—Ken!

The routine was identical to that on my previous visits—completing the *same* paperwork I had submitted *twice* already! *Does anyone bother to enter my personal information into a computer?* I wondered after I turned it in. *Sigh.* And we waited . . .

Penelope eventually appeared and began speaking with the front desk. I knew it was only moments before my name was called. Then she turned in my direction. "Hi, Apryl!"

"Hi, Penelope!" After giving my husband a quick kiss, he assured me he wouldn't move until I returned.

After slipping on the infamous frock, I followed Penelope into the procedure room. She then began to prep me for the biopsy—and this is where the spa retreat came into play. I felt as if I were having just another spa treatment. I put myself in the frame of mind that it was electrolysis *I had decided* to have done. It's not any more painful than that type of procedure. (I hope.)

"The Breast Investigator will be taking two to three samples of the lymph node, and then you'll be done." No sooner did Penelope finish her sentence than the door opened and in walked the doctor.

While greeting me, Penelope handed the Breast Investigator a paper draping. Placing it over my chest, its opening revealed the offending portion of my underarm. Seating herself on a stool she informed me, "I'm going to start with the numbing shot," and out came the needle. *It's just electrolysis. It's just electrolysis,* I silently chanted to myself as she gently poked me.

"Okay, let's give that a few minutes to completely numb the area. In the meantime, Penelope will cue up the angry little guy via ultrasound." The Breast Investigator then left while the anesthetic took effect. *Wasn't so bad,* I thought to myself.

Soon the Breast Investigator returned. "You should be completely numb now. Can you feel this?"

"No," I replied, knowing she truly wanted me to be completely relaxed and comfortable. Then she and Penelope began to speak another language. I know it was English, but I didn't understand a word.

"Okay, I'm going to insert the needle. If you feel any pain at all let me know immediately. You may feel a bit of pressure, but there should be no pain." I felt absolutely no pain whatsoever, but yes, oddly, I did feel the pressure. To get my mind off of what was happening I turned my attention to the monitor.

WOW! *How cool!* On the black and white screen I could see the needle going into my underarm. I didn't allow myself the opportunity to consider that what I saw on the monitor was actually happening to ME. We all watched the angry little guy and the needle moving its way towards him.

The Breast Investigator then informed me, "You're going to hear a loud clicking sound as I take the samples." And just as she said—*Clap!* "Okay, there's one," and out came the needle. "Now for the second." The needle went painlessly in again—*Clap!* "Since I'm getting such good samples I'm going to take one more." *Clap!* It was over.

"We're all finished! Penelope will clean and dress the area. We'll send the results to your doctor once we receive them. Please, no strenuous exercises or lifting of heavy items for about one week. There might be some bruising but that's normal. Do you have any questions?"

Hmmm, bruising, I don't remember that from the last time, I thought. "No, I can't think of any." *Dang ... how I wish it wasn't Dr. KnowItAll giving me the results.* He's so clinical and has a tendency, in a very rapid cadence, to prattle on in what I consider to be a different language. Forget about asking questions; they quickly dissipate as you're attempting to assimilate his next few sentences. No, I'd prefer to hear the results from my Gynecologist. *Oh well, it is what it is.*

"Tell your husband you're to be 'Queen for the Day'—absolutely no cooking. Now he can take you out for a much deserved breakfast!" And with that the Breast Investigator left the room. *This woman has no idea how much I trust her. She instills confidence which in turn keeps me calm.* I thought as Penelope took her vacated spot.

We again made idle chitchat as she dressed the biopsied area. And then came the tape. She must have considered me to be some sort of present minus the bow! "You're all finished—you can get dressed. Can I get you anything to drink? Apple juice, orange juice, water?"

"Mmm . . . apple juice sounds great!" I replied, following her out into the small hallway. As we walked through the door to the waiting room, I began removing my gown.

"No—not here!" Penelope chided. "The changing room is there," and she pointed to another small room. "This is just the waiting area."

"Oops! I'm so embarrassed!" and I silently chastised myself as I entered the changing room. *What am I thinking?!*

"I know, these rooms are so small — don't worry, people do it all the time," she said in an attempt to lessen my mortification.

Once inside the changing room, I hurriedly removed the gown and happily put on my own shirt. As I opened the door Penelope greeted me with a boxed apple juice. I followed her back through the hallways that made no sense whatsoever to the room where this all began. There, where the *real world* awaited with my loving husband. I looked into his eyes, which held many questions.

"Let's go to the car," I said saving the details for later. I was feeling a bit self-conscious and it felt as if all eyes in the waiting room were on me. Once outside I let out a breath I didn't realize I'd been holding. It was over — another mammogram and biopsy completed and I *won't* be returning until next year! At least that's what I told myself.

On our way home I called Adelaide to let her know how the biopsy went. "Apryl, Clíona is not doing well." Our friend had gone in for what was supposed to be a routine hysterectomy on Friday. However, due to complications, on Sunday evening she returned to the emergency room and was admitted for two days.

"My family and I are leaving first thing tomorrow morning for our vacation and Clíona needs someone to pick her up at 10. Can you do it?"

"Of course, no problem; is there anything else I can do?" *Anything to keep my mind off the relentlessly slow time clock ticking away to an arbitrary moment when the phone rings and I receive the results of the biopsy.*

"Yes, if you can check in on her during the week and maybe even spend the night with her — I don't feel comfortable with her being alone. I'm going to the hospital tonight to take her some things. How did your biopsy go?"

"Great, just waiting for results now. Let me know if there's anything I can do tonight."

"Will do . . ." and we said our goodbyes.

After telling Ken about Clíona he reminded me, "Honey, that's when my appointment is to have my heart monitor removed."

"Oh, I completely forgot. Well, Clíona needs our help. Would it be too much of an imposition to help her? She doesn't have anyone else," I pleaded.

"I didn't realize that, of course we can. As soon as my appointment's over I'll meet you there." I knew I could count on *Mr. Wonderful!* That's what my mom called him when she first met him. Actually, it was a nickname my friends gave him and, well, it just stuck!

Shortly after returning home, the tape from my biopsy started irritating my skin and I decided to remove it. When I took my shirt off we couldn't believe the amount of tape that was used. You would have thought I had major surgery.

"Dang . . . I forgot about the tape and how much it loves my skin," I said, lamenting the removal of it.

"I'll help you take it off," Ken offered and began doing so as gently as he could, but *Ouch . . . it HURT!* My stomach was in knots and nausea began to set in.

"Honey, I think I'm going to have to remove it myself. Can you get me a washcloth please?" After soaking it in hot water I wrung most of it out and placed the warm wet cloth on the bandage, drenching it. I then began peeling the tape off inch by inch. After doing so my skin was left with bright red welts. I placed some face cream on them, then dressed myself in comfy cozy attire and joined Ken in our media room for a much needed distraction.

At 10 o'clock the next morning, while parking, Ken phoned. "I'm here; it didn't take any time to remove the monitor." While gathering my things, he appeared opening my car door.

Together we walked towards the entrance of the hospital and its sliding glass doors. They opened swiftly and the all too familiar smell engulfed my senses as we walked through them. *Dang, I hate the smell of hospitals*, I thought as all of the memories of my mother came flooding back. I had to force myself to suppress them — now wasn't the time.

After all she'd been through there was no diminishing Clíona's beauty. Of course it took a couple of hours to get her discharged from the hospital. As the nurses were going through her exit procedures they handed me her prescriptions. I looked at them, then handed them back to the nurse. "Can you please call this in to her pharmacy?" I inquired.

"No, sorry—we can't," the nurse replied.

"What do you mean you can't? Of course you can. It will save us a lot of time and we'd be incredibly grateful." I added the last words purely for effect.

You'd have thought I asked the nurse to cut off her left arm by the look she gave me. Realizing I wasn't going to take no for an answer she took the scripts from me. "I'll see what I can do."

After providing her with both the phone and fax numbers to the pharmacy, it only took her 40 *minutes* to get the prescription phoned in. At this point we were all starting to get hungry.

As we collected Clíona's belongings Ken offered, "I'll get the prescription from the pharmacy and lunch too, then I'll meet you at her house."

"Perfect!" I responded.

Once at her home I helped Clíona settle in and busied myself organizing while she showered. Afterwards, I assisted with the bandages as the nurses had dictated. While doing so I told her of my run in with the tape. Sliding a drawer open, she reached in and pulled out a roll of white medical tape. "I have the same problem; this is what I have doctors use. It's hypoallergenic tape. Here, you can have this roll," she offered.

Knowing she might require it again, "I won't be needing it anytime soon, but I'll take the packaging if you don't mind?" I said as I ripped off the portion that indicated the brand and type of tape. I'd pick some up the next time I was at the pharmacy. *Only for future use of course—I won't be needing it anytime soon!*

Ken arrived with lunch and her medication, then immediately left for home to shower and ready himself for the day; I'd meet him later at the office. Removing the bottles from the bag I handed them to Clíona as she sat down at the table. Once we were both settled, after serving lunch, I started babbling about lord only knows what, when I saw a look flash across her face. "Are you okay?" I asked with concern.

"Yes," she replied, nodding at the same time, and immediately followed her response with a deep breath in through her nose. "I think I just need to sit quietly for a while," she said, silently letting her breath out.

"No problem," I said, understanding. And there we sat soundlessly together and began eating our lunch.

Rudely, our reverie was interrupted when my mobile phone began urgently ringing. Picking it up with the intention of silencing the ringer I looked at the incoming number. "Hmmm . . . I don't recognize this number; I'll just see who it is. Hello?"

"Hello, Apryl, this is Iris from the Breast Investigator's office. We've faxed your results to Dr. KnowItAll and I always like to do a follow-up call to ensure it was received. However, it says his phone number is out of order. Is he still in business?" she inquired worriedly.

"Yes, we were just there a week or so ago. That's odd . . . I know they put the phones on night ring from 12-1 for lunch. Was it maybe his answering service you got?"

"No, it definitely said it was out of order and I tried it three different times. What number do you have for him?" she asked.

I quickly looked up his number and read off each digit. "That's exactly what I have," she concluded. "Well, since we're unable to reach him, the Breast Investigator would like to give you your results." Without waiting for my response Iris placed me on hold.

Wow, this is really nice of them to call with my results, I thought—not noticing the flashing neon danger sign hovering overhead. No doctor calls with good news, and that's when I was struck by lightning!

"Hello, Apryl, this is the Breast Investigator. We got your results back and, honey, I'm sorry to tell you this, but it came back as cancer."

"What?!" *Obviously, I didn't hear her correctly.*

"Yes, I'm sorry, honey."

I felt myself crouch down towards the floor in efforts to steady myself. The room was not just spinning, but tumbling in all directions. Eventually I found my breath as words formed on my lips. "So, what do I do now?" I asked the Breast Investigator.

"We need to get you in for an MRI and find out where exactly the cancer is coming from."

"Okay, I'll call back to schedule it. Thank you for taking the time to call with the results," and I ended a phone call that I never thought I'd receive during my lifetime. How ironic that I had told Ken I wished the Breast Investigator would be the one to call with my results. Be careful what you wish for—right?!

Looking to Clíona I felt my world begin to crumble. "Clíona . . . Oh Clíona . . . what do I do? I don't understand . . ." tears began tumbling down my cheeks.

I didn't quite fathom how Clíona kept herself so calm. She sat for a moment, then placed her hands on either side of her plate. Spreading her fingers wide she closed her eyes and inhaled. As she slowly let out her breath she brought her fingers back together and I watched as she slipped her hands from the table. It was as if I were watching life in slow motion. She slowly stood, walked over to me and gave me a *ginormous* hug.

Standing with our arms wrapped around one another, time came to a standstill. Finally, one by one my senses came back and I pulled myself together. As the world around me started to come back into focus it dawned on me, *Apryl, get a hold of yourself; Clíona has just been through a horrible experience herself.*

When we finally released one another, Clíona took both my hands in hers. "Apryl, I've been here twice with my mom. One thing I know for sure is that you will be just fine."

"Yes, I will . . ."

"You need to call Ken now," and she tenderly squeezed my hands.

With tearful eyes and shaky hands I pick up my phone. *How could I have forgotten about Ken?* After a big breath I pressed the few buttons it took to dial our home phone. "Hi Honey, the Breast Investigator called with my results. It came back as cancer!" I heard myself repeat the ill-fated words.

"Oh, Apryl—NO!" I could feel his heart literally burst over the phone. Thank God he had the heart monitor removed; otherwise it surely would have imploded at that very moment. "I'll be right there."

Ending the call, I decided to get the MRI scheduled *immediately* and rang Iris back. She had an opening the next day, July 3rd, at 10 o'clock. I figured I was under the gun and needed to get things going—*I mean, why wait?!*

"Are you claustrophobic?" she inquired.

"No, I don't believe so."

"Okay, then nothing to eat or drink tomorrow morning until after the appointment. Now that we have the MRI scheduled we should probably schedule the biopsy of the nodule in your breast." *Wow, is this really happening?* "The earliest we can get you in is on July 9th due to the Fourth of July holiday and everyone taking long weekends. Does that work for you?"

"Yes, what times do you have available?" Because I had to fast, I wanted to make sure the biopsy was scheduled first thing that morning.

"Does 7:30 work?"

"It's exactly what I was hoping for." And there it was, everything was set for the MRI and the biopsy of my—*gulp*—cancerous nodule.

At some point Clíona had slipped away into another room. When she came back she was carrying her phone and said Adelaide was on it. "Hi, Adelaide, can you believe it?"

"NO! Oh, Apryl."

"I know, I really thought it was going to be nothing."

"So did I—I was so sure of it."

"I know . . ." What else is there to say at this point?

"What are you going to do now?" she asked.

"Well, I just scheduled an MRI for tomorrow and I guess now I need to find some good doctors. I'll call you later, okay?" Reality was starting to sink in as I handed the phone back to Clíona. She again disappeared with it into another room.

Not knowing what else to do, I picked up my phone and started dialing. The first call was to our friend the Shape Shifter. His assistant Brianna informed me he was in surgery. "Okay, well, I have some news . . ." How exactly do you tell people about *"your news"*? But the words spewed from my lips like lava from an erupting volcano. I felt as if I were someone else witnessing this abominable event taking place. *This wasn't really happening, I'm healthy!* It was like watching someone picking through carnage left over from a disaster and now calling the authorities for help.

"Oh, my gosh. Apryl, I'm so sorry. When did you say you were diagnosed?"

"Now . . . just within this last hour." My mind was reeling—*cancer*.

"What?!" She was completely flabbergasted. "I can't believe you're this calm."

"I guess I must be in shock." *Reality*—exactly what is *reality* and where is it at this *very* moment? It eluded me.

"The minute the Shape Shifter is out of surgery I'll let him know. He'll be heartbroken to hear this."

"Thanks, Brianna," and we ended the call.

Clíona had been coming and going in her kitchen but at the moment she was nowhere to be found. I sat back in my chair and took another deep breath. *Okay—now what?* Numb—absolutely *nothing*. I had been shaken to my very core, riveted with an insidious vice-like grip from a single word—*Cancer. Get a hold of yourself Apryl. Who else can you call? What's the next step? Doctors—who else knows doctors?* Then a light went off—*our friend Samantha!*

Samantha was always talking about her doctor friends. Maybe she knows someone who could help point me in the right direction. I picked up my phone and dialed her number. After two rings, one of her sons answered it. "Hi, may I speak with your mom? This is her friend Apryl."

"Yeah, hold on a minute," and I listened as he set the phone down. I could hear voices talking in the background but no acknowledgement of my call. *Nothing*. Like the sickening void I had deep down in my belly—*absolutely nothing*. I sat for I don't know how long until it occurred to me whoever answered didn't mention to Samantha I was on the phone. So I hung up, thinking, *okay, I'll give it a few minutes until her phone disconnects and call back*. Still Clíona was nowhere to be seen.

Once again I pressed the buttons for Samantha's mobile phone—*one ring, two* . . . "Hi, Apryl." This time it was the melodic voice of Samantha greeting me. I heard myself reiterating the ill-fated diagnosis I was given.

"Let me make some calls and I'll get back to you. Apryl, I am so sorry to hear this."

"Yeah, me too." Ending the call, I felt empty inside.

Clíona was now seated next to me at the table again. Lunch was forgotten. I think I had taken three bites prior to the call.

Heartbroken I implored, "Oh, Cliona, I don't understand . . ."

Calmly she looked into my eyes. "We don't always understand why something happens—what's important now is that you focus on healing."

Her words brought an amazing calmness to me. "Thank you, Clíona—I'm so sorry I got this news when you're in the middle of needing to heal yourself."

"Everything happens for a reason," she replied.

And there it was, even though the word hadn't been spoken. *Fate* silently imposed itself on my world and was spreading like wildfire.

After clearing the table, I offered, "Since I don't think I'd be good company for tonight, is there anything more I can do before I leave?"

"No, don't worry about me, I'll be fine." I felt horrible leaving her like this.

Then Ken walked in the door. From the moment he entered the room our eyes locked. With no hesitation he walked directly to me and protectively embraced my entire being. We held to one another for several moments then, looking into each other's eyes, stood completely frozen in time. Our eyes never veered from one another while unspoken words filled the space between us and the entire room. Words of love, compassion and heartfelt sorrow. After all, it wasn't only me this was happening to, it was *us*! The moment was surreal—one of us was broken and we both shared in the devastation.

Finally, I tore my eyes from Ken and turned my attention to Clíona. "Are you sure you're going to be okay?"

"Yes. Are *you* okay to drive home?" she asked, clearly having more concern for me than her own well-being. I was so embarrassed that I learned about my cancer while she was dealing with her own traumatic health issues. "You can leave your car here if you need to," she offered thoughtfully.

God, this was the last thing she needs. "No, I'm fine—I can drive home." After gathering my things I gave her another big hug. "If you need *anything* at all, Ken and I are just a phone call away. Please don't hesitate to pick up the phone no matter what time it is."

"Thank you, I will."

Dazedly, Ken and I climbed into our separate vehicles and headed for home. In retrospect, I probably shouldn't have been driving because after making the first left turn out of the cul-de-sac, I made an incorrect turn.

Immediately my phone rang. "Honey, are you okay?"

"Yeah, sorry, I'll turn the car around. I just got a little confused." Eventually we made it home, although I don't remember much about the drive. My world had literally been turned upside down and inside out.

Later that afternoon I received a phone call from the scheduling department at the Imaging Center. The voice on the other end informed me, "Your insurance, ACME, has a five-day waiting period for approval on MRIs."

"What? Are you serious?"

"Yes, so five days from today will be next Wednesday, July 12th."

"That seems so far away. How about if I pay for the procedure and then submit it to ACME for reimbursement? I'd really rather keep the appointment I have tomorrow," the CFO in me said taking over.

"Oh . . . okay, we can do that. I'll put you in here as 'Self-Pay' then. You're all set for tomorrow." As I hung up the phone I thought to myself, *I'll run this like I do our business!*

3
Rumor Has It
Adele

I woke myself breathing. I know it sounds odd but I was taking deep breaths in through my nose and slowly releasing the air through my mouth. Instinctively my body was attempting to release the stress from my recent cataclysmic diagnosis while I was sleeping! Or was it that my body was beginning the healing process while in a dreamlike state?

And now . . . how exactly do you start your day after receiving news such as this? Eventually Ken and I found our rhythm and as *he* was having coffee, the phone rang. It was Dr. KnowItAll. He was calling with the news of my recent diagnosis, but we informed him I had already been told.

"How are you holding up?" he asked over the speaker phone.

"I'm doing well but still in a bit of shock, I guess." We then told him I'd scheduled the MRI for later that day.

"I assume *they* will be calling you with your results?" he inquired with what seemed to be a not so thrilled tone.

"No—I don't believe so. When they attempted to contact you yesterday they received a message saying your number had been disconnected. That's why they contacted me directly."

Of course he completely dismissed the fact his phone was having problems. "I'll phone you when I receive the results from your MRI."

After we hung up I said to Ken, "So he waits to call until the next morning with catastrophic news such as this? I know he received the fax yesterday. You'd think after a life-threatening diagnosis *our doctor* would have the decency to contact us the first moment he had!"

Ken agreed wholeheartedly. But it was water under the bridge at this point. I found out from whom I wanted and *almost* exactly the way I'd envisioned it, only my version had a better ending.

Shortly after Dr. KnowItAll's call, Iris phoned. "Apryl, I notice you're down as 'self-pay.' I thought you had insurance?"

"I do, but your scheduler called and said our insurance has a waiting period. To avoid delaying the procedure, I figured I'd go ahead and pay for it and then submit the bill for reimbursement later."

"Who's your Doctor?" I could hear the wheels spinning in her head.

"Dr. KnowItAll."

"Let me make a phone call to his office. He should be able to authorize this and get the approval pushed through immediately." With a mission, she hung up the phone.

How fortunate am I to have someone willing to take the initiative? I thought. About 20 minutes later she phoned back, saying the approval was in place and returned my status back to "Insurance Paid."

Sometime later my friend Samantha called regarding doctors. "I checked with all my doctor friends and two out of three gave me the same name for an oncologist. I'm not sure what other types of doctors you'll need but this sounds like a good start."

Not knowing what an oncologist was, after we hung up, I immediately googled the meaning and, spelling it correctly the first time, this is what I found:

> **Oncology** (from the Ancient Greek *onkos* (ὄγκος), meaning bulk, mass, or tumor, and the suffix *-logy* (-λογία), meaning "study of") is a branch of medicine that deals with cancer. A medical professional who practices oncology is an *oncologist*.
>
> **Oncologist** a doctor who specializes in diagnosing and treating cancer using chemotherapy, hormonal therapy, biological therapy, and targeted therapy. A medical oncologist often is the main health care provider for someone who has cancer. A medical oncologist also gives supportive care and may coordinate treatment given by other specialists.

Lovely—just the type of doctor I want in my address book. I then googled the oncologist's name and was thrilled to see his office was 10 minutes from our home. Dialing his number I was transferred by the operator to his assistant's extension. Receiving her voicemail, I left a message to schedule an appointment.

Ringing back a couple of hours later, the voice on the other end of the phone was expressionless. Regardless, I now had an appointment for July 19th at 10:45. I felt rather numb when I hung up the phone.

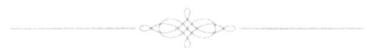

Ken cleared his schedule for the morning of my MRI. In retrospect I'm glad it was scheduled so quickly. There wasn't time for me to think about the procedure. Arriving at the Imaging Center, attempting to sound upbeat, I exclaim, "Okay, let's get this bad boy over with!"

After being greeted I was asked to sign in and "Please complete the following paperwork." That's right, they were requesting the same information they had received from me *three times prior*. Why can't they have the paperwork prefilled with my information and ask me to make changes only if it's required?

While scribbling monotonous information on the page, I paused. "Ken, I wish you could come with me," knowing full well they wouldn't let him.

"I know honey, me too. Just know I'll be waiting right here."

Unexpectedly Iris walked into the waiting room. "Hi, Apryl!"

What is that pink thing she has in her hands? I thought to myself. *Oh dear God—don't let that be for me. Not here. Not now. Not in front of all these strangers!*

With a huge smile on her face, Iris thrust into my hands a Pink Beany Baby Bear! Tied around its neck was a white ribbon with the Imaging Center's name printed on it, and embroidered in white thread over its heart was the breast cancer ribbon logo.

"This is a gift from all of us here at the Imaging Center!" she said kindheartedly.

"Oh, how nice. Thank you so much Iris." Taking it, I try to keep an appreciative smile on my face, knowing she has the best of intentions. I then stood, as it became obvious there was more to this gift. She then wrapped her arms around me, enveloping me in a HUGE hug! After she left the waiting area, and with everyone's now sad eyes on me, I didn't quite know what to do with the bear. I had my smaller purse that day and couldn't easily hide it away.

I fumbled with it a few moments until Ken lovingly offered, "Here, give it to me, I'll put it in my briefcase." *Whatever would I do without him?* I thought as I attempted to gather my senses and realign myself from the "smack me dead in the face" announcement that *I have Breast Cancer!!!*

Of course my name was called at that very moment. "Apryl Allen?" just in case anyone wanted to know who I am.

As I attempt to stand on shaky knees I can no longer feel, I hear myself utter the words, "That's me." *Yep me! The one who was just handed the PINK BEAR! The one who has Breast Cancer!!! And now that I have all of your attention, wait for it . . . wait for it . . .*

"So this is the Apryl everyone's been talking about with the beautiful smile!" the tech announced enthusiastically.

A little of the stress, along with my heart, melted at that moment. "Oh . . . how nice of you." Truly, I was appreciative. Reluctantly I followed her through the myriad of halls to yet another changing room and into the ill-famed gown.

Once in the treatment room, I felt as if I had stepped into the futuristic sci-fi feature of the week. The room was entirely white. "This is the MRI machine. I'll need you to lay face down first and place your breasts through the holes in the bed. Once there I'll use my hands to correctly position them for the procedure."

Is she serious? Holes?! Position me?! "Okay," I replied meekly.

"I'll then roll you in for the first portion of the procedure. When I bring you out I'll be placing the IV in your arm and position you again for the second half of the MRI."

"What?! I'm going to have an IV? But I'm terrified of needles . . . I'm not sure if I can do this."

Heartfelt empathy reflected within her eyes. "Apryl, we'll go real slow and take our time. If for any reason you feel uncomfortable we can have you come back at a later time. Honestly, the IV is a non-event, plus I'm *really* good with needles. I promise it will be relatively painless."

Maybe it was because of her compassionate demeanor that I started to calm down. "I'm still a little nervous. If I knew about the IV, I would've asked to take something."

"Let's just take our time and see how it goes. Lay down and we'll make sure you're completely relaxed before we start." Once I was in place, with my breasts hanging through the holes, she began manipulating them until they were *hanging* exactly where she wanted them.

"Okay, don't move. I need you to stay exactly as I've positioned you. Now look straight ahead, do you see the opening at the end?"

"Yes," I replied halfheartedly with a touch of terror in my voice.

"I'm going to push this button and it will take you into the machine. While the bed is moving, I'm going to run to the other side to meet you. I'll be holding your hand before you know it."

"Okay, let's give it a try," and I shut my eyes as tightly as I can. While this was happening I envisioned her at the other end. Just as she said, before I knew it she was holding my hand.

"Oh, what a lovely wedding ring you have."

"Thanks!"

"What are they—sapphires and diamonds?"

"Yes."

"It's quite lovely and so unusual. I wish I'd have thought of something like this."

"Actually my husband thought of it. I agree it is lovely and I get tons of compliments on it," I replied, knowing full well she was attempting to divert my attention. *Okay, I'll play the game.*

"All right, I'm going to leave you now and go into my little room over there. If you need anything at all just let me know. I can hear everything you say. You're going to hear some loud sounds but try to relax. It will be over before you know it." I believed her.

Once again, fate inserted itself. While in Sedona I had brought my Jambox so Adelaide and I could listen to music.

Suddenly I was thrust back into time . . . Adelaide took my phone. *"Let me see what songs you have on there—I feel like dancing!"* After scrolling through the list of albums, Adelaide picked *21* by Adele. Second song on the playlist, *"Rumor Has It."* It starts with a fantastic drum beat and that's when Adelaide began dancing! There she was with her beautiful dimples that are insanely contagious! I couldn't help but join in the dance.

Now, fast forward to the MRI machine. Believe it or not, the pounding sounds the machine made immediately took me back in time. Closing my eyes, I saw Adelaide and her beautiful dimples dancing to the beat of the drums. That's what got me through the 20 minutes of, well, quite frankly, the first part of hell! Then the voice of the tech interrupted my reverie. "I'm going to bring you out and get you set up for the second portion of this MRI."

I closed my eyes as she brought me out of the machine. *Why do they have you go in headfirst? What's wrong with feet first?!* I thought to myself. I sat up as she prepped me for the IV. While putting the needle in, she told me the solution they were injecting me with would be eaten by any cancerous nodes. "They'll light up like Christmas lights for me on the screen." She was incredibly gentle and, as I mentioned before, *compassionate.*

The needle went in easily. "When you lie down, don't bend your arm. You'll need to keep it straight for the entire time, so try to get comfortable. If you'd like, I can give you this pillow for your head to help with the positioning. Once you're in place, I'll be positioning your breasts again."

Soon I was gliding back into the MRI machine. As before she met me on the other side and immediately grabbed my hand. She helped with positioning me on the pillow so I could comfortably lay with my eyes in the direction of the opening. She then retreated to her protected room.

This time, with my right arm extended straight, my hand dangled out at the end of the machine. I envisioned my mother standing there holding it. Her beautiful comforting demeanor shrouded me completely and I could feel a glimmer of her strength. Once again the beat started and Adelaide and I danced our way to the end of the procedure.

The music stopped when the voice of the tech came over the speaker. "I'll be with you shortly to help you off the bed." As the table came to a stop from within the tunnel of terror, it felt as if I was breathing fresh air again. The tech then helped me sit up and removed the dreaded IV. With her assistance, I carefully stood. Once vertical, and knowing I had my balance, I flung my arms around her and cried tears of relief that the MRI was over.

"Thank you! You made this unexpected and terrifying experience somewhat palatable. I can't tell you how much I appreciate what you've done for me." I believe she was taken aback and at a loss for words and, quite frankly, I think shocked I was hugging her. I will *always* remember her kindness.

After I changed out of the gown, I returned to my beautiful husband awaiting me. Once again he took me to a late breakfast—*or was it an early lunch*—at our favorite Mexican restaurant. Yet again fate dealt another card—one I will not soon forget . . .

4

Keep It Loose, Keep It Tight
Amos Lee

For our trip to Sedona, I had changed out all the CDs in our SUV so Adelaide and I would have some great music to listen to during the drive. Driving up there we talked to her mom on speaker phone so we didn't have the opportunity to listen to music. However, on the drive back we did. One of the CDs I decided to bring was given to me by a dear friend who's like a brother. I had recently rediscovered the gift—the self-titled album by *Amos Lee*.

Now fast forward to Ken and me leaving the Imaging Center. As we were driving out of the parking lot, the disk changer switched CDs and the song "Keep It Loose, Keep It Tight" began playing. This CD would pretty much be the only one I listened to during this ludicrous period—*six months to be exact*. And the first song on the album became my mantra—I listened to this one tune over and over for the next four months. Primarily because of this particular riff in the song:

> I'm in love with a girl who's in love with the world
> though I can't help but follow
> Though I know some day she is bound to go away
> and stay over the rainbow
> Got to learn how to let her go
> Over the rainbow

When I heard this part of the song, all I could think about was Ken. He fell in love with a girl who, yes, is madly in love with the world. *How can I let him follow me? He doesn't deserve this.* We've been through so much together, most recently the wicked economy over these past few years. *Why this? Why now?* And the worst thought of all—*What if I actually did go over the rainbow?*

When we returned home I pulled the CD from the truck and took it into the house and loaded it into our home stereo for future listening. Sometime later that afternoon I decided to change into my "only to be worn at home" lounge clothes for the evening. Standing in front of the mirror, I watched myself undress. Once I was completely naked I stopped and looked deep into my eyes and then into my very soul.

This woman standing before me was stripped of *everything*! Stripped of life, of dreams, of a future that was now anything but certain. It was at that moment when this song called to me. Feeling vulnerable and exposed I walked to our living room, turned on our stereo and pressed Play.

The sounds of Amos Lee's guitar began strumming sweetly over the speakers. They were soon followed by the lightly accented piano notes played by Nora Jones. And there I stood in front of our picturesque window in our living room that looked out to the Praying Monk on Camelback Mountain and the world. I began to cry.

The day had turned to a beautiful dusky sunset which reflected orange on the red rocks of the mountain. Amidst all that beauty all I could feel was the cold, dark reality of an emptiness that had paralyzed me.

Ken heard me and came in from the kitchen. He tenderly placed his arms around me and cloaked me with love. He then placed his lips on the back of my head and inhaled my scent. My face was tear-streaked as I reached up with both hands to gently hold the forearm he had placed protectively across me. Bending my head down, I held onto his arm as my tears fell uncontrollably.

He gently turned me around and placed his lips lovingly on my forehead. I could feel his agony as his mind searched for a solution to fix this horrendous turn of fate. Tormented he clung to me, but in spite of his yearnings there was nothing he could do. I was broken.

I buried my face into his chest and wept. I cried for him, for me, for our life together and for our future. *Why this? Why now? Did I do something to cause this? What do I do? What will we do?* I clung to him with piteous desperation while my entire body wept with undulating emotions I never knew existed until that moment. Nothing would *ever* be the same—*nothing!*

The next morning, as we were having our first cup of coffee and reading the papers, the phone rang—it was Dr. KnowItAll calling with the results of the MRI. I quickly placed him on speaker phone so Ken could also hear the conversation. In his usual rapid cadence Dr. KnowItAll prattled off my results. "Only one nodule had been found in your left breast at the 10 o'clock location, if you were facing me. The right one was completely clear of cancer." *Thank God!* "The nodule is three-quarters of an inch in size. Call my office when it opens later this morning to schedule an appointment so I can examine you. I'd also like to discuss the direction you plan on taking, along with potential doctors."

We got in to see Dr. KnowItAll a couple days after his call. His assistant, after weighing me, asked me to change into the lovely gown with the opening in the front—*big sigh*. In came Dr. KnowItAll and after taking my blood pressure and temperature, he asked me to lay down for a quick exam.

He attempted to find the nodule, and even though we knew its *almost* exact location, he could feel nothing. "What's this mark here on your breast?" he inquired.

"Oh, the girl who bandaged my biopsy used a ton of tape and tape loves me. This is the battle scar that remains after a failed attempt to remove it," I informed him.

"Here, I'll put a Band-Aid on that; you should keep it covered until it heals," he said while reaching for the box.

"Ooo . . . I'd prefer it if you didn't. Tape *really* sticks to me." I couldn't bear the thought of another piece of adhesive being placed on my newly healed skin.

"You just don't know how to remove bandages. As you pull the edge of the tape keep it as close to the surface of your skin as possible; that way it won't tear your skin." As he was saying this he placed the Band-Aid on my breast—*terrific*. "You can sit up now," and I watched as he jotted a few things down in my file. "Your breasts look really healthy and at this juncture it's imperative you keep them that way. Stay out of the sun to avoid sunburns and so forth."

He then handed me a single sheet of paper. "This is a list of oncologists..."

"Thank you, but I have a friend who inquired on my behalf and was given the name of a top oncologist here in town..." and I told him the name. "I have an appointment with him on July 19th."

"Hmmm... you must be pretty connected because usually this list of doctors is the first line of defense." Slipping the paper from my hand he continued, "The oncologist she recommended is who people see if their prognosis worsens. If you're going to him I'm fine with that. Have you decided on a breast surgeon?" he asked before handing me the next sheet of paper.

"No, we don't have any names. Actually, we're not quite sure what types of doctors we'll be needing." He handed me another list with four names on it and I quickly perused it. "Is there any one in particular you'd recommend on this list?"

"Any of these surgeons are very good. I've actually had patients go to this surgeon and this doctor here was a fellow classmate in college," he said with a hint of pride in his voice.

"Cool, I'll definitely meet with both of them," and I folded the paper and placed it in my purse thinking, *I'm thrilled he knows one of them personally*. Before leaving, Dr. KnowItAll wished me well and asked I keep him abreast of the situation—my words, not his, and no pun intended of course.

Later that evening the Band-Aid started irritating my skin. "Ken, let's just take it off, I can't stand how it feels."

"Okay, here let me help you, we'll do it just like Dr. KnowItAll said." As Ken attempted to peel the edge of the Band-Aid back *it wouldn't budge*. Vile remorse churned within my stomach; the welts on my skin had barely healed and Dr. KnowItAll had to go and put a Band-Aid on it—*argh!*

"Why did I let him put a Band-Aid on me? I know better. Please hand me another washcloth and I'll soak it off." As I slowly and painstakingly removed it, the welts that had finally disappeared once again flushed bright pink and red where the Band-Aid had become so attached to me. "So much for pulling it evenly across the skin—obviously that's not the problem. Why doesn't he ever listen to me?" I asked Ken, who shook his head disappointedly. What's the saying? First time shame on you, second time shame on me—*there won't be a third time!*

Researching information is not as tedious as it once was—thank heavens for the Internet. I googled all the doctors on the list. The two surgeons Dr. KnowItAll pointed out had good ratings with patients on various rating websites. I also looked up the recommended oncologist and found his rating was three out of five stars—the middle of the road—but I felt confident in who I had chosen for my oncologist. Obviously doctors thought highly of him. Besides, what do patients really know? I place more weight with doctors.

After reviewing the surgeons, I picked up the phone and dialed the number for the *female* Breast Surgeon. Initially I received the voicemail for her office and left a message. My phone call was returned shortly thereafter by Mabel and we instantly hit it off. We spoke for quite a while on the phone about, well, *everything*, not just breast cancer.

She even revealed, "In the past I was a Professor of Classical Literature and am still doing so, but only on a part-time basis."

"How on earth did you go from being a Professor of Classical Literature to running a surgeon's office?" Talk about opposite sides of the spectrum.

"The doctor and I are sisters and she needed help here at her practice. We're a two-woman show. Me being basically everyone but the surgeon," she stressed.

I'm not quite sure how the topic came up of nationalities, but after informing her I was Comanche she proudly exclaimed, "We're Choctaw!"

"You're kidding! Were you born in Oklahoma?" thrilled to hear they were kindred spirits.

"No, we were born and raised in Connecticut."

"Hmmm . . . another thing in common, we're east coast babies!" I chimed back.

And the conversation continued with the fact that their office had been set up using Feng Shui and the doctor's favorite color is purple. "Yes, our entire office is painted lavender, which is considered a high-energy color." Of course hearing this, I made a mental note to look up the significance of colors and the role they play in our lives.

She went on to tell me, "*Saguaro Magazine* ranked my sister one of Arizona's 'Top Docs' in the April 2013 issue."

How perfect—the month of April! I thought to myself and then my mind quickly started spinning, Native American, east coast baby, Feng Shui, and even the month of April was in there. *If this isn't an omen, I don't know what is?!* Not to mention I now *adore* Mabel! She's easy to talk to and we connected on so many levels. I believe I may have found my surgeon—and not just a surgeon . . . my Medicine Woman!

"Prior to your initial consultation with the Medicine Woman you'll need to schedule an appointment with a nurse navigator. We recommend contacting one of the two employed by Imaging Center #2 across the street from our office. Basically the purpose of a nurse navigator will be to educate you on what you can anticipate over the next several months. They'll also explain the various terminologies. This in turn will enable the Medicine Woman to skip the explanation on the basics of breast cancer and get right to your reason for being here." Okay, that makes perfect sense. Being a professional, I completely understand time wasted on explaining remedial information when others can do it for you. *Smart woman!*

Thrilled with the initial phone call, I scheduled a consultation with the Medicine Woman for Thursday, July 25th, and was given the number to contact the nurse navigator. I felt totally on track! It was my goal to take on this horrific life-changing event with as much bravery and intellect as possible!

"Oh . . . and one last thing, Apryl. Back when I had cancer I was told by our Medicine Man I needed to name it. Once you do, talk to it, listen to it, and when the time comes, say your goodbyes and tell it never to return." *Wow!* What a powerful affirmation.

Shortly after my call ended with Mabel, I scheduled an appointment with the nurse navigator for Tuesday, July 16th at 10:00—*everything* was lining up perfectly.

Later that day the phone rang. It was Iris calling. "Hi, Apryl, the Breast Investigator asked me to tell you about a medical board she belongs to. They're called The Round Table and they only meet with individuals who've been diagnosed with breast cancer for the first time."

"Really?! That's so kind of her. What does the Round Table do?" This sounded like a great first step in this unknown, alternate world.

"The Round Table is a nonprofit organization consisting of medical professionals who are considered breast cancer experts. Their goal is to educate women about their specific type of breast cancer, which in turn helps you make informed decisions on the various options you have for treatments. And the best thing about this is *it's completely free of charge*. If you choose to schedule a meeting with them, the Breast Investigator will give them your results, reports and films from your biopsy, MRI and any other records we have on you for their review. In turn they'll give you their professional opinions on various options they consider to be appropriate *specifically for you*. There are no expectations of you whatsoever. Is this something you'd be interested in?"

"Yes—of course! How do I schedule an appointment?"

"Contact their patient advocate to schedule your appointment—her number is . . ." reading off the digits I quickly write it down.

"This is fantastic! I'm thrilled the Breast Investigator is including me in this opportunity. Please thank her for me." After we hung up, I googled the Round Table. I liked what I read. Feeling a bit anxious, I picked up the phone and dialed the number for the patient advocate. Receiving her voicemail, I left a message.

The next day, my phone rang while Ken and I were running errands. "Hi, Apryl, this is the patient advocate for the Round Table. I'd like to start by telling you I'm a 10-year survivor of Breast Cancer myself and know *exactly* what you're going through. I'd like to add that anything you need at all, someone to talk to or help with deciphering information or any questions you might have, I'm here for you." The voice on the other end of the call was extremely kind and sympathetic.

She then explained who made up the Round Table. "There is the Breast Investigator, a Breast Surgeon, a Medical Oncologist, Radiation Oncologist, a Reconstructive Surgeon, Breast Pathologist and a Rehabilitation Oncologist. I believe there's even a Naturopathic Oncologist." She then prattled off the group's Mission Statement and a few other details I had read on its website.

"Okay, what exactly do you do for the Round Table as its 'patient advocate'?" I was probing, looking for someone who could help decipher the numerous titles of doctors and the various procedures that I didn't even know existed.

"I'm exactly what my title says. I'm an advocate for you, the patient. I will sit in on all the meetings they have pertaining to you. Afterwards we'll go over what was discussed and I will answer any questions you might have at that time. If I can't answer them, then I'll present them to the Round Table. And, should you require it, I'm here for counseling, support and I am a great resource for information." Wow, after this explanation I felt as if I found the golden key.

My heart swelled with gratitude and appreciation. I had absolutely *no clue* at all what to anticipate or expect from the curveball life just threw at me. I felt completely blindsided and wished someone could literally take my hand and walk me through this terrifying nightmare.

We scheduled the Round Table appointment for Wednesday, July 10th at 8:00 a.m., the day after the biopsy with the Breast Investigator. After ending our call, I felt I had found someone who could help guide me through whatever I would be facing.

On Monday the patient advocate phoned confirming my appointment on Wednesday morning. "I'm so glad you called; I have a few questions I'm hoping you can answer for me."

"What can I help with?" She didn't sound as sympathetic today as she did on Friday.

"Well, I want to make sure I understand exactly the different types of doctors I require. I'm not quite sure if I have a full understanding of what each one does or what I should anticipate." Silently I added *because you're speaking to a neophyte who absolutely has no clue about breast cancer.*

In a very matter-of-fact tone she replied, "Basically you'll have your surgery, then chemotherapy, followed by radiation."

"Wait a minute—I lost you at chemotherapy. I'm going to need chemo?" My voice started quivering and my entire body started shaking, not to mention I just felt as if someone sucker punched me in the stomach. No one had mentioned chemo at all.

"Yes—because the cancer went into your lymph node you'll require chemo."

Oh my God . . . and I just wanted to know about doctors and what their titles meant—I wasn't expecting this! "Okay . . . I'll . . ." attempting to catch my breath, "see you Wednesday morning." I couldn't hang up the phone quick enough.

I just sat there in disbelief. *Chemo . . . Chemotherapy . . . My hair's going to fall out from poison I'm willfully going to allow into my body. Oh holy crap what is happening to me?* I tried calling Ken but he was with new clients and the last thing he needed was me interrupting him once again to cry. He'll get enough of that tonight. *Who do I call?* And then I thought of Mabel, the Medicine Woman's sister.

I picked up the phone and dialed her number. "This is Mabel," the voice greeted.

"Hi, Mabel, it's Apryl Allen, I just scheduled an appointment with you last week."

"Yes, Apryl, how can I help you?" I crumbled. She listened attentively as I recounted my phone call with the patient advocate. With a sympathetic heart she began to effortlessly eliminate my fears one by one. "First, no one at this point can tell you what your future treatments will be, let alone a patient advocate. So don't worry yourself about anything. Second, more than likely chemotherapy is something you'll have to do. But I've seen many women come into our office who have lost their hair. Don't worry; it grows back and in most cases thicker and lusher than it was before!"

We chatted a bit longer—actually quite a bit longer—and somehow she returned the smile to my face. I was so grateful to her, especially because she spoke my language. She understood and shared my fears, perceptions and most importantly conveyed, "You are going to be just fine!" Afterwards I thanked her for taking the time to speak with me and alleviating my fears of the unknown. *She's right, I am going to be just fine!*

5

My Way
Los Lonely Boys

*P*ouring *his* first cup of coffee, Ken and I dismiss the patient advocate's distressingly bleak opinion from yesterday. Instead, we decide to take it one day at a time with today being the biopsy of my left breast. In truth, I know Ken's heart is literally broken with the knowledge of what my future potentially holds. Attempting to hide his heartbreak and fear, he instead conveys only courage and inner strength.

The biopsy's a little more than an hour from now so I leave him to shower and mentally prepare myself for the inevitable procedure. While standing in front of the mirror arranging my hair, I stop and contemplate my reflection. I look deep into my eyes, into depths untouched by any human being. Depths only accessible to me and me alone in this horrid nightmare.

I never thought I'd feel this type of heart-wrenching fear. It's the kind that leaves you completely stripped of everything, while attempting to hold onto something—*anything*. It's as if you're standing on the edge of a cliff surrounded by dense impenetrable fog and the only thing you can see is your physical being. You know the world is out there *somewhere*. Yet it's completely out of your reach. The reality of your life is now but a figment of your past. *Is there even a future out there?* You so desperately want to believe there is.

God . . . how can this be happening? What could I have possibly done to have caused this? What's more inexplicable is I'm not alone in this nightmare; my loved ones have been dragged into the trenches of this hellhole with me! *Apryl, you've got to stop this type of thinking, it's not going to do anyone—especially yourself—any good.*

My nerves start to kick in and I tell myself it won't be any worse than the previous biopsies I've already been through. Just the numbing shot is all

I'll feel. Plus, I trust the Breast Investigator *implicitly*. She has only my *very best* intentions at heart. Finally, my confidence began to return.

I force a smile on my face and tell myself *you can do this—you're not alone!* I have to be strong, for my husband, the people working on me, and most importantly that little girl deep within. At this moment I have a choice: I can either be a train wreck, or put these energies into *healing*. I choose healing.

Not forgetting the tape saga the last go-around, I brought the remnants of the medical tape Clíona so highly recommended. I had planned to grab a package, *or two*, the next time I was at the pharmacy. Of course, being that my attention was on more *pertinent* matters, I neglected to purchase it. Thankfully Ken offered to get it while I was in my two-hour *treatment*.

After signing in and seating ourselves in the waiting room, I began fumbling in my purse for the torn piece of package. Finding it I present it to Ken. "This is the tape Clíona said she uses . . ." and I start to point where it indicates *hypoallergenic*.

Ken became agitated. "Apryl, I'm not five-years-old. I think I can figure out what kind of tape to get." Of course he could, but he was in one of his moods. He was behind at the office because of the time he was spending with me and his patience was wearing thin.

"Okay, I'm sorry honey. I just want to make sure . . ."

"I know Apryl," he said impatiently.

Okay, he's right, I'll quit. And I turned my attention to—yep, you guessed it—the paperwork they once again asked me to complete. What is this, the fifth time now? After turning it in, Ken and I sat in silent anticipation for my name to be called.

As if on cue Penelope appeared. "Hi, Apryl, are you ready?"

"I suppose I am," and I look to Ken.

"Honey, you'll be *just* fine. I'm going to run to the store and pick up the tape; then I'll be waiting right here for you," he offered as reassurance.

I informed Penelope of the intended purchase and inquired, "Whom should he give it to when he returns?" She told one of the girls in reception, who then assured us the tape would be brought in promptly. And off I went for my second biopsy of the year.

Through the labyrinth of halls we went. I already knew the routine and quickly changed into the special folded frock. Once in the procedure room, Penelope began prepping me for the biopsy.

"We plan on doing the same procedure as we did before. However, we've been unable to locate the nodule on your mammogram. If we can't find it using the ultrasound, we'll have to do an MRI biopsy."

"What? That sounds complicated." Now panic-stricken, I couldn't begin to imagine how they'd accomplish that kind of biopsy—nor did I want to.

"Yeah . . . it is," Penelope admitted.

"I'll tell you what, if you can't find the angry little guy, hand me that wand thingy—I'll definitely find the little sucker!" I was dead serious! Both of us began laughing at the thought.

It was then the door opened and in walked the Breast Investigator. "What are you two giggling about?" she inquired quizzically.

"Penelope just informed me she was having a difficult time finding the nodule," and I filled her in on the punch line. Then, somewhat humiliated, I added, "I guess I'm in this predicament due to the fact I have breast implants."

This had been a lingering thought since I opted for them because someone I looked up to at the time—upon hearing of my surgery—said to me in a judgmental and arrogant manner, "*You know you're going to get breast cancer now—don't you?*"

No sooner did the words leave my lips than the Breast Investigator immediately dismissed my vague attempt at penance for a wrongdoing. "Apryl, implants have nothing to do with breast cancer. As a matter of fact, with all the research that's been done, there is no scientific data that links breast cancer to breast implants. The statistics remain the same for women regardless." She smiled kindheartedly, taking her place next to me on the stool. "Besides, if a woman requires a mastectomy, what do you think they put in afterwards?" Silently I admonished myself, *why did I allow myself to brood over that uneducated, insolent judgement all these years?*

Picking up a shot needle she then began the first step of the biopsy. "You know the routine. We'll start the numbing process first."

While the Breast Investigator injected me with numbing solution, Penelope squeezed a glop of gel onto the magical wand. And there we were, all of us, with our eyes glued to the monitor.

"*Ah-ha*, there's the angry little guy," Penelope pointed out. *Whew! Thank God!!!* I wasn't about to go back into that MRI machine.

Just then the door opened and the receptionist handed Penelope the hypoallergenic tape. Now our focus was solely on the task at hand. We all watched as the needle made its way, this time to the cancerous nodule. And, as before, *Clap!* Out came the needle with the first sample. And in it went again with absolutely no pain, just the same pressure as before, and *Clap!* Out it came and in it went for the last sample—*Clap!*

"Now I'm going to clip a titanium marker to the nodule. You'll hear a clicking sound as I do this." In again went the needle and, even though I felt no pain whatsoever, I could feel the movement as she pierced the angry little guy with his new piece of jewelry. I found myself letting out a breath that once again I didn't realize I was holding when the needle came out for the final time.

The Breast Investigator stood to leave the room. "Now, Apryl, I don't want you being a repeat offender, so when you leave the building today plan on not returning for any more biopsies." I couldn't agree more! "Penelope will get you cleaned up and then we'll have a couple of mammograms taken of your breast now that it's been marked with the titanium clip." She then said her goodbyes and vanished behind the door.

Penelope quickly filled her vacant chair and, using the *hypoallergenic tape* Ken had purchased, began to dress the recently biopsied area. As she pulled a *long* piece of tape off the roll she exclaimed, "This is the strangest tape I've ever seen!" Then attempting to rip it, "Hmm . . . I'll have to use scissors I guess."

I looked at the tape and had to agree, it wasn't white like what Clíona had, *or had it been white?* This tape was a solid nude color—at this point everything was all a blur. "Yeah it is strange," I agreed but quickly dismissed it because *I knew* Ken had purchased the *correct tape* for me. Again, she used the same amount as before to secure the treated area.

"Okay, we're all finished. Follow me and we'll get those mammograms taken." *God this is never-ending* I thought as I followed Penelope through the gaggle of halls into a different mammo room. After introducing me to the tech, Penelope disappeared through the doorway and the woman began positioning me on the machine.

"This is odd-looking tape they've used on you," she pointed out.

"Yeah, regular medical tape loves me, so my husband purchased the hypoallergenic kind."

Appearing puzzled, she walked over to her somewhat of a desk and picked up a white roll of tape. "I keep that kind of tape here too and it looks *nothing* like that."

Hmmm . . . she's right, but Ken purchased this himself. "It must just be another brand," I replied, shrugging my shoulders.

Dismissing any concern, she returned to aligning the machine for the mammogram. While doing so she blathered on about a vacation she had just returned from, but I really wasn't listening. When she began twisting my breast this way and that, something inside me said she wasn't doing it right.

"I just had a biopsy and I don't think the Breast Investigator wants this kind of mammogram done." The tech took a step back, then excused herself.

When she returned she informed *me* that, since I just had a biopsy, "The Breast Investigator said you don't require a regular mammogram, so you're finished."

Following her to the changing room I rid myself of the ridiculous gown. I then followed the tech back to the reception desk, and just as I locked eyes with Ken, Iris foiled my escape.

"Apryl, the Breast Investigator would like to see you again."

"Sure, can my husband come too?" I inquired.

"Yes." Ken quickly followed but then excused himself into a nearby restroom.

Of course just as Ken closed the door, almost instantaneously the Breast Investigator materialized and took me into the MRI tech's office across the hall. Together, both of them began talking about their findings on today's 3D mammogram versus the MRI, but I wanted to make sure Ken was part of the conversation.

I politely requested, "Can you wait until my husband joins us? This way we won't have to repeat anything."

The Breast Investigator, appearing a bit harried, acquiesced. "Sure."

Dang . . . can Ken take forever or what?! What is he, Niagara Falls? Finally, the door opened and introductions were quickly made. "As I was saying before, I attempted to find the cancerous nodule on the 3-D mammogram we just took. I've turned that sucker every which way, but no matter what I did, I couldn't find the angry little guy. Yet on the MRI he lights up like a Christmas tree." While still studying the printout she inquired, "Have you decided on doctors yet?"

"We met with Dr. KnowItAll, who gave me a list of surgeons, and have narrowed it down to two. As for the oncologist, a friend recommended a top oncologist here in town," and I gave her his name.

"Iris, could you please get me the list of breast surgeons we have on file?" As asked, Iris immediately brought the list for our perusal.

"Oh, this makes me happy," I exclaimed, feeling the anxiety of choosing yet another doctor slightly diminish. "The two surgeons I've narrowed it down to are on your list as well!" I pointed to their names.

"Both of the surgeons you've chosen are very good doctors. As for the oncologist, he's a good pick as well," she replied.

"If you were choosing between the two surgeons, is there one you'd prefer over the other?" I was looking at a life and death matter and wanted only the best working on me. *Who wouldn't?*

"We're really not allowed to recommend just one doctor. But I can tell you this, both of the surgeons you have chosen are very good." Of course she responded with a politically correct answer—*thank you attorneys.*

"I understand but if it were *you* going through this which one would *you* choose?" How exactly do you word this so doctors will give you an honest answer that doesn't hold them accountable? Surely they have a particular doctor they'd *personally* go to or at minimum a preference.

"Let me put it this way, I would be very comfortable with either of the doctors you've chosen." Her answer did ease my nerves a bit. "Tomorrow you're meeting with the Round Table, correct?"

"Yes, we have an 8:00 appointment. Will you be there?" I inquired.

"Yes, but only for the meeting with the Round Table to discuss your diagnosis. I have a surgery scheduled afterwards. I'll bring the films to the meeting and give them to the patient advocate for you afterwards. Once you've decided on your surgeon, you'll need to give them to that person."

"Thank you, I truly appreciate you giving me this opportunity." I genuinely like her.

"If you need anything at all, please feel free to call us. Be strong, and stay up on your future mammograms. This might have been avoided. But don't beat yourself up over it. It is what it is and thankfully we caught it." Saying our goodbyes, the Breast Investigator gave me a huge hug, and Ken and I left, anxious to return to our world.

As we drove out of the parking lot, I felt numb. Numb from *everything*. Numb primarily from all the "What-ifs." *Could this whole crazy episode have been avoided?* As if he read my mind, Ken pleaded, "Apryl, don't beat yourself up over missing a mammogram or two." He then pointed out, "They may not have caught anything during that time, *and* didn't she just say they couldn't see the nodule on today's mammogram? It was the lymph node that caught their attention."

I knew he was right. "That's true, thank heavens for the lymph node! But in the future, I won't be missing any of these appointments."

"And I'll be driving you to each and every one of them. And honey *please* . . . don't beat yourself up over something that's really only speculative. We've caught it and that's the important thing." I truly am fortunate to have a supportive husband.

Returning home Ken settled me in the family room to watch some much needed—please take me away from reality—movies. On Netflix I had come across a TV series called *Fringe*, a futuristic sci-fi program. The series ran from 2008 to 2013, with 100 episodes. I really hope we like it—I could use some mind-numbing, take me away from everything, shows!

We watched the first episode and loved it! But as Ken was queuing up the second show I became agitated; the tape on my skin felt funky.

"Dang it! I can't believe this hypoallergenic tape is problematic too!"

"Let's go take a look and I'll help you take it off," Ken offered.

Facing the mirror, we inspected the wrapping job Penelope had done for the second time. *Holy Cow!!!* She had gone crazy with the tape. Maybe she thought it wasn't going to stick. Inhaling deeply, Ken once again attempted to peel it off starting at the corner just like Dr. KnowItAll showed us.

"Honey, I'm sorry to tell you this . . . the Band-Aid was difficult, but this tape is not budging." Literally I felt my stomach do a triple somersault!

"Okay, let me try," I said begrudgingly. Ken was right; I couldn't even get a corner up. I stood glaring at it in the mirror, feeling nauseous.

"Oh Ken . . . this is horrible. I think I'm going to be sick. My skin just healed from the last go-around. Can you please hand me another washcloth? I'll do what I did last time and soak it off with hot water."

That attempt proved futile. "What the heck . . . the water isn't even penetrating this tape. Are you sure you purchased the *hypoallergenic* tape?" I inquired, knowing the question could potentially cause an argument.

After throwing a bit of a fit he stalked off towards the kitchen to find the packaging he purchased to prove me wrong. When he returned he flung it into my hands.

"See, it's the exact tape Clíona recommended."

After examining the package, and recalling my ill-omened forewarning, I pointed out to Ken, "Okay . . . you bought the correct *brand*, but see here—*what I attempted to point out to you this morning*—the little print that reads WATERPROOF TAPE? This is where it should have read HYPOALLERGENIC TAPE!" He grabbed the packaging in disbelief and, after reading it twice, realized his blunder.

What could we do at this point? There was nothing he could say or do to make the situation go away. His reaction said it all—*anger!* Anger over the fact he was in too much of a hurry and didn't pay attention. The fateful mistake had been made and now I would attempt to remove it from what I knew was going to be a battleground of ravaged skin.

Ken was so enraged. I knew it was really anger directed at *himself*. He then excused himself from the room, from the house, and disappeared for an attitude adjustment walk around our neighborhood.

And there I stood . . . staring at myself in the mirror. A*ngry* too about his tantrum and haste to purchase the tape. *Angry* that I have to deal with this . . . this *bullshit* cancer. *Angry* at life for throwing me yet another curveball while others get to walk through it unscathed. I looked at myself in the mirror as tears welled up in my eyes. *Oh God . . . this is the last thing I need right now*, pleading, *help me get through this—please!* Sighing, I leaned against my bathroom counter for support. Then, mustering all the courage I could, I readied myself for the inevitable.

As my mom used to say, *"There's no use crying over spilt milk."* It really wasn't Ken's fault. It was simply a mistake. *Now, what is the most logical way to get this damn tape off?* I contemplated. Then baby oil came to mind. And there I stood for the next *hour*, peeling, applying baby oil and using a hot wet cloth to remove the bandages. Once finished, I stepped back and viewed myself in the mirror. My breast was nothing but red welts with skin missing in various places. *And Dr. KnowItAll said I needed to keep my skin as healthy as possible!*

Attempting to look on the bright side, I thanked my lucky stars I didn't wait until that night to check the bandaging. Relieved to be done, I had just finished washing my tear-streaked face when Ken returned. He wrapped his arms around me, apologizing profusely for his inept stupidity. And then told me how sorry he was *again*.

I of course told him it was just a mistake and asked him to put some gauze over the biopsy. "And please use the smallest Band-Aid you can find to secure it." I then dressed in my most comfy shirt and we retreated once again to our family room for another episode of *Fringe*. We both vowed as we left the bathroom that this would not happen the day of surgery. We would be armed with the *correct* medical tape. *And I'll make sure to ask they use as minimal amount of tape as possible. No need for yards of it.*

When the patient advocate phoned, confirming my appointment, she had asked we arrive 15 minutes prior to our scheduled meeting. However, on the morning of the appointment we arrived at 8:00 straight up, 15 minutes late. We checked in at the front desk not knowing where we were supposed to go. At first the receptionist had no idea what we were talking about. But then, as if a light went off, "Oh, you mean the *Round Table!*"

"Yes, I'm Apryl Allen. I have an 8:00 appointment with the *Round Table*."

"Okay, please have a seat in the waiting area and someone will be with you shortly." Ken and I turned in the direction of the foyer and were astounded to find it was half the size of a football field. We seated ourselves in the most secluded area we could find in this vast waiting room. And we waited.

No one came for more than 20 minutes, so I went back to the reception desk and inquired, "Did we cause some sort of problem because we arrived at 8:00?"

"No. The patient advocate knows you're here. She should be out shortly."

Returning to my seat I noticed a thin blonde woman sporadically appearing at the front desk. I had a sneaky suspicion she was the patient advocate, because she had glanced over in our direction. Not sure of the protocol we continued to wait, all the while attempting to do so *patiently*.

We had been waiting for an hour when a face we recognized finally stepped through a door—it was the Breast Investigator. She acknowledged us by waving her hand and started in our direction, but was thwarted after three short steps by another doctor. We watched as they began an animated conversation. Moments later, she again was heading our way. When she reached us, she warmly greeted us both, then offered me a much needed and welcomed hug.

She then handed me all of the items in her hands, with the exception of her purse. "Here's your films and reports from your recent procedures. They've been presented to the Round Table and we've discussed what we believe to be an appropriate protocol for you."

"Thank you. Just so you know, we haven't seen the patient advocate yet."

Seeming indifferent, "Oh . . . well, she should be out here soon." She then apologized. "I'm sorry I can't stay longer, I have a surgery I have to get to," and we said our goodbyes.

I looked at Ken. "This is a bit strange." Neither of us were very happy at this particular moment, primarily because Ken had to move a breakfast meeting to accommodate me. And worse, it appears no one cares. Once again, we seat ourselves.

While we're waiting, another couple arrives and sits in a bank of chairs about 30 feet from us. I guessed the woman to be in her early 50s, and by the way she's dressed appears to be from India. She looks extremely tired and is wearing a scarf on her head. I did my best not to stare, but all I could see was my future. Each time she looked in my direction, I'd glance away, attempting to appear as if I were looking at something, *anything* else. But deep down inside I think she knows I was looking at her.

At last, the patient advocate appears to be heading towards us. Suddenly she switches her course and stops to speak with the couple. They then stand and we watch as the patient advocate directs them through a door. With her eyes focused on the stack of papers in her arms, she once again is headed our direction.

Coming to a halt in front of me, she finally makes eye contact. I now have her full and undivided attention. I can't believe my first impression of this woman was "kind and sympathetic." I couldn't have been more wrong! She was somewhat arrogant and made us feel as if we were beneath her social status.

Offering no apology upon greeting us, she urgently says, "I need to get you back for your meeting with the doctor."

"We don't meet with the Round Table?" I asked, a little taken aback.

"No, that's what I'm for. I speak with them on your behalf and tell you their findings." I now realize she messed up. We were supposed to arrive at 8:45 for a 9:00 appointment—it was the Round Table that was scheduled to meet at 8:00. *I can tell this isn't going to work for me*, I thought as we hurriedly followed her through a maze of halls and into an examining room.

"Am I going to be examined?" I inquired feeling ill-prepared.

"No, it's just a meeting with one of the doctors." Offering no other information, she then excused herself and closed the door.

While awaiting Dr. Mysterious, it feels as if the room has no air circulation and grows uncomfortably warm. Just as Ken reaches for the doorknob, to allow fresh air in, the doctor arrives and introduces himself. Talk about an unexpected happenstance—he was, in fact, the other surgeon who I planned on interviewing.

The doctor was extremely nice, I mean *really* nice, but I like Mabel so much and I'm already sold on the Medicine Woman. Plus, her office is closer to our home than his, and we like the hospital we'll be going to as well.

"Funny . . . we've narrowed it down to two surgeons—and you're one of them!" we inform him.

We then mentioned Dr. KnowItAll, his classmate from college. "Really . . . Dr. KnowItAll," he smiled, "Please give him my regards the next time you see him."

It was now time to get down to the dirty details. He began, "First, I want to start by saying no cancer is the same and this *Tango* you're about to embark upon will happen in steps." My hands were literally shaking while taking notes. The world he's describing is completely *different* from the one I'm accustomed to. I stop him frequently and ask for explanations.

Then we discussed what my future looked like through a nonexistent crystal ball. "Nothing is written in stone until you have the actual surgery. Up until that point everything is just speculative; only educated guesses based upon cases similar to yours. I recommend all my patients have a genetic test prior to surgery. Have you scheduled yours yet? It can take several weeks to get in."

"No, I didn't realize I needed one. I'm just now starting to interview doctors." I scribbled on my notepad—*Schedule a Genetic Test.*

"Once you decide on your surgeon, it will be that person's responsibility to request this test. I'd look into it right away as it will dictate what type of surgery you'll require." *Note taken and consider it done.* "Based on your reports, the Round Table is recommending surgery—a lumpectomy and lymph node dissection—followed by chemotherapy and radiation. Then you'll be placed on hormonal therapy, a pill you'll be taking daily for five years. The radiation oncologist here today feels you should probably have radiation first, but ultimately you make that decision. Whatever your final treatment ends up being, you'll be placed on the prescription drug *Tamoxifen.* Right now there is some controversy as to whether it should be taken for five or 10 years, but either way you'll be on that for a while. Do you have any questions?"

"Just one. A few of my friends are concerned I'm taking this diagnosis too lightly." If anything I felt drained and quite frankly, numb about everything.

"I noticed on the form you completed you were diagnosed with melanoma back in 2002. That's when you faced your mortality. I would say your current demeanor is perfectly fine." He beamed a warm genuine smile. "Any other questions?" he inquired.

"No, I don't have any," and looked to Ken as he shook his head too. "You've shed light on quite a few things for us. I greatly appreciate your input and taking the time to meet." We all stood.

Reaching out to shake his hand, he politely shook his head. "No, we don't shake hands here. For someone like you and what you're about to go through . . . we give *hugs!*" and he gave me a wonderful heartfelt squeeze. "Okay, if you'll wait here the patient advocate will be in to answer any final questions you might have and then tango get you on your way."

Once again we found ourselves waiting for the arrogant woman who seemed so pleased with herself and everyone, except for me and Ken. Eventually she appeared, but only to give me forms to complete. I reluctantly took the paperwork from her and began filling it out. Once finished we waited some more. It was going on 11:00.

Disgusted, Ken took matters into his own hands. "I'm tired of waiting for this woman. Let's get out of here." We exited turning left out of the room and, as we did, passed another examining room with its door open. I made eye contact with the patient advocate sitting at a table across from the couple we'd seen earlier.

She abruptly stopped their conversation. "Did you finish the paperwork?" she asked, appearing concerned we were leaving.

"Yes, and we don't have any more time to wait," I replied, thrusting the paperwork in her direction.

Taking the paperwork, "I have a few questions I need to go over with you before you leave, and there's also a gift bag . . ." Reluctantly we followed her back to the room we came from. Finally, she apologized, but only offering, "Sorry, this couple is taking a little more time than I anticipated." Then, switching gears, "How are you doing, Apryl?" she inquires using a sing-song mushy voice.

Was she serious? "You know, Patient Advocate, to be honest I've been handling everything pretty well until our phone call on Monday." Why hold back, this is how I talk in business, and I'm treating cancer exactly as that—a business.

"What do you mean? I don't understand," she quizzically asked in a congenial manner.

"Okay, to be frank, I don't appreciate you predicting the outcome of my cancer when you're *not* a doctor." I couldn't have been blunter.

"I never did that!" she squawked, having the audacity to act confused.

"Yes, you did! You told me exactly what I could anticipate. 'First surgery, and then chemo followed by radiation.' The surgeon we just met with said all cancer is individual and I believe my outcome could be different. Besides, I'm here for the Round Table's recommendations—not yours!"

"No, I know what I'm talking about. It's in your lymph node and therefore you *will* require chemo. I'm sorry to have been the person to have told you this, but I've been doing this a long time and that's exactly how it goes with a diagnosis such as yours." She even had the gall to incorporate a smile on her face while saying this!

"Well, I don't agree with you. I believe it could possibly be *different* for me. Not every story has the same ending. Thank you for your time." I wasn't about to let her dictate my future; I was going to do this my way!

Standing, she watched as Ken and I proceeded out the door of *her* examining room. Following at our heels, she quickly passed us in the hallway. When she came to what looked like a nurse's station she reached over the counter and pulled out a gift bag. Then, putting on her sweetest smile, she held the bag out in my direction as we approached.

"This is for you. Just some special goodies to help you on your *journey*. And if you need anything at all, please know you can call me anytime day or night. If you have questions or need help with decision making, I'm here. I've been where you are and know *exactly* what you're going through. Even if you just need someone to talk to, please feel free to call."

Yeah right . . . you're exactly the person I'd call.

When we returned home, I opened the goody bag. It contained a bunch of pamphlets and a small heart-shaped plastic container with fake pink rosebuds in it. I read through some of the literature, which consisted mostly of advertisements for wigs, creams, potions, clothing and a store called Lulu's Loot located in one of the hospitals. *Humph . . . what kind of name is that? Strange for something so serious—way too cute for me.* I threw out pretty much everything, keeping only a few pamphlets I thought I might need later down the road, placing them in a location I would remember but definitely out of sight.

6

Face the World

Apryl Allen

"Normally we don't schedule the genetic test until after your consultation with the Medicine Woman. But since you've decided she'll be your surgeon . . ." Mable began shuffling papers. "You'll need to call the following number," meticulously she enunciated each digit. "Have a pen ready because initially you'll get a recording with instructions to the website. Once there you'll download a questionnaire and, after they receive it, you'll be contacted to schedule the appointment."

As instructed I called the number and, just as Mabel said, the recording directed me to a link for the "Cancer Genetics Risk" assessment program. Navigating my way to the form, I downloaded what was called the "Family History" questionnaire. *Okay, sounds simple enough* — that is, until I printed it.

They wanted to know in depth every detail of my family's health — both my maternal and paternal grandparents, my immediate family consisting of my parents and children. It was never-ending . . . they wanted to know about my siblings, their children, my aunts and uncles — on both sides of my family — and cousins. *Really, my cousins?!* I leaned back in my chair; I was in disbelief.

This black and white form sought the name of each and every one of my family members, my relation to them, their gender, current age or age at *death*, if applicable, their cause of *death*, did they have cancer, and if so, what type and at what age were they diagnosed. They also wanted to know what countries my ancestors originated from.

Are you kidding me? I thought they'd want to know about me personally — my habits, where I was raised, stress levels, and so on. I hadn't planned on contacting *anyone* in my family until I myself understood exactly what I was dealing with. And now they're asking me to give them health information on family members? I'm the youngest of 11 children. Most of my siblings have multiple children, and they want me to include aunts and uncles, and *their* children too? We're talking around a 100 people here!

I picked up the phone, thinking to myself, *surely they don't really need all this information.* Somehow, don't ask me exactly how, I ended up speaking with the genetics counselor directly.

"My family is huge. Do you really need me to obtain all this information?" *Please don't say yes,* I silently pleaded.

"The more information you can provide, the better we'll be able to assess your genetic makeup. In essence, whatever you give us will help all the more in determining your risk factor."

After we hung up I stared blankly at the form. One other ever-so-minor-detail I didn't mention was this could cause catastrophic repercussions to my heart while attempting this feat. You see, I'm considered the black sheep of the family. Attempting to have a voice hasn't fared so well over the years.

Picking up the phone, I call Ken at the office. "And it only gets worse . . ." I started.

His advice, "Honey, this is your decision to make, not mine. If it were me I'd say screw it and put down whatever information you know," attempting to be as sympathetic as he could.

After ending our conversation, I contemplated, *is it worth it to contact these individuals at this particular moment in my life? Why couldn't my mother be alive right now? Then it would be just one call and she'd collect all the information for me. That's it! Who do I know in the family that can do this for me?* Ringing a couple of nieces, I left messages informing them I required help on a project.

With time being of the essence, and not knowing when I'd receive return calls, I decided to contact a couple older siblings to see what information they had readily available. I started with one of my sisters and I ended up leaving a nondescript voicemail for her. Then I tried one of my brothers whom I knew had health issues. Surely other siblings have shared their "you should know for your own personal health" with him.

To make a very long story short, no one individual had all the juicy details on everyone's health, and some had pretty serious ailments I was unaware of. So I took the plunge and for three days nonstop I spoke with every family member willing to speak with me about their health issues. Talk about *dreadful*. I attempted to keep conversations light, but inevitably found myself searching for my mother's strength. It was just awful hearing about everyone's woes. And just when I thought I was finished, a sibling would prattle off a health issue of another sibling. When I attempted to get the details, he or she would respond, "I'm not sure, you'll need to speak with them." *ARGH! This is insanity!!!*

These calls started at 8:00 in morning and ended around 8:00 at night. After the last call of each day, I literally melted into our sofa. I was both physically and mentally drained. Not to mention a few scrapes and bruises I received when a couple family members attempted to make me feel bad about myself.

I ended each call stressing I didn't want to receive phone calls at this time, explaining that, "Everything is so overwhelming at the moment."

As for our grandparents? Everyone seemed to have a different version to tell. And let's not forget about how exactly they passed! *Big sigh— too much information!*

Having contacted the majority of them, with the help of my nieces, I now had all the intimate details on my siblings and *their* children. As for my aunts, uncles and cousins on my mom's side, I obtained their information from her sisters, who seemed to be up on everyone's ailments. And, thankfully, my dad had only *one* sister, who had a family of *three* children, so only one phone call to a cousin got me their health history. Quite frankly I was now at my breaking point. I had spoken with far too many people. I was feeling horrible about myself, my relatives and their ailments, and sad about my family. Simply put, I was spent.

When it was finally over, the family history was so complex that I had to recreate the questionnaire. There was no way I was going to handwrite all this information on the form—besides, there wasn't enough space.

In retrospect, I received good information. I found out that a few of my siblings had deep vein thrombosis which could potentially have detrimental side effects, *including death*, during surgery or when taking certain medications. After I compiled the final report, I printed and faxed it over to the genetics counselor.

Afterwards, I decided to ring the counselor and inform her I didn't contact all my cousins personally. She answered on the first ring. "Hold on, let me get the fax and see what you sent." A few moments later, "Apryl, this looks fantastic. There's no need to get more information; we can definitely work with this." *Thank heavens*, I thought.

She began directing me to call the number I was originally given to start the scheduling process, but then decided to cut out the middle man and offered to personally take down my information.

"What's the next step after this?" I inquired after I satisfied her need-to-know interrogation.

"Someone will be contacting you to schedule an appointment. You probably won't get in for a couple of weeks," she informed me.

"Rats . . . I was hoping to get this done sooner so I can get my surgery done and over with." It was out of her control.

Surprisingly, after we hung up, she phoned back moments later. "We had a cancellation for next week and I can get you in on Thursday, July 18th at 10:30. Does that work for you?"

"Absolutely, I'll take it!" *How lucky am I?* Once again, I phone Ken to clear his schedule.

Ever since I had spoken with Mabel from the Medicine Woman's office, floating in the back of my mind was our conversation about naming my cancer. How exactly do you start? How do you pick a name for something you *never* wanted? It was time to name *him* and only I and I alone could do it.

I was told once that my body protects my heart. That thought has always stayed with me and I believe it unequivocally. Truthfully, I have experienced an inordinate amount of heartache during my lifetime. An Elder of my tribe once said, *"We all have a story to tell."* I understood exactly what she meant. There are things people have experienced that I don't think I could have physically or mentally handled.

I guess we learn to deal with it and find a balance by looking to the future and, *hopefully, ultimately* learn from the experience itself. No matter what the fallout or damage, we simply gather ourselves together—or maybe not so simply, but we *attempt* to do so—and we make it work—relatively speaking—and find a way to face the world. We then continue on to some unknown—or could it be pre-determined?—destination.

Interestingly, in my heart I find I don't hate *him*. I'm not angry with *him* nor do I have ill feelings towards *him*—*he* simply . . . is. And then the name came to me—*Jorge!* For many reasons—too personal and painful to share—I have chosen this name. It was time to let go.

I look at Jorge as a culmination of all my heartaches, heartbreaks, tears shed, lonely nights and loss of not only dreams but those individuals I loved, still love and will continue to love for the rest of my life, but for whatever reason they've chosen not to be in mine. He's gathered all those pieces together and held them, ironically, over my heart, intact for a day when I was strong enough to let go.

I want to make it very clear . . . I'm not cutting people out of my life. I'm simply letting go of the heartaches I've been holding onto. Heartaches I've chosen not to carry anymore.

And now I'm ready to move forward . . . to a future filled with love, kindness, happiness and most importantly *health*! I'm not perfect, nor do I even in the slightest bit portend to be. However, as best I can, I am going to live my life to the fullest. I will look to my past as the foundation that made me who I am today while surrounding myself with those individuals who truly care and have only the best intentions towards me.

It's been difficult for me to repeat *over and over* my various activities involving Jorge to loved ones. The meetings with doctors, tests, the test results, the waiting and my overall preoccupation with "How am I doing" since Jorge has taken a starring role, is starting to take its toll on me. I'm exhausted at day's end, not wanting to speak with *anyone*. However, my behavior leaves people feeling neglected and concerned. I find all I want to do in the evening is melt away from reality and my current life. (Thank you *Fringe*.)

Clíona had mentioned she sent e-mails to her inquisitive minds. Instead of rehashing unwanted experiences, in one retelling, my loved ones would know firsthand the intimate details of my tango with Jorge as it unfolds.

From: *Apryl*
Sent: *Saturday, July 20, 2013, 4:53 PM*
To: *The Inquisitive Minds*
Subject: *ADA (aka Apryl D Allen) – it's all about me!!!*

To The Inquisitive Loving Caring Individuals In My Life Who Want to Know!!!

Thanks for all the phone calls, texts and e-mails . . . I apologize if I have not responded. It's been difficult repeating over and over the various events of the day, etc., and I end up exhausted at day's end. Therefore, I have decided to send an e-mail informing you what the heck is happening! I'll send e-mails as events unfold and please forgive me if I don't return calls; some days I'm on definite overload. Don't get me wrong, I enjoy hearing your voice and speaking to you, feel free to call and say "hi" ANYTIME! Just know some days I'm exhausted and don't feel like rehashing . . . well, you know.

Big Hug & Kiss,

Apryl

Everyone understood of course, all too well, and the phone stopped ringing. I don't know if that was a good or bad thing.

After our initial greeting, the Medicine Woman's nurse navigator invites us back to her office with no windows. Taking our seats, in her earth-toned room filled with florescent lights, we watch as she closes the door to her private space and maneuvers past her desk, behind our chairs, to a cabinet. Opening it, she begins flipping through various paraphernalia, pamphlets and booklets, returning some to their shelves, while others she hands to me.

"Hold on to this pamphlet. Set this one aside," she instructs.

Appearing to be satisfied with the deluge of paperwork, she informs us, "The items I've asked you to hold onto we'll be discussing. The others are literature you can peruse at your own leisure."

Closing the cabinet, she then peers into a cardboard box on the floor. "We haven't had a chance yet to put these away." Reaching into the box, she produces a pre-wrapped cellophane bundle of approximately 300-plus pages, pre-tabbed and three-hole punched. She then pulls out an empty 7 x 9-inch binder labeled "C101." *Great ... someone's being awfully cute about something I wanted to know nothing about, and now I'm getting a crash course in it! Cancer 101—just lovely.* Lastly, she gives me a bag to place all this unwanted and superfluous information in. At least the bag doesn't advertise I have breast cancer; it simply says "Imaging Center #2"—*thank heavens!*

Settling herself at her desk, the nurse navigator picks up one of the pamphlets. "This is an extremely informative piece of literature," and she begins taking us through the A to Zs of Breast Cancer. We talk about the fact I not only have Jorge but the Lymph-Along-Kid too, explaining exactly what that all entails. In detail, and using only the kindest of manners and demeanor, she briefly highlights the pertinent parts of the pamphlet, including showing me what a PETA Scan machine looks like. I listen intently as we discuss the more-than-likely scenario that will unfold in my not-so-distant-future.

This woman was so kind and moreover, *compassionate* while discussing Jorge, I couldn't help but wonder if she too had gone through this experience. "Have you had breast cancer?" I inquired, wishing to connect with someone—anyone—who had been haphazardly thrown into this same nightmarish hellhole. Someone who was able to attain a sympathetic yet peaceful outlook—something I desperately desired. You know ... the proverbial light at the end of the tunnel.

With heartfelt empathy she replied, "No, but my niece has. She's currently going through chemo. She's a hairstylist and decided to shave her head and forego the wigs." Taking the opportunity, she then pulls out a brochure advertising wigs and informs me of a few places in town that take insurance. "There's even a place that you can purchase used wigs since you will only need one for a relatively short period." That's when I noticed the room was a little warm and squirmed a bit.

Lifting a colorful brochure from the pile with "BRCA Gene" written across the front, she inquires, "I'm sure you've read Angelina Jolie recently had a double mastectomy?"

"Yes, I've read about it, but honestly I don't know much more than she tested positive for a gene and opted for surgery." I wondered *what exactly does that mean—a "double mastectomy?"*

"This is the genetic test she had done that came back positive. Testing positive for a BRCA gene means you're at high risk for breast and ovarian cancer. Do you have this appointment scheduled yet?"

"Yes, Thursday morning," I reply numbly. *Dang . . . this is really happening and I'm having this same test done.*

"Are you familiar with what a mastectomy entails?"

HUGE gulp! "No, I'm embarrassed to admit my mother had a mastectomy but I don't really know the intricacies of the surgery."

Fingering through the pamphlets, the nurse navigator finds what she's looking for and pulls it from the stack. "This is what a mastectomy is." She starts turning the pages. "The surgeon removes your entire breast, nipple and all . . ."

"Holy crap . . . nipple and all? I thought it was just your breast tissue." Suddenly feeling nauseous, I'm finding it hard to breathe and the room slowly begins to spin.

"There've been so many advances made towards reconstructive surgery. They're able to tattoo the nipple back on your breast and even rebuild a nipple. Would you care to see the before and after photos of this particular doctor's surgeries?"

No, I don't want to look at it! God, why am I here, this shouldn't be me! I find myself slightly nodding my head, knowing full well my face has turned white. I quickly glance at the photos, then bow my head as tears begin streaming down my face.

Ken reaches for me and tenderly wraps his arms around me. "Honey, it's going to be okay. I love you so much."

The nurse navigator, realizing how fragile I am, quickly folds the pamphlet back together. "I know this is difficult, but I've seen a lot of women requiring this type of surgery and it truly is amazing what doctors can do. We'll leave that for now, but if you'd like to discuss this in more depth at a later time, you have my card. Feel free to call me *any* time. And

Apryl ... you're going to be fine," she said tenderly touching my hand, attempting to remove the sting from the reality of breast cancer.

Unlike the patient advocate, the nurse navigator was prepared, *extremely* informative and *compassionate*. She hands me a list of about six local reconstructive surgeons and, not wanting to cause more anxiety, casually discusses them. Afterwards, we say our goodbyes.

Once in the car, "I can't believe Angelina Jolie opted for that type of surgery. She is *incredibly* tough; I don't know if I can do it."

"Luckily we won't need to make that decision until we obtain the results from the genetic test. Yours could be negative, Apryl ... remember that," Ken implored. Silently I again thanked my lucky stars for having such a supportive husband.

I keep hearing over and over how cancer is as individual as the person themself and just because one person had a particular experience doesn't mean you will. I understand certain things are a possibility but, at this particular moment, I'm attempting to digest everything that's being thrown at me. I can only take in and consider those possibilities that are imperative at this moment. Don't get me wrong—I'm mentally preparing myself for the worst-case scenario, but deep inside I'm praying for the best. I've been told we won't know 100 percent about Jorge, including his stage, until I have surgery. What I do know is I've been diagnosed with Invasive Ductal Carcinoma, Intermediate Grade 2-3. *Whatever that means ... more homework for me.*

The genetics counselor had given me detailed directions to her office, so once inside the facility we went directly there. As we entered, we were greeted by the counselor herself who looked a bit perplexed. "You're supposed to check-in downstairs first. They'll let you know when I'm ready."

Oops! I thought the main desk was for another area of the hospital and assumed the office we were going to had its own reception area. I felt a little foolish, especially because I like to consider myself extremely efficient, organized and someone who follows directions well. Regardless, we headed back through the maze of halls, down the elevator and to the front desk, where we checked in for our appointment. It was easy to miss the innocuous sign that read "Check-In."

Only a few minutes passed when my name was called; the counselor was ready for us. "Do you need directions on how to get to her office?"

"No, we know where we're going, thank you."

Having salutations for the second time that morning, we followed the genetics counselor into a spotless white room with a window. In the middle of the room, furnished complete with white cabinets and a sink, was a stark-white round table.

Once settled she inquired, "Do you understand what genetic testing is and why you require it?"

"Somewhat, yes. So we'll know whether I'm at high risk for breast cancer," I replied, a bit unsure of the hows and whys.

Confidently she responded, "That's correct, but more specifically, we want to find out if you have the BRCA 1 or BRCA 2 genes."

"This is the gene Angelina Jolie was recently in the news for, correct?" holding my breath, I awaited her educated response.

"Yes, that's correct. The odds of getting breast and ovarian cancer—which are closely related—jump to about 85 percent when a woman tests positive for the BRCA 1 gene. She tested positive for this gene and they estimated her risk of developing breast cancer at 87 percent, and ovarian cancer was estimated at a 50 percent risk. However, percentages of risk vary for each individual. Only a fraction of breast cancers result from an inherited gene mutation. Those with a defect in BRCA 1 have a 65 percent risk of getting it, on average." And there were those words slithering silently as a snake—*cancer is as individual as the person themself.*

"That's why she opted for a double mastectomy, to reduce her risk factor to 5 percent." She then inquired, "I noticed on your paperwork that you had a hysterectomy. Do you know if your ovaries were left intact?"

"Yes, because I was only 35 at the time, they suggested I keep my ovaries to avoid hormone replacement and early menopause." Now I was questioning myself, *should I have had them removed?*

We continued on, laboriously pouring over the extensive family health history I provided. We then moved on to the test itself.

"You have two options in terms of which laboratory does the testing. Laboratory A costs $3,000 and you'll receive the results in two weeks. Laboratory B costs $1,500 and results will be provided within four weeks."

Is there even a question? "I'll take Laboratory A." Regardless which I choose my insurance will cover it. This was the easiest decision I've been asked to make since this whole convoluted diagnosis occurred. And then I silently wondered what type of test it would be. I watched as she walked over to the cupboard above the sink and pulled out a small kit.

After placing rubber gloves on her hands she removed its contents and, as if reading my mind, "I don't want to taint any of the contents of the test with my genes." The test consisted of a glass vial and Scope mouthwash. *Mouthwash?!*

"You'll swish the mouthwash around in your mouth for 30 seconds, then spit it into the vial. There's enough mouthwash in there for two swishings."

"Really, mouthwash?" Now I'm curious.

"Yes, believe it or not, the genes within your mouth are the best to use for genetic testing. The mouthwash helps to hold it in a particular status while it's shipped to the laboratory, where the testing will be completed. We'll FedEx the vial today overnight for delivery tomorrow. Your results will be received two weeks from the day the lab receives it. But since tomorrow's Friday, let's plan on two weeks from Monday of next week, just to be on the safe side."

"And we want the results to come back *negative*, correct?" I reaffirmed.

"Yes—negative."

Hummingbirds have been a constant in my life since my mother passed away. I've had several very special encounters with them. One in particular occurred shortly after my hysterectomy in 2003. Being housebound, I noticed something flitting around our atrium tree while I was reading. I ignored it for the first couple days, but when it continued I decided to investigate the source. To my surprise, I found a hummingbird had built a nest.

Thrilled, I grabbed a nearby chair with hopes to peer into the tiny little home. And there they were, three itsy bitsy eggs nestled deep inside, providing a much needed lift to my spirits! Every day I looked in on our new little family. Most of the time the Mama bird sat atop the eggs, but on occasion she'd leave—I assume for nourishment—allowing me to check in on the little darlings!

On Mother's Day of 2003 I watched as the little babies left their nest for the first time. Of course Mama protectively lingered nearby. At first I felt complete joy and elation, but then disappointment and sadness dampened my spirits as I longed for them to stay. Sitting on the floor next to the glass atrium door, I watched as they began short fly-hops—first one branch at a time, then two, then to the treetop and . . . *poof* they were gone! I felt *empty*. Something else to disappear completely from my life.

Suddenly the Mother hummingbird returned and flew down to where I was sitting on the floor. She was looking directly into my eyes, hovering in front of me for several moments. It was then she softly spoke to my heart. *I'm not leaving, this is only the beginning*, and off she flew. Every year thereafter our atrium had hummingbirds and nests.

Fast forward to when I was completing research for my *Shape Shifter* musical in 2011. During my research of animals, I read somewhere that hummingbirds teach us to find joy in what we do, thus restoring health and balance within our lives. These birds have the ability to move their wings in the pattern of a figure eight (my favorite number) which, as we all know, is a symbol for infinity. *Infinity* . . . linking the past, present and future. When we moved I was concerned we wouldn't see hummingbirds anymore. I couldn't have been more wrong. They're a constant in my life!

Once more let's fast forward, this time to the moment when I was actually writing the story for my musical. For whatever reason I had awakened early on that particular morning. I normally work inside our home, but on this day I was drawn to sit outside in our middle courtyard. So I prepared a makeshift desk on the patio table, and once seated, the words began pouring out of me.

Engrossed in my work, I was vaguely cognizant of a humming sound. Preoccupied with my project, I simply dismissed it and continued with my writing. Yet the pulsating sound engulfed my senses to the point that it could no longer be ignored. When I finally looked up, there was a hummingbird *literally* 12 inches from my face! Soon another joined in and together they performed a *Round-Dance* around my head three times! I was in awe as they faced me hovering, all the while moving in quarter increments of a circle. At the time Ken was still asleep, so sadly I experienced this other-worldly event on my own. It was *incredible* to say the least!

A *Round-Dance*. I was elated as a child when my family joined this type of dance at powwows. It's when both men and women, young and old, join hands in a circle moving clockwise, in a sidestep fashion, harmoniously together to the beat of the drums. If there are enough people two circles are then formed, with the second moving in the opposite direction. The origins of this dance lie in the healing dances of the Plains Indians and its spiritual core inspires joy and happiness.

Since the appearance of *Jorge*, I've been given an inordinate amount of printed material labeled with various titles that include such words as "Cancer," "C101," "Breast Cancer," *etc.*, *etc.* I *really* don't need, nor want, the daily reminder of *him*. As far as I'm concerned *he's* already gone. However, I do need *something* to keep all this paperwork in rather than stacking it on the desk. Then it came to me—create my own book. I grabbed a two-inch, three-ring window binder that would allow me to create my own front and back covers. I then decided to pull from the vast amount of photos I have from my past when I was younger and *healthy!*

While flipping through the pages of photos, looking back at my past life, I couldn't help but fondly reflect at their beauty. I ran my hand gently over one of the images. *God . . . why did I allow myself to put on weight?* Chastising myself, I quickly retracted the statement, remembering what the blonde, skinny, vapid, 10-year survivor of breast cancer patient advocate had said during our initial phone call: *"I've always eaten so healthy and it didn't matter—I could have had the French fries!"* No, cancer doesn't have a face. It goes after anyone, at any age, no matter your lifestyle! *Please God, let a cure be found soon!* I silently pray.

Eventually I came to a black and white brochure and a color flyer from a past photo-shoot for a gun holster company. Each photo displayed my perfect figure. In fact, in both photos I looked like one of *Charlie's Angels*, expertly brandishing a gun while looking for the bad guy, only at the time I didn't know his name was *Jorge! These images are perfect for the front and back covers of my book—even better—my Warrior Book!* I thought, admiring them.

Making copies of the photos, thus avoiding any damage to the originals, I proceeded to change the wording of the ad for the holster company to my own. I took to my computer and methodically chose the perfect font. After doing so, I reversed the black and white lettering so the letters appeared white, just as they did on the flyer.

Then I asked myself, "What do I choose to create?" It was at this moment I quieted myself and listened to my heart. After a few moments my fingers began typing the words: Health ♡ Love ♡ Happiness ♡ Peace. That's all I've ever really wanted from life.

At the beginning of the Warrior Book I placed magazine photos used in a "dream book" I created back when I was in my early 20s. The dream book consisted of items I longed for in my life. They weren't necessarily material objects, although there were a few of those; the majority of the photos were of a more spiritual nature. For instance, there was a glass of wine that wasn't completely filled, leaving room for knowledge and life experiences yet to come. A garden of flowers I often envisioned myself walking in. Photos depicting health and fitness. A child holding onto a woman in the backseat of a car representing the family I hoped I would have one day. And a woman standing with her back to the camera in a shower as water cascaded from the top of her head down her body, reflecting the ability we all have to wash away our worries.

In my younger years these photos were meant to help me create a full and peaceful life. I couldn't think of a more befitting time than now to blow the dust off of them and revisit the future I had dreamed and longed for. I also included one past and one present photo of myself. The past photo was a head shot I used during my acting days; the other was a photo that had been taken for my *Shape Shifter* album of me laughing; it captured my love for life. Of course this section wouldn't be complete without a photograph of my handsome and loving husband.

Next was a plastic page with slots for various business cards to place my doctors' contact information. I then added tabs for the various paperwork given to me by doctors. However, I didn't want to use their titles or names on the tabs, and thus the naming of my doctors was born—1) Breast Investigator 2) Genetics 3) Mad Scientist 4) Medicine Woman 5) Radiation Man and 6) Shape Shifter. The book was now complete.

The next morning, while enjoying my first cup of coffee, I allowed Hugo, our sweet but naughty 6½-month-old little devil of a Havanese, to play in our courtyard. As I stood next to the open door I could feel a storm brewing. We were about to have one of those amazing monsoons Arizona is famous for. I love days like this, when the sky darkens and moisture fills our arid climate. I waited anxiously to breathe in the smells of the first droplets I knew would soon fall. Then I realized that Hugo had never heard thunder and I wondered what his reaction would be?

As if in response to my unspoken question, and with no warning whatsoever, *KABOOM!!!* Hugo leapt into the air and as fast as his little legs could carry him, high-tailed it inside the kitchen door. He was scared! Quickly by his side, I began coddling him when I noticed something on the floor next to his paw. I picked it up and examined it closely. *Holy Cow—it's a wet hummingbird feather!!! What are the chances of that?!* I knew at that very moment my mom was with me!

Carefully I cleaned and dried this tiny delicate feather. Then protectively I displayed it on a dry paper towel to show Ken. Amazed at how fragile it looked, I stood in awe at its beauty. As it dried, numerous iridescent colors could be seen reflecting from the lights above. There were golden yellows, silver grays, sky blues, hot pinks and lime greens. Although the feather initially looked dark gray, the reflected colors, in some instances, appeared to be *glowing!*

Meanwhile the wheels were turning in my head: *I have to do something really special with this tiny little feather.* Then it came to me — *place the feather in my hair on the cover photo of my new Warrior Book!* Carefully I taped it to the photo. Interestingly, now when you look at the feather, it appears to be something I was *wearing* for the photo-shoot. The book in my mind had now reached true *perfection!* And as Clíona refers to me, I truly am a Comanche Princess Warrior!!!!

7

Freedom

Anthony Hamilton & Elayna Boynton

The day has arrived for the long awaited—*is this really happening*—meeting with the doctor who I believe will be my oncologist. It's Friday, July 19th, and the appointment's at 10:45. It seems as if I scheduled it in another lifetime. I guess, in retrospect, it was another life ago. I'm literally shaking at my core, not because of him per se, but because he will ask me to willingly put poison into my body.

I step into my closet, *hmmm . . . what to wear*, I ponder. I don't know whether I will get to keep my breasts and I want to feel beautiful and feminine. Perusing my choices, I come across a bright and cheerful full-length summer halter dress with deep luscious brown braided ties made of a sponge-type material. The dress itself is pale yellow with deep brown flowers. Slipping it on, I focus on the fact Ken plans to take me out for a late breakfast or early lunch.

We drive to the appointment. *I don't want to be here.* Luckily for me Ken's by my side. *I can't do this.* We park in the parking garage. *Can't we just leave?* We make our way through the sliding glass doors. *Take me anywhere else but here.* Now we're standing in front of the elevator that will take us up to the oncologist's office. *I can't do this without you.* We stand silently in the elevator as it rises to the fourth floor—it begins to slow . . .

Rewind to when I initially made this appointment. I'd gone to the gym and ran into our friend Alec, whose wife had lost her long-term battle with cancer. He offered advice that day about the office we were walking into at this very moment. *"Apryl, I want to prepare you and there's no way to delicately put this. Everyone claims they know one, but there's no such thing as the 'Best Doctor in a field.' The reality is it's who you feel comfortable with. Truthfully, what you're about to experience will not be your usual doctor appointments. You'll walk into an office and some patients will look as if they're from a war zone."*

What did he just say? I felt as if I were at the end of a tunnel struggling to decipher his words.

"People will look as if they've literally been on a battlefield. It's not a pretty side of cancer." It was then I noticed tears welling up in his eyes.

What do you say to that? My God, what this man and his wife must have gone through. I'm only sorry I didn't have the opportunity to meet her.

"Thanks Alec, I appreciate you preparing me for it. You know, I never even gave that a thought." My throat tightened to the point I wasn't sure if I could speak another word.

"I know, sadly, this is one of those hidden and shocking truths of cancer." His voice cracked and he excused himself to get a glass of water. Although I was left standing there, attempting to keep my chin up, I was incredibly appreciative of his candidness. And because of this conversation, I feel that much more prepared for . . . oh yeah, the oncologist's office.

The elevator doors swing open with a big *Thug!* We step off and look to our left. There to greet us are two large sliding glass doors, anticipating my arrival, ready to welcome me to my new life. Ken takes my hand and together we walk through them. Thankfully, I'm greeted by a cheerful woman who genuinely asks, "How are you on this beautiful morning?"

While scribbling my name on the sign-in sheet I put a smile on my face. "Great, thanks, and yourself?"

"I had a wonderful week so no complaints and best of all today's Friday!" This is a good sign. "Please have a seat. We'll be calling you up momentarily."

As promised, my name was called shortly after I was seated, but only to collect my co-pay. About 10 minutes later, we're invited back to *another* waiting room.

As we sit familiarizing ourselves in this second waiting area, I find myself feeling self-assured. I completed the forms the Oncologist sent me which I've placed in my Warrior Book, along with the redundant "see attached" information and anything else I thought they could possibly require. Hands down, this is absolutely the most information I've ever been asked regarding my health and state of well-being.

Another 10 minutes pass and we're asked by the same person to follow her again. This time we're taken through a maze of halls and into the office of none other than the oncologist himself.

"Please have a seat. The doctor will be with you shortly." Now I feel a bit nauseous as we're left to contemplate his highly anticipated arrival.

"Apryl, have you looked around the room yet?" Ken inquires as I sit on pins and needles.

I lift my eyes from my hands clutched nervously together on my lap and scrutinize the room. His office isn't anything special. Big clumpy pieces of furniture in cherry red are lined along the walls. A computer monitor sits atop his L-shaped desk a few feet away from the chairs we're currently occupying. Mounds of paper in messy piles adorn his desk.

Books have been placed haphazardly on shelves, but then a wooden figure atop his bookcase catches my eye. As I look closer I notice several of them around his office. They're hand-carved hummingbirds, to be exact. This has to be a sign I'm in the right place. My mom's with me at this very moment.

As if reading my mind, Ken says, "Your mom's letting you know she's here with you!" I feel the stress in my shoulders relax a little and inhale. Ken reaches over and takes my hand, giving it a squeeze.

At that moment the door swings open and in walks a jovial round man who seems, amusingly so, to match the office. He's wearing tan suit pants, a white button-down shirt and a maroon colored tie. Bringing the ensemble together is a doctor's knee-length white coat. And within the left breast pocket of his jacket are several pens. Although his clothing is neatly pressed and clean, he appears a bit disheveled.

"Good morning, Apryl. Welcome," he drones with an almost deadpan but somewhat lyrical lilt to his voice. He seats himself in a leather chair across the desk from us. Introductions are made to Ken and niceties exchanged. Immediately he begins rummaging through my paperwork. "It says here you have copies of your past surgeries and a family history completed separately from our paperwork."

"Yes." He watches as I pull from my Warrior Book copies of all the paperwork in chronological order. He looks expressionless as he scrutinizes the many pages of history pertaining to my health. He stops at the page about the current state of my well-being.

"You've written here you currently have lower back pain?" he questions, glancing over the edge of my paperwork making eye contact.

"Yes, but I think it's from Pilates. It's been bothering me for a couple years now. Although, it's not bad enough to schedule a doctor's visit for," silently I remind myself, *don't forget your right index finger.*

"Is there anything else that's bothering you?" he queries.

"Well . . ." I started meekly, "since you've asked, I noticed the tip of my right index finger hurts, but I don't remember smashing it on anything."

Again a deadpan look that turns into a subtle curled lip and then a stifled chuckle. "Right now your mind's on heightened awareness. You'll notice the slightest of things you normally wouldn't, due to your recent diagnosis." *Oh, good, someone who makes perfect sense,* as I giggled inwardly to myself. I like this oncologist man—and you won't believe this, he actually reminds me of a *Mad Scientist!* Go figure.

Reaching the end of my historical health facts, the Mad Scientist proposes, "I'd like you to have blood work done today here at my office." *Rats! I hate needles.* "Along with a PET/CT scan to ensure there's no cancer elsewhere in your body, and an echocardiogram to test the strength of your heart."

"Strength of my heart?" Panic sets in.

"Yes, chances are you'll require chemo and I need to know what strength your heart can handle." *GULP!* I watch as he scratches something down on a pad of paper, then continues, "I'm also going to request an *Isinthis* scan . . ."

A slightly panicked gasp escapes my lips. "What type of scan is that?"

He looks at me quizzically and chortles, "What do you think I said?"

Realizing I obviously misunderstood, I joined in his laughter, although I still wasn't sure what kind of scan he was talking about.

"Can you please repeat what you said?" I asked with a nervous laugh now trilling from my throat that's suddenly constricted by an unknown lump—*the lump is obviously nerves, nothing to concern yourself with, Apryl.*

Instead he insisted, "No—I want you to tell me what you *thought* I said." Now Ken joins in the laughter too.

Embarrassingly so, while squinting my eyes and shrugging my shoulders—preparing myself for the metaphorical *crash* about to happen—I laboriously repeat the word exactly as I heard it syllable by syllable, "*I-sin-*

this?" My inflection holding out for what I hope to be the correct version of what was said.

The Mad Scientist reels with laughter. I look at Ken nervously, not quite knowing what to say, and end up joining in on the gaiety! Eventually the Mad Scientist gains his composure and replies, "My assistant's told me I've been mumbling my words lately." Clearly repeating his words, "What I said was I am going to order a scan from your *Eyes to your Thighs!"* Oh . . . *thank goodness! I couldn't bear another crazy "never heard of it before" procedure!*

He then asked us to gather our things. "Let's get your blood work done."

Did I mention how much I detest needles yet? *I so want to skip this part.* Begrudgingly, we follow him out of his office and back to the waiting room we had previously occupied. However, instead of entering the waiting area, the Mad Scientist stopped at an administrative workstation equipped for two people. He began speaking to a woman in scrubs at the desk while I stood familiarizing myself with the surroundings.

The Mad Scientist then motioned to me and Ken. He directed me kitty-corner to a nurse's station across the hall equipped with what reminds me of four pedicure-spa chairs. At the same time, he caught the attention of one of the techs. "Please have the following blood work completed on Apryl." Handing the tech my file, he adds, "Once you're done, please show her to an examining room." Turning back to me, "I'll see you shortly."

Meanwhile, I watched the two people currently occupying the spa chairs. A construction worker probably in his late 40s, who evidently earned his living from being outside, looking sun-drenched and sweaty, had a tech hovering around him. Seated next to him was a woman in her early 50s, dressed in business attire with her lovely purse sitting on the floor next to her. The woman sat helplessly awaiting her fate with wide-eyes reflecting *exactly* what I was feeling inside—*I can't believe this is actually happening to me!* All too soon it was my turn.

The blood work was relatively painless. I think the anxiety of waiting for the needle to be thrust into my arm was the most difficult part. As I felt the needle go in, I flashed back to a memory of my mom in the hospital when she required a shot in her stomach. I stood helplessly by as she begged the nurse not to give it to her. I'd never heard my mom plead with *anyone* before. My heart wrenched and tears immediately began to fall.

The nurse, concerned she'd hurt me, asked, "Are you okay?"

Taking more than a moment to find my voice, I reply, "Yes, sorry, I was just thinking of my mom, who passed away from breast cancer."

"I'm so sorry . . . this will be over shortly," she said sympathetically. I did my best to regain my composure and think about something else. As quickly as she could, the nurse took *six* vials of blood. She then placed a cotton ball and purple bandaging around the compromised area.

We were then shown to an examining room and I was asked once again to place the gown on with the opening in the front.

After she left Ken inquired, "You're in a *dress* — how exactly are you supposed to do that?" *Darn . . . maybe this outfit wasn't the brightest of ideas.*

Thank goodness I'm creative; Ken watched as I undid the halter portion of the dress and dropped it down. After tucking it into the lower half of my skirt, I slipped on the paper vest and precariously positioned myself on the examining table. Ken silently applauded my ingenuity.

Shortly thereafter, the Mad Scientist rapped on the door and joined us in his examining room. After inspecting my breasts, he scribbled notes into my file. He then handed me an order for an echocardiogram and inquired, "Do you have a cardiologist?"

"No, I don't — but Ken does." Ken reached for his phone.

"Since you personally don't, here's the place *we* recommend. We've worked with them in the past — not negating yours, Ken — but we know this group. They're efficient and prompt, and if for any reason we don't receive something, we know exactly who to contact."

Without asking I knew Ken agreed. "Great! we'll use yours."

Handing me the contact information he noted, "There's a couple of locations to choose from." After glancing at the paper I handed it to Ken to file in his briefcase. He then continued, "I'll be staying in close contact with your Medicine Woman throughout this entire process and will be speaking with her prior to your Thursday appointment. I'll let her know your test results at that time. Now, if you'll excuse me for a moment, I'd like to introduce you to my nurse practitioner."

When he returned and greetings were exchanged with Patience, he directed, "Order a PETA/CT Scan for Apryl. Let them know she'll be calling and give her their number." Patience left to attend to his instructions.

"We're finished for today. Do you have any final questions before I go?" he inquired.

"Just a couple," I said, looking to Ken for much needed support. "I'm feeling a bit anxious at times about *everything* I'm going through. And do I have all the doctors I require in place? Also, what exactly will the procedures you've scheduled consist of? I feel a bit lost at this point."

"I know just the person who can help with that." Once again he disappeared, closing the door behind him.

When he returned introductions were made to *his* nurse navigator. She too wore a white medical coat which she left open over a printed summer dress. Pleasantries were exchanged, then the Mad Scientist turned to her. "I'd like them back in a couple of weeks to review Apryl's test results." He then turned to me. "At that time we'll discuss your game plan. In the meantime, here's the number to schedule your PET/CT Scan." Glancing back to his nurse navigator, he said, "Please show her the scheduling desk where she can make future appointments prior to leaving." He then excused himself for the final time.

As he opened the door just enough to allow himself through, three people could be seen excitedly awaiting him. *His groupies*, I thought as he attempted to gently shut the door behind him.

The Mad Scientist's nurse navigator stood facing us in the middle of the room. Then, deciding to get a little more comfortable, she leaned against the examining table I had previously occupied. She began with, "I *completely* understand what you're *feeling* and know *intimately* the process you'll soon be going through," pausing for effect. Then with an air of clarification, "I too have been diagnosed with breast cancer and am going through it for the *second* time."

Oh good . . . someone I can relate to. Maybe she can lift a little of this fog. "I'm so sorry to hear that." Then realizing what she just said, "How terrible you have to go through it a *second* time." Then it registered what I was saying—*Wait a minute . . . how does that happen exactly?* A chill ran down my spine. *Doesn't she work for the Mad Scientist?* Looking to my notes for guidance I attempt to realign my thoughts on the more pertinent matter at hand—*ME!*

"I'm hoping you can help with some of my concerns. First, I'd like to make sure I've contacted and scheduled all the doctors I'll be requiring.

And, is there anything I've missed or don't know I need?" Continuing on with my list of questions, "I'm also interested in the details of my upcoming PETA/CT Scan and echocardiogram—I don't like surprises. I have a slight fear of needles, not to mention quite the imagination . . ." I was about to tell her how it freaked me out I required an IV during the MRI when I noticed a glazed look staring back at me.

Completely dismissing my questions and concerns, the nurse navigator began with *her* tale of breast cancer. She started by reiterating, "I probably wouldn't have gotten it a second time had I stayed on the prescribed Tamoxifen. You're required to take it for five years, but I couldn't handle the side effects after the first two and decided to go off it. I was known as 'the bitch from hell' here at work, with my husband and our family and friends. I couldn't take it anymore—not to mention the toll it was taking on me personally. So I went off it."

Ken and I sat paralyzed while she regurgitated—in colorful detail— her *hour-long* rehearsed calamity of the absolute worst outcome I could possibly imagine. Both of us, exchanging glances, read each other's thoughts, *maybe there's a reason she's telling us this. After all, the Mad Scientist did suggest we speak with her.* And worse, *is there something they know we don't or that the Mad Scientist couldn't find the courage to tell us?*

Ignoring our heightened concern, she continued her morbid saga. "Shortly after I started chemo I got up one morning to take a shower. Now I knew my hair was going to fall out, but what I didn't anticipate was *how* it would happen. I started washing my hair and suddenly clumps were coming out in my hands. My husband came to comfort me, and after calming me down, rid the shower of my recent episode. Most people don't realize this," she added smugly, "It's not just limited to the hair on your head—*all* of your hair falls out!"

She began cackling and, for whatever unknown reason, we joined her fearful chortle. You know the kind when you narrowly escape a near-death experience. Did we really need to hear this? I so desperately wished I could cover my ears and run out of the room yelling *"TMI! TMI!!!"*

Unrelentingly, she continued taking us into the deepest depths of the double M she was *personally* in the middle of. Then, apprising me of the various surgeries I could choose from, she graphically detailed each option. The most horrific experience of this mind-numbing nightmarish voyage was that *she personalized it!* This was an up-close detailed experience of everything *I* was personally and unequivocally—leaving no stone unturned—about to embark upon myself.

At last I found my voice. "But I may not have to go through any of this, right? I mean, I only have it in one breast and unless the BRCA test comes back positive, I won't require the double mastectomy—*correct*?

"Well, yes, that's true. I'm just letting you know what *could* happen."

"Okay, but I'd rather focus on the moment than the 'what-ifs.'" I don't think this woman is aware of what she's doing. Isn't she supposed to provide support and help *me* get through this emotionally? Instead I feel as if she's pandering to her health crises. And they consider her a nurse navigator? She's more like a *Nightmare Navigator!*

"Understood" she said, but it was too late, the damage was done. Then, trying to sound upbeat, "I just want to let you know I've been through it all and am an *excellent* source should you need *anything*. In the future, when they prescribe medications, you can contact me directly and I'll make sure they get filled. You can even contact me to schedule future appointments. Basically I'm here to help with *all* your needs. I'm also the 'go-between' for you and the Mad Scientist," she added with a smile. "Now let's get you checked out. This is how you'll leave after each visit," and she opened the door, allowing much needed fresh air into the room.

We couldn't gather our belongings quick enough and were more than pleased to follow her out the door. Turning right down a hallway, I could literally taste freedom before us. At the end of the hall were three stations, each separated by a partition on the countertop for privacy. Three vacant chairs stood idly in front of each station.

"This is the scheduling desk." She then turned to a woman manning one of the stations. "Please help Apryl schedule her next appointment with the Mad Scientist." She then turned back to me. "Apryl, should you need *anything* at all, I'm here for you. It does help to have *someone* to talk to who's already been through what you're currently facing." *Gee thanks . . . you'll be at the top of my list, right up there with the patient advocate.* She then gave me a hug and *finally* left Ken and I to our own devices.

Scheduling my next appointment proved difficult as well. I gave the approximate date when the Mad Scientist wanted us to return. However, when the scheduler handed me the appointment card, it was for more than a week *past* the requested date. I kindly pointed out the error.

"Oh, oops, you did say the second, not the 12th, didn't you?" She quickly changed it and completed a *new* appointment card for me. Yes, I double-checked the date and time and would from that point forward when scheduling appointments. She then pointed us in the direction of a frosted glass door to exit the office.

By the time we got to the car I was a train wreck. Tears uncontrollably streamed down my face. "Ken, I really don't think I have it in me to go through this. I *really* don't. How do people find the strength to do this? God—why can't my mom be here? I need her so badly right now!"

"I know you do, honey. If there was any way I could make that happen you know I would!" Then he paused for a moment. I knew that he was attempting to fix me, fix the situation ... fix this whole sordid nightmare! Then with his sweet, calm voice said, "I think what you have to do is try and put everything that woman said out of your mind. I should've stopped her long before, but I thought there was a purpose for what she was telling us. I don't understand why the Mad Scientist brought her in. There was no need for her. And you said it yourself, we'll know *nothing* about what your treatments will consist of until *after* we receive your test results." He was right, but I was melting fast right before his eyes. "Maybe you should call Clíona. She's a good source to help put things back in perspective."

Yeah ... Clíona—he's right! I picked up my phone and dialed her number. *Rats, voicemail,* and I left a message I can only imagine she'd need a translator to decipher.

Afterwards Ken tried to cheer me up. "Let's go to your favorite spot for lunch. I think we both need a drink after that diatribe."

"Okay, but Ken ... I think I might need something *more*. I think I'm having what they consider an anxiety attack. This has to be what they are, and I can't face this without *something—I don't think*. Maybe Valium because there's no way I'll go on anti-depressants. I refuse to do that. Plus, I know myself; I'll only need something *occasionally*."

"I agree." He then suggested, "Why don't you call Dr. KnowItAll. Get him to prescribe something for you and we'll pick it up on the way home."

"Great idea!" and I dial his number.

I felt relieved when Ruford answered the phone. He knew of my recent diagnosis and I wouldn't need to reiterate everything from the beginning. But after telling him of my dilemma, he said, "I'm sorry, Dr. KnowItAll is out of town for the next week. If you can wait until then we can get you an appointment with him." *Rats!* I forgot, he did tell us at our last appointment he was going on vacation. I ended the call disheartened.

Then an idea flashed before me as I recalled the offer of the Nightmare Navigator to help me. Digging for her business card in Ken's briefcase, I find it and dial her number.

"All I'll need is *maybe* five tablets of Valium. I'd ask my internist, but he's on vacation. Do you think you can get the Mad Scientist to prescribe something for me?" *Please say yes!*

"Let me see what I can do," is all she offered.

"Okay, but honestly, I don't do drugs and all I'm asking for is *five* pills." I was pleading from the very core of my being. If I require more than that I can get them from Dr. KnowItAll when he returns.

"Do we have the number for your pharmacist?" she inquired.

"Yes, you do."

"I'll call you back shortly." When she did I was in the middle of lunch, so she quickly said they had called a prescription into my pharmacist for the requested Valium. "Let me know if there's anything else I can help you with," she implored. *Absolutely, I'll do just that.*

After lunch we drove directly to the pharmacy to get the prescription. The pharmacist himself came out looking a bit worried and handed me a bottle with a quantity of *50 pills*. Whispering to Ken, "I told her five, not 50!" Surely it was a typo on their part.

"Don't argue, Apryl; just take them," was Ken's whispered response out of the corner of his mouth—and I did.

Of course, the pharmacist cautioned, "These pills are highly addictive. Be very careful you don't get too attached to them."

I can't help but think about my beautiful mother during this time. I cannot imagine what it would be like to go through something like this on your own without your spouse. I am so very fortunate to have my husband by my side. The only real fear I have now is fear of the unknown.

That night after dinner, and a much needed *Fringe* episode, I took my first of 50 Valium. Within 15 minutes I drifted off to another place, another time, and slept like a baby without a care in the world.

8

Qué Sera Sera
Pink Martini

The Medicine Woman shares her waiting area with another doctor but it's currently empty of patients. Its room contains two separate windows, allowing you to peer into each workplace. One window is open and I watch the administrative staff busily buzz around. The glass is closed to the other, but through it two women can be seen talking at the far end of the room with their backs to the window. Its walls are painted light purple. I knew immediately which office I'd be entering.

In front of the closed window a clipboard is precariously positioned lengthwise on the counter. Upon closer inspection, the Medicine Woman's name can be seen in large lettering at the top of the sheet. Signing in, I take my place next to Ken. The flowers on display aren't real but offer somewhat of a cheery atmosphere to this otherwise dreary room that's painted vomit brown.

Moments later, a woman slides the window open and calls my name. When I approach she asks if I have my completed paperwork.

"Yes." Handing it to her I add, "Instead of writing down my past surgeries, I've included copies of the procedures themselves. I've also included the family history I was asked to complete by the genetics counselor."

Taking the paperwork, she begins assessing it. With her eyes glued to the forms, she instructs me in a preoccupied tone, "Have a seat and someone will be with you shortly," and slides the window closed, turning her back to me. Her demeanor was not particularly welcoming.

I returned to my seat, and using a very low tone, informed Ken, "That's definitely not Mabel; she has a distinctive voice. She also told me their office is staffed with just the two of them. That has to be the Medicine

Woman checking me in." Not to mention she appears to be a bit unaccustomed to normal administrative duties.

Ken and I patiently waited for the window to roll open again. When it did I was asked to come through the door to the left. They would be around shortly to open it. *Really? A locked door? Are cancer patients problematic?* I mused.

When the door opened, using more of a statement rather than a request, "I'd like to have my husband join us as well." The Medicine Woman nodded her consent and we followed her down the short hallway.

Escorting us into an examining room she handed me a rose-colored paper frock. "Please change into this from the waist up with the opening in the front." *Yes, I know the drill,* and she left us to comply with her orders.

While changing, I inform Ken, "Mabel said the Medicine Woman doesn't like family members asking questions so sit quietly while she examines me." Ken chuckled to himself and agreed to comply. Immediately I realized how obnoxious I sounded and retracted the request. *What the heck am I saying—Ken's nothing but respectful to doctors.* My mind feels as if it's spinning out of control when I climb onto the examining table.

There's a light rap on the door and the Medicine Woman enters. She's trailed by a laptop computer atop a table with wheels. No sooner does she seat herself at her makeshift desk, then she starts firing off questions. Once through the interrogation she stands and readies herself.

"I'd like to examine you now," she says pushing her computer on wheels to the side. "Please lie back on the table."

She starts the—*oh how I hate it*—examination, attempting to feel for Jorge. Unable to do so, she moves over to my underarm where the Lymph-Along-Kid resides and starts poking around there. *Ouch that hurts*—and I flinch.

"Oh, sorry," and she moves back over to where Jorge supposedly is. Placing her index finger on his general location, "It says he's here at the 10 o'clock position." She presses down hard with her finger.

"Okay, I feel a little pain there," I respond.

Then she pushes her finger a little deeper and says, "I believe this is him."

Agreeing, "Yep, I think you're right." *Youch!*

"You may sit up now and get dressed. Meet me in my office, which is to your right out the door. I'll be waiting there to discuss my prognosis," and we watch as she and her computer on wheels disappear behind the door.

I quickly change, and, as instructed, Ken and I enter her purple office. Of course he chooses this moment to inquire, "Do you have a restroom I can use?" and leaves me to face this woman alone.

The Medicine Woman immediately begins discussing the details of surgery, ignoring the fact that Ken just left the room. I listen intently, while feverishly taking notes, as she spews the various procedures she deems suitable for someone in my predicament.

Can't Ken go to the restroom prior to these appointments? I hate it when he leaves. I didn't dare ask her to wait, thinking *she'll just have to repeat it when he returns.* I mean, I'm not going to sit quietly staring at the walls, with *this* woman, in *her* office. I can't believe the amount of information she's prattled off while in Ken's absence.

Not skipping a beat, "After the surgery we wait to hear whether the margins around Jorge are clear. If not, we schedule another surgery. This process continues until we're given the 'all clear.'" She then pulls out a diagram of a woman's torso when Ken returns. "To better explain your surgery, this is the location where the lumpectomy will occur. As I mentioned, you'll also require a lymph node dissection. At that time, I'll be taking a few lymph nodes to verify only the one is cancerous."

"How many lymph nodes will you take exactly?" I inquire.

"You never know; it could be 10 or 15. We'll want a good sampling is all I can say with certainty." She seemed confident in her conclusion.

I then asked her a few personal questions. "Why is it you decided to become a breast surgeon?"

Taken aback that I asked a personal question, she took a moment to respond. "Because of all the different types of surgeries I've been trained on, I found this is what I love to do best." *Okay, I like that answer.*

Then I touched lightly on the topic, inquiring about a *double M.* "Should the BRCA testing come back positive would you recommend I have a double mastectomy?"

"Absolutely YES!"

"Even though I only have cancer in one breast?" I felt my throat start to constrict.

"Yes, that would mean you're at *high* risk and I don't want you back in here due to another Tango. Why would you want to take that chance?" She looked blankly at me as if to ask, "*Are you a fool?*"

"So that would mean you'd take both my—*gulp*—nipples too?"

"Yes, since you've been diagnosed with Jorge there is a strong potential he could come back through the nipples . . ." She continued on, yet I drifted off to another place, brooding over *how* exactly I came to be sitting in this chair.

I returned as she finished her much unwanted informative speech. ". . . So, to answer your question, *yes* I would recommend you remove both of your nipples as well. But that's *only* if your BRCA gene tests positive." *Thank goodness she ended this on an up note.*

"So what you're saying is, if it comes back negative I won't require a double mastectomy, correct?"

"Correct. Of course you can always opt for a double mastectomy, which will negate any concerns of breast cancer returning in the future but that's a decision only you can make."

"I'll tell you right now, if it's negative I'm going to choose the lumpectomy and lymph node dissection. I don't want to put myself through an unnecessary or unwanted surgery when there's the possibility it may never return." And I made a silent promise to myself *I'll focus on creating negative results!*

"The last thing you'll need to decide on, besides what type of surgery you'll have, is a reconstructive surgeon. Because you have breast implants you'll need to discuss whether you will keep the implants in or have them removed during your chemo and radiation treatments."

"Does it make a difference to you during the surgery?"

"No, it makes no difference at all to me. Besides the implants, a reconstructive surgeon will make you look esthetically correct, filling in any indents left after the removal of Jorge. You'll need to make this decision prior to picking a surgery date because I'll need to align my schedule with that doctor. Do you have a particular surgeon in mind?" she inquired.

"Yes, a personal friend, our Shape Shifter."

"Well, just in case for whatever reason he doesn't work out, I'll have Mabel give you a list of surgeons I particularly like to work with." *Hmmm . . . she really is particular,* I thought, then quickly dismissed it as I'm the same way when it comes to my music. "Also, I'll be on vacation starting the first week of August and will return on the 12th. Once we learn the results from your BRCA test," pushing her chair back she stood, "we'll know what type of surgery you'll require and can schedule it at that time. I'd like to introduce you to Mabel now."

Following the Medicine Woman out of her office, we stop at Mabel's desk. As I said before, it's as if I've known Mabel forever. I gave her a huge hug and thanked her again for realigning me during my "OMG" moment.

Mabel then handed us the paperwork we had discussed, reiterating, "As soon as you receive the results from the BRCA gene test, phone our office immediately. We'll be on vacation, but calling in for messages. Knowing the results will help us determine the type of surgery we'll need to schedule upon our return."

"Thank you. I'll let you know as soon as I hear anything. Supposedly we'll have the results on August 5th," and inwardly I finished the sentence, *I'm confident they'll be negative.*

Taking the elevator down I smiled. "Ken . . . I like her a lot, especially Mabel! I think we just found my surgeon." He agreed.

"And best of all, now you can take me away for our anniversary! Since she'll be on vacation until the 12th, we know the surgery won't happen until *after* the 15th." Ken had wanted to take me away . . . away from everything—especially Jorge! This was a much needed boost to the outlook of our not-so-distant future.

The next day I decided to enlist the help of my Inquisitive Minds with a very important request:

From: *Apryl*
Sent: *Saturday, July 27, 2013 7:05 PM*
To: *The Inquisitive Minds*
Subject: *ADA Update – BRCA Gene Testing*

To The Inquisitive Loving & Caring Individuals In My Life Who Want to Know!!!

Please keep me in your prayers, thoughts and wishes. AND, whatever ability or pull you have in the spiritual or otherworldly sense . . . NOW would be a good time to call in some favors and ask for help! We need my BRCA 1 and BRCA 2 genes to come back NEGATIVE!!!

So until next week, keep a smile on your face as I will have one on mine. Please know I'm in a very good and positive place! I'll let you know how it goes after I speak with my Mad Scientist! Most importantly Monday, August 5th will be a pivotal day for me as I should learn of the results from the genetic test, along with it the positive aspects of what my future has in store!!! Until next time . . .

With all my heart, a Big Hug & HUGE KISS!

As you recall, I had contacted our friend the Shape Shifter the day I was diagnosed with Jorge. He phoned, of course, offering, "If there's anything at all I can do let me know; any advice or questions you might want to bounce off of me." He was so sorry to hear of my little visitor and wanted Ken and I to know he would be here for us anytime day or night.

His kind-hearted message spoke of my inner strength and having more spirit than anyone he knew. He also offered some great advice, of which I took to heart: "Pick someone who you don't mind visiting a few times. You should feel very confident and trust in their ability to guide you. Most importantly, you have to feel they are sincere in caring for you. That's all you can ask for." He ended with, "This is going to be just a little bump in the road, one that you can beat easily. I feel you're very well equipped for it and you've got great support."

Well, now I'm in need of him—a reconstructive surgeon. It was time to play my *Get out of Jail Free* card. "Brianna, I'd like to speak with the Shape Shifter about my upcoming surgery. It appears I'll need a reconstructive surgeon to close up after Jorge's removal. Do you think he'd be willing to do it?"

"I'm not sure. I know he normally doesn't take cases like this. And another major problem is he doesn't take insurance . . ." *Well, that puts a wrench in my plans.*

Rewind back to 2003 ... The Shape Shifter had hired Ken and his partner to design his office. During their first meeting he told Ken how he got his initial start working in the ER with top doctors in the field of reconstructive surgery. He worked on people who had been in *crazy* accidents—literally rebuilding faces, hands, you name it. From there he decided to become a reconstructive surgeon—cosmetic surgery soon followed.

When I was told I had a second melanoma on the inside of my left knee, I asked him if he'd be willing to remove it. *"No, I'd prefer not to have anything to do with cancer,"* was his reply.

Really?! "Neither do I!" I said, looking at him incredulously. Literally I saw him melt before my eyes.

After a long pause, looking deep into my eyes, he acquiesced. *"Okay, call my office and get it scheduled."* Honestly, he has one of the hugest hearts I know. I was so very thankful to have him in my life at that moment, not realizing what the future held for me, nor the role he would play.

Fast forward to 2013 and my conversation with Brianna. "Honestly, he doesn't do those types of surgeries, nor does he like to perform them in tandem with another surgeon. But I'll definitely ask him for you. Maybe there's another Shape Shifter he would recommend." *Double Rats! Another Shape Shifter?!* "Also, I don't know when we'll hear from him because he just left today on vacation and won't be back until August 5th."

"Oh—I *really* don't want to bother him while he's on vacation."

"It's no problem; he's concerned about you and wants to help in any way he can. I'll leave a message and we'll see what he says."

"Okay, but I *really* hate troubling him with this . . ."

"It's no problem. I'll let you know when I hear from him." I felt bad for asking and truly didn't want to impose on our friendship *again*—especially if he didn't do this type of surgery.

Apryl . . . think, think, think . . . what do I do? This is quite the conundrum I'm in. It seems like nothing's easy. That evening my mobile phone rang; it was the Shape Shifter himself.

"Apryl, I got Brianna's message. Listen, my best advice is get the surgery done and forget about the reconstructive part for now. We can deal with that at a later date." I agreed. That advice seemed to make sense and I do *trust* the Shape Shifter implicitly.

Phoning Mabel, I received her voicemail. Leaving a message, I told her of the conversation, and my decision regarding postponing the reconstructive portion of the surgery until *after* I was through all the treatments. Of course this would only be the case *if* the genetic test came back *negative*. If it didn't that would mean a completely different type of surgery and a *different* Shape Shifter.

Mabel phoned back, informing me the Medicine Woman felt it would be in my best interest to have a reconstructive surgeon present during the surgery. "Maybe it's a good idea you get another opinion." My mind was reeling at this point. I didn't want to look deformed, and honestly, I really didn't want to have a second surgery. *What do I do???*

All I want is the surgery scheduled and, truth be told, over and done with. Ken and I had scheduled our anniversary trip and I wanted my game plan figured out *before* we left. I pulled out the list of reconstructive surgeons both the Medicine Woman and her nurse navigator had given me. I began scrutinizing them.

Three of the same names were on both lists. I thought to myself, *Maybe I should get a second opinion since the Shape Shifter doesn't want to deal with Jorge; what would it hurt to meet with someone who actually does these type of surgeries?* I decided to start there. I googled all three doctors and quickly narrowed it down to two. I did as much research as humanly possible on both of them.

With the research behind me, it was time to schedule consultations and once again show my breasts to yet more strangers. I'd be meeting with two Shape Shifters, primarily for the infamous *second opinion* from doctors who deal with patients in my predicament. My game plan was, after meeting with the two of them, I'd contact our friend the Shape Shifter and let him know he was off the hook for my surgery and, more importantly, get his feedback on my decision. I was feeling pretty optimistic!

Since the Medicine Woman said she worked with the Male Shape Shifter several times and thought highly of his work ethics I contacted his office first. "Good afternoon. I'd like to . . ." *blah, blah, blah*—my story was getting old, even to me.

"Let's see, the first consultation appointment he has available is on September 25th," his scheduler replied.

"What?! But that's so far away . . . I was hoping to have my surgery the first week of September. There's nothing sooner?" I pleaded.

"No, I'm sorry. I can put you on a cancellation list if you'd like?" she offered with sincere empathy.

"Yes, please, I'd greatly appreciate it."

After our call I decided to enlist the help of both the Medicine Woman and the Mad Scientist with my war cry. Let's see how much pull they actually have.

I dialed the Medicine Woman's number and spoke with Mabel. "Let me call over there and see what we can do," she offered, "I can't promise anything but we can try."

I attempted to contact the Mad Scientist, but he and his staff were at their other office. Since it was late on a Friday afternoon, I'd try next week — worst case at our appointment on Friday.

In the meantime, I called the *female* Shape Shifter's office. Her first consultation appointment was on August 21st. *Dang . . . I didn't realize how much in demand these Shape Shifters are.* At this point it was out of my hands — there was nothing more I could do. I let go of the anxiety of having to wait for an October surgery. If it was meant to be there'd be a cancellation.

As if on cue, fond memories of my mother fill my senses. I drift back to when I was a little girl — there with my mother cooking in her kitchen. She began singing one of her favorite songs, "*Qué Sera Sera, whatever will be will be . . .*"

Foreboding unease has taken center stage. My appointment for the PET/CT scan is rapidly approaching and I feel ill-prepared. *God, another procedure I have no idea about.* I asked some acquaintances who'd personally experienced this type of procedure what it was like, but it was so long ago and they couldn't recall the details.

"It's nothing to worry about," one friend informed me.

"Yeah, well, I thought the MRI was nothing to worry about and I ended up with an IV in my arm for half the procedure."

Why didn't I ask when I scheduled it? Oh, wait . . . I did, I asked the Nightmare Navigator! Why is it so difficult to get information? I like knowing what to expect during treatments so I can prepare myself mentally.

Why can't they offer a detailed handout prior to these procedures? I hate surprises.

Since I couldn't find anyone that knew definitively, I took matters into my own hands and decided to inquire at the imaging facility. Maybe someone would take pity on me and give me all the dirty details. I phone the number I used to schedule the PET/CT scan and a sweet voice answers the phone. "This is Malaika. How can I help you?"

After explaining my dilemma, I inquire, "Do you know, by chance, what the procedure I'll be having consists of?"

"Hmmm . . . I don't, but if you hold for a moment I'll see what I can find out."

Since I have a great imagination, I began to contemplate the type of response I'd be given. Would it be that she has no idea and would transfer me to a questionable catch-all voicemail that never gets checked? Or would it be she couldn't find anyone and simply says, you're having a full body scan? Or worse, would she prattle off another mind-numbing procedure as quickly as she could, all so she could get off the phone and back to whatever it is that's occupying her "me-time"? God forbid I interrupt a personal text—it's not as if I have a life-threatening disease I'm attempting to rid my body of!

Ending my bluster of "what-ifs," she picks up the receiver. "Hello, Apryl?"

"Yes," *wait for it . . . wait for it . . .*

"We don't have anything written down with a detailed explanation." *I knew it—so which response will she choose?* "So I asked the head technician and he'll personally speak to you about it."

What?! I actually found someone who didn't have the *"I'm going to get rid of this caller as fast as I can"* attitude? This woman actually seemed to *care*.

"One moment and I'll transfer you to Benny."

Once he realized I'd never had this type of procedure, Benny spilled the beans. "You'll first be injected with a radioactive solution, then after about 45 minutes of non-activity you'll be taken in for the PET/CT scan."

"Okay, so an injection is involved. Will the needle be staying in my arm during the scan?" *I really don't think I can stomach another IV.*

"No, *before* the procedure is when the injection takes place. We'll then be doing two different scans. The first will take three minutes and the second 25."

"Okay . . . but just to let you know, I have small rolling veins. Is the person doing the injection good with needles?"

"Let's see, what time is your procedure scheduled for?" I could hear him plucking away on his keyboard, attempting to ascertain who my tech would be.

"It's at 6:30 tomorrow morning," I offer in an attempt to help with the search.

"Why are you having it so early? If you come in at 11:30 I can personally do it for you."

"I'm supposed to fast prior to the procedure, and I don't want to go without food for half a day."

Benny insisted, "Why don't you come in at 11:30?" I had a feeling he wasn't going to take no for an answer. Besides, you can't ask for more than the head tech working on you. Before I could respond he changed my appointment time.

Sighing, not sure if it was from relief or because I get to ask Ken yet again to change his schedule around for me, "Okay, fine, 11:30. I'm supposed to fast before this procedure, correct?"

"Actually, there's more to it. I don't want you working out 24 hours prior to this procedure. Have you worked out today?"

"No . . ." *The past few days I've been a bit preoccupied, and workouts have been at the bottom of my list of things to do.*

"Good. Tonight I want you to eat a very light meal, meaning no carbs. And most importantly, I want you to be a couch potato until I see you. And, yes, you're correct, don't eat anything six hours prior to the procedure. You can have water, but nothing else. This way when the radioactive glucose—glucose is sugar—when it's injected, it will quickly be devoured by the cancer. Because of your inactivity the cancer will be the first to eat the solution; it will then light up like stars on the scan."

"So if cancer's attracted to sugar does that mean I should stay away from sugary foods?"

A slight chuckle erupts from Benny. "Interestingly, all cells depend on glucose for energy and growth. And although there is some controversy over sugar, just remember, everything in moderation."

"*Whew* . . . you had me a bit worried there." Laughing, we wish each other well for the evening and say our goodbyes. After the call I felt much calmer about the procedure.

We arrive 15 minutes early for the PET/CT scan. Signing in at the reception desk I'm greeted by the most beautiful, full of life smile I think I've ever seen.

"Good morning, Apryl! I see Benny changed your appointment this morning to 11:30 so he could do it himself."

"Yes, you must be Malaika?" My face lit up with recognition of her voice.

If her smile could have gotten any brighter it just did. "Yes, I hope you feel a little more prepared for today."

"I do. Thank you so much for actually *listening* to my concerns. I was so nervous about this appointment—truth be told I still am—but not nearly as much as I was yesterday."

"Good, I'm glad to hear it." After collecting my co-pay, she told me to have a seat while she notified Benny I was here.

When Benny arrives I ask if Ken can join us. "Of course, he's more than welcome to." Benny shakes Ken's hand and we follow him down the hall into a 10 x 12-foot room. Inside the room is a Barcalounger and a chair comfortably positioned between it and the wall.

"Please make yourself comfortable in the reclining chair and Ken, you can have the seat next to Apryl."

After we're settled, Benny instructs, "I'm going to start by first checking your blood sugar level; it should be under 120." Pricking my finger, he takes a sample of my blood. "Perfect, it's 93. Now I'm going to inject the radioactive glucose solution. I'll do so by using a syringe attached to this IV."

The process is exactly how my naturopath injects vitamin IVs. I had a few in efforts to boost my immune system from my bout with mono in 2011. When I first heard of vitamin IVs I'd envisioned an IV drip, but this process uses a syringe which is manually injected by the person holding it, in this case Benny.

"Okay, you're going to feel a little pinch . . ." and that's about all I felt.

"Wow, you're pretty good at this. I hardly felt anything." Relief calmed my weariness.

"Yeah, not to boast, but this *is* my forte. People with diseases such as Parkinson's ask for me to do their blood draws and injections. This is nothing compared to that; imagine trying to take blood from someone who has no control over their limbs. They don't just shake, they flap wildly." *Wow . . . I never thought of that.*

"Okay, we're almost halfway done." We talk a little more, about anything to take my mind off the needle in my arm. Then, "We're all finished!" and he delicately removed the needle and bandaged it. Then he offers, "Let me help you recline your chair." Up came the footrest and back went the chair; he then covered me with warm blankets. I couldn't have felt more cozy in my own home. Turning off the lights he implored, "For the next 45 minutes I want you to quietly relax. Try not to move."

"May I read?" thinking I'd be allowed to do so.

"No. Any movement you make is where the solution will go. I want you to lay as still as possible."

"Really?! Okay, I'll just relax then." And he left us with the door open to our room.

Sitting next to me, Ken uses the hall light to read while I drift in and out of consciousness. I so want to sleep and escape from the stress of it all, but because of all the stress I can't.

After 45 minutes, although it felt like 15, Benny appears. "It's time for your scan. Ken, you can join us if you'd like. Feel free to leave your belongings here. I'll shut the door. No one will bother them." I silently thank Benny. Knowing Ken would be in the room made me feel that much stronger!

We follow him down a short hall and into a huge room, about 30 feet by 30 feet. And there, in the middle of the room, stood a VLM (Very Large Machine)! It felt as if we walked through a portal and entered the future. The machine is completely white with a bed that slides into the opening of the contraption. *Please help me find the inner strength for this procedure* I silently plead.

"There's a restroom over in the corner. Please empty your bladder. When you return, lie down on the bed face up."

Washing my hands, I observe a fearful woman staring at me from the other side of the mirror. Looking deep into her soul I implore, *you're strong. You can do this. There's nothing you can't do!*

Almost as if it were a hushed whisper, echoes from the past reverberate throughout my entire being and I sense the soft, gentle love of my mother. Closing my eyes, I hear her voice, "*I love you Apryl D—I'm here with you.*" Taking a deep breath, I open my eyes and look at the woman staring at me from her unknown world. *I'm not alone* I remind her and open the door to the futuristic threshold.

A bit on the nervous side, I attempt to mount the scanner bed gracefully while six eyes watch me. "Apryl, this is Thomas, he'll be assisting me with your scan today."

Thomas took over. "Apryl, please place your hands over your head and get into a comfortable position, you'll be in it for a while."

As instructed, I place my arms over my head and clasp my hands together in prayer position, crossing my thumbs as you do in some yoga poses. A plush pillow was provided for my head and Thomas places a triangular pillow under my knees. The bed itself has a relaxing cushion on it and, unlike the MRI machine, this bed is surprisingly comfortable.

The scanner itself is open at both ends and its size, if the bed were rolled into the machine, is the length of my body, allowing my head and feet to stick out at each end. The height of it extends almost to the ceiling. The machine itself hardly makes any noise, and I'm actually able to hear music playing in the background.

After I'm settled, Benny informs me, "I'm going to let you take a ride to make sure you don't feel claustrophobic." As my head reaches the middle of the machine, "Apryl, you can open your eyes to see where you're at if you'd like." I do, but quickly close them as I'm very close to the top of the scanner and feel a little scared. After closing them I find I'm good again!

"Since you're doing so well, we're going to perform a quick three-minute CT scan." It went by faster than I thought three minutes would, primarily because my mind drifted to another place in time. The Beach Boys was playing in the background and it took me back to my early 20s, when I was asked to introduce the famous band at a concert. My recollection was interrupted by Benny's voice. "Apryl, if you're doing okay, I'd like to continue with the PET/CT scan. It'll take about 20 to 25 minutes. Or, if you'd prefer, I can bring you out for a quick breather, but you can't move. You'll need to stay exactly in the position you are."

"I think I'm good . . . we can keep going." Having allowed Ken in the room, knowing he's here with me—just a breath away—gives me all the confidence I need. I know he won't let *anything* happen to me.

"Okay, we'll continue on then," and we proceed with the Isinthis scan—*from my eyes to my thighs*.

These two scans combined will allow the Mad Scientist to see inside my body in 3D. COOL! *I hope they let me see it!* The bed moves to and fro a few times but as long as I kept my eyes closed and mentally drifted to another place, I was good. Finally, it's over!

Benny returned to help me off the bed. Once both feet are firmly planted on the ground I take his hand within both of mine and gently squeeze it as tears fill my eyes. "Thank you so much! You've been so kind; I appreciate *everything* you've done for me!" My hand squeeze quickly turned into a hug.

Benny hugged me back, "You're welcome."

Next up on my list . . . Echocardiogram. Ken once again drives me to the appointment. I feel so selfish of his time, but appreciate the fact he's with me more than he'll ever realize. Arriving at the facility, I sign in.

"Thank you, please have a seat and someone will be with you shortly," we're told. Ken and I turn to face the small waiting area.

Fifteen people are waiting for their appointments; all have white hair and a few of them require oxygen tanks. *God, I don't want this to be our future.* Two seats are currently unoccupied and we quickly fill them. Looking around for the overly-used and outdated magazines, none are to be found. Thank goodness for technology; we'll catch up on our e-mails then.

About 15 minutes go by when the tech appears. With what I assume is a Russian accent she calls my name, "Apryl Allen?"

"That's me," I respond and walk towards her. When I'm close enough to ask, without alerting the entire room, I inquire, "Would it be possible to have my husband join us?"

"No, I'm sorry. It's a very small room and there really isn't any place for him to sit."

Returning to Ken he hears the slight fear and concern in my voice as I tell him he can't accompany me. He quickly assures me, "This is an easy appointment, honey. Everyone we've spoken with says it's just an ultrasound." Begrudgingly I hand him my purse and Warrior Book and give him a quick kiss.

"Thanks, honey, I'll see you in a few minutes," and he watches as I disappear with the blonde woman through the door.

She was absolutely telling the truth; the room I follow her into is very small. What looks like a gurney on wheels occupies most of the room. To the right of it, squeezed in between the bed and the wall, is a stand with a boxy computer monitor perched atop, and placed in front of that is a stool. The tech steps out of the treatment room to allow me to change into my favorite gown. No sooner do I wrap it around me than she raps on the door.

"Come in." Feeling a bit panicky I quickly scan the room for any signs of needles or IVs. Thank goodness, none were visible.

Asking me to lay down, she seats herself next to me. Then she became Miss Talkie, Talkie . . . about everything *except* my procedure. I don't mind, though; it's a welcome change from the numerous appointments I've been dealt so far. Picking up the magic wand, she glops gel on the end of it and unties my gown.

"Sorry, this'll be a bit cold," she warns prior to starting.

YIKES! The gel is really cold! The monitor soon distracts me from what she's doing and I'm instantly captivated by seeing my heart beating inside me for the very first time. Technology is amazing! I watch as it performs its duty *Thump-Thump, Thump-Thump, Thump-Thump.* She moves the wand over my chest, attempting to capture a good picture of my heart, all the while avoiding my breast itself. She accomplishes this by pressing the wand up under the crease of my breast and pushes the mass of it up high. It feels as if I'm wearing some sort of lopsided bustier contraption.

Squeezing more gel on the end of the wand, she then places it on my upper left rib cage to capture my heart's side view. *Talkie, Talkie— Talkie, Talkie.* Again, I really don't mind the conversation. Suddenly I feel an ever-so-light electric shock. You know the kind, when you touch someone or something with your fingertips and you shock them or yourself. But it wasn't even that, well, shocking. It was so light it almost went undetected.

"Does everything look normal?" I query, not wishing to interrupt our interesting tête-à-tête, but my Inquisitive Minds will want to know.

"I'm not the person who reads these, but from what I can see it looks healthy." I always love hearing good news. And we continue on with our *Talkie, Talkie*. "Okay, we're finished," and she plucks several tissues from a box and hands them to me. "You can go ahead and change back into your blouse. Would you like me to step out of the room while you do so?" At this point she's seen my entire torso; besides it seems I'm becoming desensitized to all the viewing and handlings of my breasts.

"No, I don't mind." By the time I utter the words I'm putting my blouse on. She makes her way to the end of the bed, leaving room for me to stand and follow her out, through the short maze of halls, to the door where my husband's waiting on the other side. Mentally, I take my imaginary checklist and mark off another procedure from the now seemingly endless agenda.

9

Time in a Bottle

Jim Croce

*W*aiting, Waiting, Waiting—This is maddening!!! Since my appointment with the Mad Scientist is on Friday—the last day of the actual two-week timeframe required for the BRCA testing—I thought I'd be proactive and contact the genetics counselor in hopes the results would be ready. Hence yesterday morning I left her a message. It's at this moment she returns my call, just as Ken and I are pulling out of the parking lot after my echocardiogram.

"Apryl, I'm sorry, but the test has not been completed. It's still pending approval from ACME Insurance. When I received your call yesterday, I phoned the laboratory to inquire of its status. They just now returned my call. I know you were hoping to have the results prior to your upcoming appointment."

"You've got to be kidding me?" I'm flabbergasted! The stupidity of it all—I would have paid for it myself had I known this. I'll have to pay for it anyhow if my deductible hasn't been met.

"No, I'm so sorry. Honestly I've never seen this happen before. I've asked them to put a 'RUSH' sticker on your sample and was told we could have the results as quickly as one week—of course that's one week from the time they receive the approval from your insurance." *Seriously?!*

Ken, after hearing my end of the conversation and seeing my grief-stricken face, receives a watered down version of what was said. "Waiting for approval?" Enraged he repeats the words. We both agree it's absolutely absurd! To think there's a waiting period for approvals on health issues, but no required waiting period when you purchase a gun? Something is really wrong here!

While driving home, Ken and I attempt to look on the bright side of life, you know the "everything happens for a reason" scenario.

"Well, I guess this means I'll have more time to get my body and mind prepared for the surgery." As I finish the sentence we pull up to a stop light. There on the car in front of us is a license plate that reads "PLSBELVE."

Yes, I Believe! I believe life is a gift filled with dreams waiting to be discovered. I believe change is inevitable; you can choose to be part of the change or fight it every step of the way. I believe in the choice we make every day when we climb out of bed and look in the mirror and choose to face whatever our future holds.

More waiting, waiting, waiting ... but I'm no longer awaiting the *authorization* from ACME Insurance. The genetics counselor called me with the news. The laboratory received the approval from ACME, YESTERDAY, July 31st—*Insert expletive here!!!!* But before I get into the details of the phone call I'd like to fill you in on some pertinent information.

First, let's look past the fact our company (also known as a small business) pays an astronomical amount annually that is slightly north of six figures for health insurance for 15 employees. That's $6,600 plus a year or $555 a month per employee! That's outrageous considering two-thirds of our employees are 35 and under. With the exception of my tango with Jorge, we're a relatively healthy group of people!

Second, unbeknownst to me, the laboratory I chose to complete my genetics test attempted to patent the BRCA 1 and BRCA 2 Genes, claiming it owns the rights to them. Of course, a lawsuit was filed on behalf of researchers, genetic counselors, patients, and anyone else offended by this claim. It stated the genes could not be patented because all people have them and testing for this gene is solely to determine whether a mutation can be detected, ergo how could they be patented? Other laboratories were wanting in on the rights—*and monies*—to test for these mutations as well. Remember I had mentioned earlier I had the choice of using *another* laboratory? The *other* laboratory could complete this same test for half the cost; however, it would take *four* weeks versus *two* to do so.

AND third, since I'm healthy and have not paid anything towards my deductible, I knew we'd be paying $2,000 out of pocket regardless to cover medical bills. Of course I opted for the more expensive test that took half the time so I could get the results in *two* weeks versus *four*. *Who wouldn't choose that option?!*

What I don't understand is why no one told me of the small, yet potentially catastrophic fact that the laboratory is required to *wait* for approval from your insurance company *prior* to completing the test. Mind you it takes two weeks for them to complete this test, unless of course your name is *Angelina Jolie*. For that reason, after receiving the vial containing the *key to my future*, the laboratory shelved it until the approval could be obtained.

Here's the visual in my mind ... the vial consisting of Scope mouthwash and my genes were shipped via FedEx *overnight* on Thursday, July 18th, to the laboratory. Having been received on Friday, July 19th, it was shelved pending approval for payment from ACME Insurance. My paperwork was then submitted to ACME and placed in someone's limbo of lost inboxes awaiting this ruler of all rules to determine whether it's a "qualifying event." It's evidently taking the full *two weeks* for this bubble gum-chewing individual to verify that my "qualifying event" listed as #2 on their website—*and below for your perusal*—qualifies!

> *Breast cancer diagnosed at 50 years or younger. (I'm 46.)*
> *AND at least one close blood relative diagnosed with breast cancer at any age. (My mother.)*

Now let's get back to my phone call with the genetics counselor. She's as exasperated as I am. "This has never happened before. I wonder if it's due to the lawsuit filed against the laboratory on July 15th."

At this point I really don't care why, I'm more interested in *when*. "Do you think we'll receive the results within the seven-day 'RUSH' period you requested?" *Has my life really been relegated to time in a bottle?* The thought was repugnant.

Her response is peppered in frustration. "Normally I'd say yes, but based on what just happened I'm not 100 percent positive." *Lovely . . .*

Quickly I change gears and do the math in my head. *Okay, I was thinking worst-case scenario anyhow, and with that in mind, the approval was received on Wednesday and one week would be . . .* "So that means I should have the results by the end of next week, Friday, August 9th, provided everything goes smoothly?"

"Yes, but that's if they keep to the Seven-Day Rush."

"Is the laboratory normally efficient?" *Think positive . . .*

"Normally I'd say yes—but like I said, this is the first time I've ever encountered this so I can't say with 100 percent certainty it will be." Well at least she's being straightforward.

"I appreciate your honesty and all you've done. Thank you so much." I hang up the receiver and decide to think on the positive side. *As far as I'm concerned the seven-day countdown begins now!*

Being relatively of sound mind when embarking upon this unwanted *Tango*, I didn't realize you not only have to be smart and savvy enough to ask the right questions but, more importantly, you must have the ability to out-think, read minds and predict any and all possible scenarios that can arise while conducting business with our glorious healthcare system.

So what does this all mean? I get to wait another week—actually more because it's counted in business days—before I can determine what type of surgery I'll require! EVERYTHING is on hold until then. What have I learned? The next time I need to have a test, ask whether it requires authorization from my insurer. And if so, what's the most expedient method of obtaining that approval. I never knew waiting could be this excruciating.

SIDEBAR
FYI for those of you who don't own or run a small business:

Until 2009 our deductible for company-paid health insurance was $250 with a $25 co-pay. I would personally like to extend a very special thank you to everyone who put into place Healthcare Reform. Because of the *Reform*, our insurance carrier in 2009 informed us upon renewal—and in preparation of what was to come (yeah, right)—if we wanted to keep our $250 deductible our insurance would go up by 65 percent. On average, insurance for small businesses goes up 25 to 35 percent annually and has systematically done so for our small business since 1999.

I don't quite understand how this is determined since the cost of living is drastically lower. And to make matters worse, for whatever reason, small businesses don't receive the same vast discounts the huge conglomerates do. Therefore, we raised our deductible to $2,000 with a co-pay of $45, in efforts to keep our premiums to the standard 25% increase. We also had to change carriers to achieve this savings. *Whew . . . aren't we fortunate?!*

Now this is addressed to Congress. My mom used to say, *"What's good for the goose is good for the gander."* For those of you who think Healthcare Reform is all that, why aren't you signing up for it? And for the others who claim you're against it, at least have the decency to offer us The People the same insurance Congress is privy to!

And, Lastly, how exactly did these private insurance companies become so intertwined in government-regulated requirements? Something's really wrong here.

Okay enough of my ranting . . .
END OF SIDEBAR

Finally, it's Friday! Today we're to review the test results of my PET/CT scan and echocardiogram with the Mad Scientist. My heart's telling me everything will be fine but my head's working overtime on the "what-ifs" of it all!

After signing in and paying my co-pay, we wait only a few minutes before my name's called. Keeping with protocol, we follow the unknown face back to waiting room #2.

"Have a seat and someone will be with you shortly for your blood draw." *What! Another blood draw?!*

"I just had one the last time I was here; are you sure I'm supposed to do it again?" *Surely she was mistaken.*

"Every time you see the Mad Scientist you'll be having your blood drawn." *It would have been nice if someone had told me. Mental note: Ask the Mad Scientist why so many blood draws.*

Ken and I sit patiently—what else can you do?—in waiting room #2. The room consists of nine chairs placed in a U-shaped formation. You can't help but look into other patients' eyes. I know I've said this before, but cancer really doesn't have a face except, perhaps, fear. Everyone in this waiting room is from different backgrounds—young, old, male, female, social, ethnic, tall, short, large, small—you name it, we're all represented.

Waiting rooms are the true melting pots of society. *God . . . please find a cure soon!*

My name's called. "Apryl Allen?"

I feel I've become a pro at this. "That's me," and I stand to greet whomever the vampire is who will be taking more of my precious blood.

"Good morning, Apryl. How are you doing today?"

"I'm good, thank you," I respond, climbing aboard the spa chair. "Just a reminder, I have small rolling veins."

"Okay, I'll be gentle," the vampire assures me with a smile as her fangs slide out. "You're going to feel a little poke," and in goes the needle—of course I turn my head because if I actually watch it being done, I'm sure I'll faint. Once the needle's in I'm okay, and I watch as five vials are filled. Out comes the needle.

"Please hold this cotton ball here. Hmmm . . . since you're wearing such a pretty blue and purple skirt, I'll bandage you with purple so you match!" Pleased with herself, the vampire reaches for the purple roll.

"Wonderful!" I have to find humor in this, otherwise I can see myself easily becoming a blubbering mess.

"You may have a seat again in waiting room #2. Someone will be with you shortly." I find my place again next to Mr. Wonderful.

"Are you okay?" he sympathetically inquires.

"Yeah, I just wish someone would've given me a heads-up about all this." My eyes start to fill with tears, and I turn my attention to my phone and do my very best to focus on dry eyes.

And we wait for another 10 minutes, then, "Apryl Allen?"

"Yes." And we stand to follow another face down the hall and into yet another examining room.

Once in the room I ask her name. "Ramona." Without warming up to us she takes my vitals. The clip goes on my finger, in goes the thermometer, and then the blood pressure cuff inflates. Blood pressure—*perfect*, temperature—*perfect* and oxygen level—*perfect*.

"The Mad Scientist will be with you shortly," and she leaves us to wait some more. Don't doctors understand we have lives too? This is ridiculous! Every time we've been here, we've waited a minimum of 40 minutes. And just when we feel we're ready to get up and walk out, the door swings open.

"Good morning, Apryl . . . Ken," the Mad Scientist acknowledges us in greeting with a nod of the head. Trailing behind him is his nurse practitioner, Patience.

"Good morning," we respond.

"We've gone over the test results from your PET/CT scan and echocardiogram and everything appears to look good." *I like he doesn't waste time with idle chit-chat.* "Let's see, blood pressure—Normal; red and white blood count—Normal; glucose—Normal; calcium, liver, kidney, *etcetera, etcetera, etcetera*—All Normal! And you have a strong heart, so should you require chemo it won't be a problem." *I'm sure glad he said "should you require!"*

"I wouldn't have expected anything less," I reply. Then, because my curiosity's peaked, "Why do I need to have blood work done each time I see you?"

The Mad Scientist defers to Patience for the explanation. "We'll be drawing blood each time to keep a close watch on Jorge and his sidekick the Lymph-Along-Kid. We want to make sure nothing changes drastically with either of them and we gauge this in numbers. Right now you're at 13. If all of a sudden it shoots up to 90, we know we have a problem."

Speaking of Jorge and the Lymph-Along-Kid, they appeared exactly as they did at their MRI premiere. ". . . And we're still seeing only the one lymph node that's angry but of course we won't know anything for certain until after your surgery," the Mad Scientist concluded. "I see we haven't received the results from your genetics test."

"No, I'm still waiting." I feel that's all I ever say anymore.

"Unless you have questions, we're done for today."

"Actually I do have a few," I reply. "My first question is more of a request . . . It's regarding the *male* Shape Shifter I may potentially use for my reconstructive surgery. His first available appointment isn't until the end of September and I was hoping to get in earlier to see him. Would you be willing to contact his office and petition on my behalf for an earlier consultation appointment?"

"Patience, contact the *male* Shape Shifter's office and see if we can get Apryl an earlier appointment." It was a smug yet humorous request, and that's why I love my Mad Scientist, he makes me laugh!

Feeling a bit cocky myself, I proceed with my list of questions. I start by informing him, "Since my tango with Jorge began, friends and acquaintances—having only the very best intentions of course—have asked questions or offered advice for things they consider to be very real concerns or potential procedures."

It's really quite remarkable how many lotions and potions are out there claiming you should use them in lieu of treatments. Of course, there's the media with their vast pool of experts touting the latest findings and procedures. I did my best to research them all and in the end eventually posed the following questions to my entire league of extraordinary doctors. Below is an amalgamation of their responses:

Does the sugar we consume cause cancer?
There's conflicting information about the effects of sugar but no reputable data has been presented on the matter.
Interesting side-note: The brain and other cells get their nutrients from glucose!

Do "Frozen Head Caps" (similar in appearance to swim caps) prevent hair loss?
There has not been any reputable data or scientific research completed on this.
Side note: After personally reading an article in the newspaper I asked myself the following question — not knowing the Mad Scientist had posed this very question when meeting with a roundtable of oncologists. "If a frozen cap is worn to deaden the cells in efforts to prevent hair loss, does that mean the chemo too may possibly not reach those deadened cells wherein some other form of cancer appears on your scalp?" Of course no one had an answer and again, no reputable research has been done. Because of this, I'm not willing to gamble with my life in this area. Should it be my fate, I'm more than willing to go without hair for a while.

Should I go on a gluten-free diet as it could be anti-inflammatory during chemo?
Unless I'm a celiac, there is no need to go on a gluten-free diet — it will make no difference. During chemo

they'll be monitoring certain levels and may have me refrain from or eat more of specific types of foods.

A new procedure is being tried in a few states wherein a mass amount of radiation is focused in the cavity where the cancer was removed during surgery. This is done with hopes of negating the need for postoperative radiation treatments. *(The normal protocol is every day for five days each week for five weeks.)*
Yes, this procedure is currently being tested, but it's new and at this time there are no studies to back up its long-term outcome. *(But that's neither here nor there for me since Jorge's enlisted the Lymph-Along-Kid; I'll require the five days a week for five weeks visits—or whatever the methodology ends up being. Rats!)*

After the Mad Scientist answered all my questions I allow him to leave. After doing so, I realize I neglected to bring up my encounter with his Nightmare Navigator. I felt strongly someone should know of our experience and, quite honestly, I was a bit uncomfortable about bringing it up with him. Maybe my unease was because I felt sorry for her and didn't want to cause her any more grief.

But someone needed to know and since Patience was still working on my paperwork, I decided to tell her. "Patience, Ken and I want to tell you about our experience with the Nightmare Navigator. I had told the Mad Scientist I had concerns regarding these past procedures and was interested in learning the details of each test ahead of time. I also told him how I was having a bit of anxiety regarding my future and was hoping he could provide some insight as to what I should anticipate.

"Sure, I completely understand. You've been hit with a lot." Obviously this wasn't the first time she's heard someone say this.

"Well, he then introduced us to the Nightmare Navigator and left her to discuss my concerns and fears. However, instead of answering our questions, for almost an entire hour she took us into the deepest darkest moments of a double M, and shared with us all the intimate details of her experience. To say the least, I was a complete mess when I left here."

Patience's mouth fell agape during my recounting and offered, "I'll definitely speak to the Mad Scientist and let him know what happened. I'm so sorry you had to go through that."

We thanked her and left the examining room, feeling quite a bit more optimistic about my future than we did after our previous appointment. Stopping at the scheduling desk on our way out, I booked our next appointment for the morning of Tuesday, August 13th. Of course, when I was handed the appointment card, I *double-checked* to make sure the date and time were accurate.

Driving home Ken and I discussed our experience of having to deal with this life-altering situation. Our conversation then turned to the challenge of gathering necessary information only to have someone (be it a nurse, friend, family member, or you fill in the blank) decides it's his or her duty to take us down the path of no return and present us with a worst-case scenario. I know we should be aware of the possibilities, *but really*, until you know exactly what you're dealing with, there's no need to entertain the nightmarish experiences of others. Nor should you have to listen to someone else's gory details. Everyone's experience will be different; after all, they say *no two cancers are the same*. I guess we were still shell-shocked with the findings and didn't know better, but *we do now!*

After being dropped off at the house I was busying myself in efforts to divert my attention from my tango when the phone rang.

"May I speak with Apryl Allen please?" the soft, southern accent politely requested.

"This is she," I reply feeling a bit apprehensive as to what doctor's office is calling now.

"Hi, my name is Betty-Sue. I'm calling to introduce myself; I'm a nurse who works for ACME Insurance. Since you're part of ACME's network, you now have access to on-call ACME nurses. We want to let you know we are here 24 hours a day, seven days a week to assist with any medical needs or health concerns you might have."

Nurses are now on call; are you kidding me?! ACME Insurance wants *me* to discuss my medical needs and concerns with an *on-call nurse* who's halfway across the country, and who knows nothing about me or any medical conditions I may or may not have?! Glad to see our insurance dollars are being put to such good use! Of course, this has nothing to do with Jorge. But since she was wasting my time anyhow, I thought I'd take this moment and tell her what happened with my genetics test.

Betty-Sue was shocked to hear this, and sounding concerned, said, "I have to be honest, that doesn't sound right. ACME Insurance has a two-day turn-around approval period for something like this. I'm going directly to my superiors on the matter. Someone will get back to you with why this happened."

Not so politely I respond, "Thanks, but I won't hold my breath. I know I'm basically talking to a brick wall." I hang up before she could respond to my overtly rude comment.

After telling Ken about the phone call he said he received this same call, but from a different nurse a week earlier at the office. Evidently, the woman wouldn't leave a message with our receptionist about why she was calling. When Ken did finally take her call, he was, to say the least, a bit upset she interrupted his day with this superfluous information.

Now you're going to think me a bit tainted, but I'm sure this network of nurses is similar to the customer service representatives we've all spoken with. Whether you speak with the IRS, an airline, phone company, satellite or cable company or any other institution, in the end, they all have the same response: *"You can't hold me accountable for anything I say to you on the phone. AND if I don't like you, or your complaint, I'll simply transfer you to one of my contemporaries. And please, don't ask to speak with my superior, because honestly . . . there isn't one."*

I know what you're thinking . . . *taking it out on a stranger?* Well, ACME Insurance offended me! With all the money we're paying for insurance, they have the audacity to impose a waiting period when it comes to your health! Besides, venting did make me feel a little better that afternoon!

Shortly after I hung up with the ACME nurse, my phone rings again. *What now?* I ask myself answering the phone. "Hello?"

It was the scheduler for the *male* Shape Shifter's office, "You won't believe this, but we just received a cancellation and have an appointment on August 14th at 2:00."

Thrilled, I appreciatively accept the appointment. It's late in the afternoon on Friday and I'm absolutely spent, done with phone calls and, honestly, finished with my discussions of Jorge for the week. I'll call the scheduler for the *female* Shape Shifter on Monday, in the hopes of obtaining an earlier appointment at that time.

SIDEBAR

Telling people about your Tango is difficult. Sometimes you'll find yourself blurting it out at the most inopportune moment. Give yourself a break in this area since you're still reeling from the shock of it all. Although I feel I should warn you, there will be various personalities you'll encounter during this period. Frankly, it's not just limited to this particular type of scenario; you can apply it to any life-altering health misfortune. And try not to take anyone's response to heart, although sometimes it's difficult not to. More than likely the person has never experienced anything this serious and is at a loss for words. Either that or the person lacks any compassion as a living human being!

First, let's look at the individuals who forget how to have a conversation. I call them the *Side-Steppers*. In some instances people you consider friends, sadly some family members too, will attempt to avoid you. If by chance you run into them, be prepared—they may not acknowledge what you're going through. Often, even a simple greeting goes unsaid. If the inevitable does happen, and a conversation can't be avoided, they'll look at you as if you're a fragile relic. And with as much empathy as they can muster, they'll contort their face into something that reflects ghastly, monolithic pain and ask, "How are you *feeling?*"

How am I FEELING? HOW am I feeling? How AM I feeling? You find the words tumbling and swirling through your mind. I often reply, "Well, had they not found the Lymph-Along-Kid to be a little grouchy on my mammogram, I wouldn't know anything is wrong at all. I feel *perfectly* fine." The more appropriate question is, *"How are you doing?"* I mean, I'm not on my death bed.

Of course there are those who have a difficult time recognizing the realities of life; I consider them *Mere Mortals*. These types of people have never encountered anything of this magnitude before, nor do they think they ever will. I found it quite amusing when, upon hearing of Jorge, this personality responded with "Oh—Bad luck." *Hmmm . . . Bad luck.* Exactly what does that mean? Bad luck for me and good luck with the rest of my life? Or maybe, bad luck for *me*, good luck for *you*. Seriously? That's all you can come up with . . . bad luck?! This response made me feel as if life was just a game and I was losing.

Then there's the *Brazen Bully*. I truly believe these people do not have a complete grasp on life. They consider themselves *above* all others. The *best* at everything. *Nothing* can take them down! Oh yeah . . . and they hate to lose. One such *Bully's* reaction to Jorge was, "I wouldn't have expected you to handle it this well—I mean I know *I* could . . . but *you*?" Her lack of compassion and calloused remark reaffirmed she doesn't know me at all. Truthfully, I was so caught off-guard by her cold-blooded . . . I guess implication that she's so *tough* and I'm not, I was momentarily at a loss for words. My response? "I'll happily trade places with you."

Moving on to the people who attempt to relate to you by sharing horror stories. Let's call them the *Freaky Freakers*. Be leery of, and absolutely prepare yourself for them. They will materialize when you least expect it (i.e., the Nightmare Navigator). My suggestion? When people start taking you down the path of no return, stop them immediately! Remember, there's no one Tango; it's different for everyone.

Case in point: an acquaintance chronicled an experience his friend had. I think he realized in the middle of his ghastly tale as I turned completely white that it probably wasn't the smartest choice of a story. But he was too far into it and just kept going. Unfortunately, this happened only a couple of days after I was diagnosed with Jorge. All I can offer here is, don't take it to heart. Your experience will more than likely be different.

There's no dismissing the *Dismissive Dimwit*. This individual will completely trivialize you and your Tango. Usually he or she starts by telling you, "Your Tango's no big deal," and claim, "As a matter of fact, yours is the best kind to have because it has such a high cure rate." *Really? I didn't realize they found a cure for cancer!* Worse, they'll completely dismiss what you're going through with, "At least you can have it cut out by having surgery." At some point the *Dimwit* will launch into, "Now, let me tell you about the scare I had . . ." I can't quite figure these individuals out. Are they attempting to lessen my fear? Or is it the "it's all about *Me*" syndrome? As far as I'm concerned, unless you've had cancer, you don't get to talk about scares!

And speaking of the "Me" personality, we shouldn't overlook the *Forget-Me-Nots*. More than likely somewhere in your past they've done you wrong and now, in efforts to make themselves feel better, they attempt to right the wrong. They'll start off by saying, "You know what I would just *love* . . ." Of course the more appropriate question would be, "Is there anything I can do for you?" Eventually curiosity will get the better of you and you'll find yourself asking, "What would you just *love*?" Their response will be, "I'd just love it if . . ." blah, blah, blah. Be careful now, because if you don't gush over their magnanimous offer, they'll quickly turn the tables on you and belligerently shriek, "I can't help it if you want to cut me out of your life." And you never hear from them again. But is that such a bad thing?

The last personality comes in two variations. Look out because they often appear as an acquaintance of a friend or family member—or worse, *they are your friend or family!* I've aptly named them *Preacher Screechers*.

The first person starts pontificating they either know someone, or maybe they themselves, have personally rid their bodies of an ill-fated disease using the *power of their own mind*. Still others claim to have *intuitive healing abilities* that will miraculously cure you. How exactly is that supposed to make me feel? I believe in mind over matter, but are you willing to take the chance? I'm not; this is my life we're talking about here!

The second type will tout holistic remedies. They'll claim to have researched various elixirs concocted from herbs, minerals, roots, vitamins, eastern medicines and lord only knows what else. They'll also claim to know someone who has beaten Jorge using this method. I believe there is some truth to this, but I think this treatment needs to go hand-in-hand with Western medicine. Besides, how do I know I'm getting the authentic stuff and not something someone cooked up in their garage?

These individuals can be quite convincing. Again, I'm not the one who can say whether their approach is possible or not. I unequivocally believe in miracles and applaud those that have achieved success! For me, I'm going with what I know to be factual. My advice? Tread lightly and listen to your heart. All in all, I believe most people have the best of intentions. Take what they say with a grain of salt. Trust in yourself and the rest will follow.

END OF SIDEBAR

10

Morningstar

Apryl Allen

I'm up before the sun. Taking refuge in our living room, I look out the window in anticipation of the sunrise. The Morningstar can be seen, its brilliant aura manifesting the start of a new day. There's a calmness about me. I take another sip of coffee. Smiling, I fondly reflect back . . .

They always start off the same—dreams of my mother. I'm in her bedroom cleaning or sorting through items for her; that's when I feel her presence. Next, I smell her. To me, her scent is something very similar to roses. And then she appears.

When I dream of my mother, she never speaks. I never hear her say my name. Instead, what I feel is the immense bond we share. Upon seeing her I typically rush into her arms, but this time I'm already there. My arms are tightly wrapped around her with my face buried in the crook of her neck and I'm sobbing.

In this dream I allow all my fears, all my sadness and all my grief to drain from me. My disposition begins to change as she cloaks me in her protective and tender love, a true unconditional love.

As I stand locked in her embrace, I feel a sadness; perhaps it's because she's unable to physically be with me, or maybe it's because of what my future holds. Yet I feel the stoic strength she had when she was diagnosed with this same cancer. Her love envelops me completely, as if to say I have her strength and will make it through this. Encircled within her arms, within her love is where I stay.

When I awoke from this . . . *dream*, it wasn't a normal awakening. I could feel her everywhere. Nothing woke me in particular, not a sound, nor a movement, nor a voice. It was as if I was already awake. I could feel her lying next to me. Memories of the many nights I climbed into bed with her as a child, and those mornings when I'd wake with her, came flooding back.

Reaching over I feel for her, *she was here!* Deep within my heart I knew unequivocally it was *her* lying next to me. The beautiful, sweet yet powerful love I'd known was once again here. The pride she felt for me as her daughter rose within and swelled inside me. I felt both a tremendous joy and comfort knowing she was with me at this *very* moment—here next to me.

Then gently, like the first raindrops from a springtime shower, droplets began to fall. As they fell, each one that touched my skin began to remind me where I was—in the safety and comfort of home with *her*. Gradually her love began to transform itself—a masculine presence, immersed in trust and protection, can be sensed. These two types of love combine into one and, as if being passed to another, I realize I'm lying next to my husband.

Normally at this time, as in past dreams, I would feel sad, knowing I was no longer with my mother. But this time was different; I still feel her. Her presence is strong and resonates throughout my entire being. After reaffirming her certainty of my safety her love slowly begins to dissipate. But it took a long time before she left. When I awoke completely—returning from this ethereal place—I was *home!*

Sunday evenings have a way of sneaking up on me while Ken and I are enjoying the usual whatever our weekend holds. It's been our normal routine over the years; on Sunday evenings we discuss what our upcoming week looks like. Since the arrival of Jorge, it's always prompted a dread of Monday and whatever the week has in store.

It begins with a sort of dismal panic, then proceeds with me wishing I could just stay stagnant in time. Of course Monday comes and somehow I find the courage to face the day. I have to forget about the week ahead, otherwise it becomes too overwhelming. Strangely, the days seem to meld together.

It's as if I'm holding a pitcher of water, slowly watching the liquid drain away into nothingness. I'm literally witnessing precious time vanish from my life. My former self is completely on hold with no end in sight.

It's Monday, August 5th, the day I was *supposed* to find out whether my BRCA 1 and BRCA 2 genes are negative. This waiting for results is excruciating! Whoever came up with the saying *Patience is a Virtue* must have never experienced the agonizing waiting period for life-altering information.

Just in case—not that she'd have forgotten me—I leave a voicemail for the genetics counselor this morning. "I know this is a long shot, but by chance does the laboratory have my results from the genetics test?" After hanging up I attempt to put it out of mind until the end of the week.

Once again I find myself dialing for appointments. The *female* Shape Shifter has no cancellations. "You're first on our list should anything become available." *Rats!* Well, at least I have the appointment with the *male* Shape Shifter on Thursday.

You do everything you can to divert your attention to *anything* else. And that's exactly what I was attempting to do, because Friday seems like a lifetime away. I'm working on our monthly bills and balancing accounts when our home phone rings.

"Hello, Apryl?" It was the genetics counselor calling.

"Hi! I know I'm being a bit of a pest and I apologize. I was just hoping . . ."

"Apryl, we got the results!" immediately followed by, "Both genes came back negative!"

Thank my lucky stars above. "WEEEHOOOOOOO!!!" My body fills with every imaginable emotion from joy, elation, gratitude to humility. If there's such a thing as an out-of-body experience, I had it at this very moment. Once I came back down to planet earth I can hear her laughing and reveling in the moment along with me.

"This is the best news I think I've ever received. When did they call you? How did you find out?"

"I called even before you left your message this morning to see if they had the results. I didn't want to get your hopes up so I thought I'd wait until later this afternoon to call you back, just in case. They just now returned my call."

I am so very thankful she understood what a mind-numbing waiting game this has been for me. If it were up to Dr. KnowItAll to inform me, he would have waited to call the next morning, but thankfully he wasn't involved in these results.

"Truly, I can't thank you enough, you've been so kind to me!"

Heartfelt joy could be felt in her response. "Of course . . . You're welcome!"

When I hung up the phone I melted. Tears streamed down my cheeks. I know how deeply fortunate I am to have these results and am so thankful I can now move forward without the burden of this "What-If" looming darkly overhead. Then I sat, but only for a moment, pondering the past couple of months and everything I've been through.

Picking up the phone I dial Ken. With spectacular enthusiasm I inform him of the test results. At first there was just silence, then a broken voice was heard. "Oh, honey . . . that's fantastic! I love you so much!"

In every e-mail I've been sending to the Inquisitive Minds, I've asked them to keep me in their hearts, thoughts, prayers or whatever it is they do when it comes to their beliefs. All I have to say is I must have some pretty powerful friends and loved ones! Not to keep them waiting any longer, I quickly sent off an e-mail thanking them for their kindness and concern and, *most importantly*, their enlisted help.

From:	Apryl
Sent:	Monday, August 05, 2013 3:28 PM
To:	The Inquisitive Minds
Subject:	I Got the BRCA Test Results!!! GREAT NEWS!!!

WAHOOOOOO!!!!! The BRCA genetics test came back NEGATIVE and I GET TO KEEP MY BREASTS!!!! I can't even begin to tell all of you how so VERY HAPPY I am!!! I know I have WONDERFUL friends and loved ones, but I guess I'll have to add pretty dang powerful ones to the list too!!! There is no doubt whatsoever to Ken or I, because of you, all the prayers, love, and kind thoughts sent my way WORKED!!!! Thank you, Thank You, THANK YOU!!!

I will definitely be giving my breasts an extra squish tonight . . . and I'm sure Ken will be happily doing so too!!! WHEW! What a relief! Now we have something to celebrate during our trip. What a FANTASTIC anniversary present!

Now onward and upward!!! I know I have the strength to get through the rest of this Tango ... especially with loved ones like you!!! I love all of you, I love my breasts even more than I ever thought I could ... most importantly, I LOVE LIFE!!!

A Big Hug and HUGE KISS to all of you!!!

With the waiting over, Ken and I had a wonderful time in La Jolla! The weather was exquisite, 72 degrees during the day and mid-50s at night. It was the ideal place to drift away from everything, especially Jorge.

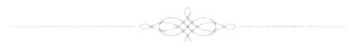

After returning from our mini-retreat, our first scheduled appointment was with the Mad Scientist. We haven't seen him since the news of my BRCA genes testing negative. The normal routine takes place upon our arrival: Sign in, complete necessary paperwork and pay co-pay. Then follow whomever the face is that greets us back to waiting room #2. Rolling up my sleeve, I watch as the vampires consume however many vials of blood they're hungry for on this particular day. And finally we're ushered back to the examining room and await the Mad Scientist to anoint us with his presence.

Forty minutes pass and it feels as if we're slowly losing our sanity. Finally, Patience comes through the door and cordially greets us. Is the Mad Scientist going to be much longer?" we inquire.

"How long have you been waiting?" she asks.

"Forty minutes. This is ridiculous! It's incredibly difficult for Ken to be absent from the office. We'd just appreciate it if our appointment is at least within 15 minutes of the actual time." *Are we really asking that much — to be on time?*

"You're absolutely right. There's no reason you should be waiting this long. I'll go find the Mad Scientist and get him in here," and she disappeared though the door I so desperately wished to exit as well.

Returning she's trailed by the Mad Scientist, who jovially greets us, "Good morning, Ken and Apryl." No apology is offered for his tardiness. "The Medicine Woman sent over her notes—great news about the BRCA genes testing negative!"

"Yeah . . . what a huge relief—it is fantastic news!"

"Based on the results, have you decided on when and what type of surgery you'll be having?"

"We're hoping for the first week of September and I've decided on an axillary lymph node dissection and lumpectomy." Correctly stated, the exile of Jorge and his companion, the Lymph-Along-Kid. "We may decide to wait on the reconstruction portion of the surgery . . ." and I fill him in on our discussions with our Shape Shifter and the phone call from the Medicine Woman asking I get a second opinion.

Neither agreeing nor disagreeing with our decision, he says, "As long as you feel comfortable I have no problem with whatever you decide." Then, as if it was an afterthought, "And depending on your cancer levels you may not require traditional chemo."

"What do you mean by my levels?" *What . . . there's something else that could bring even better news?*

"Should the levels of Jorge come back low there is the possibility we can avoid traditional chemo and instead administer it as a pill."

"Really?!" *Okay, this is something I can enlist the help of my Inquisitive Minds for once again . . . creating low levels!*

Placing his hand on the door knob, he starts to turn it and then pauses. "Schedule Apryl to come back after her surgery, when we have the results from her pathology report. At that time we'll discuss her future treatments." Opening the door, he attempts to make an early exit from our appointment.

"You're not leaving, are you?" I inquire. "I have a few questions I'd like to get your thoughts on."

Looking to Ken, "Is she always like this? So demanding?" he asks with a smile on his face, and closes the partially open door.

"Yes, but I love it! She's made me a lot of money with her inquisitive mind," Ken countered with a chuckle.

Lightheartedly the Mad Scientist surrenders. "I wish I could say the same about my wife!" Pretending he just noticed I'm in the room he gives a little jump. "All right, what questions do you have for me?" he asks smugly.

Reaching for my purse I pull from it my little green journal I refer to as my "Book of Life." I received it as one of the daily gifts from the spa that Adelaide and I had stayed at. I gave it its name due to the tree embossed on its front cover. The book comes in quite handy; I use it to write any questions or concerns I have about Jorge and the Lymph-Along-Kid.

"Oh ... this is serious, she has a book! I guess I should get comfortable," the Mad Scientist says, seating himself next to Ken while he humorously exaggerates his complete and undivided attention towards me. I begin firing off questions.

After satisfying my queries, the Mad Scientist stands to leave. "Patience, please write up the order for Apryl's pathology report and send it over to the Medicine Woman."

Inquiring about which report the Medicine Woman prefers, Patience doesn't appear to like the answer the Mad Scientist gives her. Actually, her reaction says it all. Ken and I watch as her face contorts into a sour look as if she just took a whiff of something appallingly rank.

"That test is a little outdated, isn't it?" She and the Mad Scientist then proceed to go back and forth in a language Ken and I don't quite understand. Frankly it makes me nervous they're doing this. Nobody asked *my* opinion and I obviously want whatever the best and most accurate test is that's offered.

Finally agreeing on which test to order, the Mad Scientist wishes me a successful surgery and takes his leave. Patience, after completing the order, inquires, "Do you want us to send the authorization to the Medicine Woman or would you prefer to take it to her?"

"I'll be in that area and can drop it off." *Besides, it gives me a reason to pop in and say one last "Hello" prior to surgery day.*

"Okay, if you'll excuse me, I need to go print the order. I'll be back in a moment," and once again she disappears.

Returning, she hands me one of the most important papers I know I will ever hold. With this appointment behind us, we're one step closer to the exile of Jorge. *God, I can't wait to get my life back.*

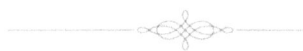

Uggg . . . regarding the previously aforementioned waiting, waiting, waiting game. Okay, so I get to eat my words about the on-call ACME nurse. She actually phoned back about the two-week "waiting for approval" period.

First, I couldn't believe she actually called and was incredibly grateful to her for doing so. Then, feeling bad for having said *"I was probably talking to a brick wall,"* I apologize to her.

"It's understood; you're going through a lot right now. I just wanted to call and let you know ACME Insurance received the faxed request from the laboratory on Monday, July 29th. As is our protocol, within 24 hours from the time it was received—to be exact, 23 hours—we faxed our approval to the laboratory for the genetics test."

So it was the laboratory's fault, not ACME's. "Betty-Sue, thank you for this information. I'll definitely let my genetics counselor know of your findings. It's horrible that the laboratory put the blame on ACME Insurance." How I despise finger-pointing—*not to worry, I won't get started on Congress again . . . that's a never-ending battle I choose not to put my energy in.*

11

I'll Wait

Taylor Dane

During past appointments I've taken numerous scribbled notes about my—no, I can't get out of it—surgery. It took a while but eventually, between the Mad Scientist, Medicine Woman, and a few other not so willing participants, I got them to explain in detail what I could anticipate.

On that glorious day I'll first go to Imaging Center #2. At this facility, a very fine wire will be connected to the titanium marker that was attached to Jorge during my biopsy. The wire remaining, hanging out of my chest, will then be coiled up and taped to my décolletage. *The very thought of this makes me queasy!!!*

Afterwards, Ken will drive me about a half mile to the hospital, where I'll have out-patient surgery. *Big breath—deep sigh!!!* The Medicine Woman, using the wire as a guide, will remove Jorge, including the margins surrounding him, to ensure all residual from my tango has been completely purged from my body. She'll then remove the Lymph-Along-Kid, along with several of his closest friends, to verify no other lymph nodes are cancerous.

After the surgery, they'll test the margins surrounding Jorge to confirm my tango is indeed over and there's no further cancer. If there is, I'm taken back to the operating table so the doctor can remove more margins until they're completely purged. A lymphatic drain will then be inserted into the area where the Lymph-Along-Kid and his friends were. The drain will be left in anywhere from a few days to a couple of weeks. At that time, after the green light is given, I'll have whatever therapies (chemo and/or radiation) is recommended by the Mad Scientist and the Radiation Man.

I'm still unsure whether I'll have a Shape Shifter present at my surgery. If one is, no future surgeries will be required. However, should I choose to have reconstruction done at a later date, I'll need to wait for my body to heal. Once it has, and I'm in the right state of mind, whoever the Shape Shifter is will then complete the final step by filling in the crevasses and dips where Jorge once was.

After reviewing this information with Ken, I reiterated what the Medicine Woman had said at our consultation appointment: *"If the margins aren't clear you'll require a second surgery and this process will continue until all tainted margins have been removed."*

"Apryl, you misunderstood; the margins will be tested *at the time* of the surgery. So stop worrying about a second operation." *How did I misunderstand?* I thought, chalking it up to too many doctors and did exactly as he suggested. The thought of a second surgery was immediately vanquished from my *"what-if"* scenarios. Thank heavens, one less thing I need to concern myself about. I keep telling myself *this will soon all be in my past . . .*

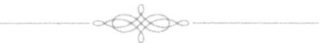

Still no luck scheduling an earlier appointment with the *female* Shape Shifter. At least today I'll be meeting with the *male*. Ken had been in meetings all day and said we'd have to meet there. I arrive before he does. *Wow, does this guy have money or what!* I thought to myself as I entered his office.

Cordially greeted, I scribble my name on the numerously signed sign-in sheet as the receptionist asks whether I have my paperwork completed. After producing all the reports and information about me they could possibly need, I was then asked to have a seat and told someone would be with me shortly.

Being married to an architect, I quickly learned how clients look for ways to cut costs when designing hotels, homes, and office buildings. But this guy had spared no expense—he was out to impress! Still, just because you have money doesn't mean you have taste. His office is heavily designed in marble, stone and tiles, expensive but teetering on the edge of gauche. He even has a full-blown water fountain in his waiting area. I much prefer the elegant office of our friend the Shape Shifter; how I wish he was the one performing my surgery.

Getting past the façade of his office, I'm now fascinated by the army of women he has working for him. All busy bees buzzing around—*is this guy that much in demand?*

Suddenly a familiar voice breaks the buzzing. "Apryl's here?"

"Yes!" one of the worker bees replies happily. That's when the door next to the reception desk swings open and a sweet-looking, short-haired, blonde woman exits the hive.

"Hi, Apryl! I spoke with you on the phone," her brilliant blue eyes twinkle as she speaks. "I'm so sorry for the reason you're here, but you're going to love THE Shape Shifter! He'll take good care of you. From our conversations I feel as if I know you and want to give you a hug!" Wrapping her arms around me, she lavishes me with a heartfelt squish. She's *darling* and her hug did actually take the sting out of why I'm here. Not to mention I'm thrilled I'm the only one in the waiting area.

"Prudence will be with you shortly. In the meantime, can I get you something to drink? Water or anything?"

"Thank you, no. I brought my own," holding up the bottled water one carries when you live in an arid climate. Shortly after seating myself in the empty waiting room, the outside door opens, allowing hot summer furnace air in the room. I look in anticipation of Ken's arrival.

Instead, two women parade in wearing obnoxiously high heeled patent leather platform shoes, one pair being bright red, while the other tried a subtler approach, white. The heels on them alone had to be, at a minimum, six inches. *These have to be hookers*, I smugly think to myself.

Once past the shock of their shoes, my eyes scrupulously make their way up their curvaceous size 10 figures that are painstakingly stuffed into very colorful size 6 cocktail dresses. In an apparent attempt to appear businesslike, they've added suit jackets with buttons stressed to the point of popping open at any second, ready to unsheathe the minutest details of their ensembles.

Wait ... what's that they're holding in their hands—briefcases?! They're sales reps attempting to acquire an appointment with the *male* Shape Shifter? *What on earth could they possibly be selling?* And that's when Mr. Wonderful walks in. The reaction on his face says it all. He sums them up with one lifted eyebrow and a curled corner to his lips. Sitting down next to me, he attempts to stifle a deep down belly laugh.

His well-trained eyes then study the office surroundings. "God, how I wish *our* Shape Shifter was doing your surgery."

"Me too," and we attempt to divert our attention to the thoroughly fingered magazines in the waiting area. *Just keep me away from stories pertaining to double Ms please!*

No sooner did we begin flipping through pages than Prudence, a thin 60ish woman—I just had a face lift for the umpteenth time, with breasts that defy gravity—appears, calling my name. Politely she asks us to follow her and we arrive at a room reminiscent of a courtier dressing room in a high-end retail store, furnished with *two* three-sided mirrors.

"Please have a seat, I have a few questions before you meet THE Shape Shifter." After her debriefing, "I'll let THE Shape Shifter know you're ready. In the meantime . . ." she opens a pair of doors to an armoire. "You may change into a robe. We'll be back momentarily." Within the antique cupboard are several silken robes. Now I'm curious, as is Ken, and we anxiously await the arrival of THE Shape Shifter.

Shortly after changing, a polite knock on the door is heard. Drum roll please . . . in walks THE—I'm barely 35 years old—Shape Shifter. I sigh because, feeling a bit on the plump side, I now get to reveal my lovelies.

"Hi, Apryl," he greets enthusiastically, "I'm THE Shape Shifter; it's nice to meet you." *Very polite, so far so good.* "I'm sorry to hear about your recent diagnosis." He seats himself in a chair across from Ken and me while Prudence takes her place next to him. Flipping through my file, "I see you've chosen the Medicine Woman as your surgeon. Do you have a date scheduled yet?"

"No, but I'm hoping for the first week of September."

"After reviewing your file I see you had a breast augmentation done by my friend the *other* Shape Shifter. We're good friends. As a matter of fact, I'm supposed to see him tonight." *God . . . how did this happen?*

"Really? Yeah, he's a good friend of ours too. Please don't mention to him I've met with you; I haven't told him yet. He doesn't care to do these types of surgeries, nor does he take insurance. You do take ACME Insurance, correct?"

"Yes, I do." Then he connects another dot. "Interestingly, I see your first augmentation completed in 1992 was done by one of my school-friend's dad. Now isn't that a small world?"

God, it just got worse ... his "school-friend's dad." Am I that old? "Yeah, he did." I feel so uncomfortable, not to mention I hate offices like these. *Again, why exactly did I allow myself to gain that additional—ahem—10 pounds 20 pounds ago?*

THE Shape Shifter, I guess reading my comfort level, quickly changes the subject. Noticing I've relaxed, he returns to the matter at hand. "So how do you feel overall about your breasts, putting Jorge aside, that is?"

"Well, I feel they're too large and I'd like to go back to the size I was in my early 20s."

"Okay let's take a look," and here it is ... the unveiling. "Hmmm, they're definitely sagging."

"Excuse me? They may have shifted a little, but they are definitely *not* sagging." *You don't have to drive home the fact I'm not 20-something anymore—nor do I want to be. Okay, maybe my figure, but overall I love my body.* Together we all laugh, with Prudence looking a bit, well ... prudish.

"What type of surgery are you planning to have?" he inquires.

"Since my genetics test came back negative I'm planning on a lumpectomy and lymph node dissection."

"Okay, in that case, what I propose is doing everything in one go. I don't like working on tissue that's been radiated, so before that all starts, I'll make your left breast perfect, void of any dents after the removal of Jorge, and finally a breast lift. At that time we'll do the same on your right breast. I'll remove your current implant and replace it with a smaller one, then give it a lift as well. All of this will be covered by your insurance, of course, since women's breasts are supposed to be the same shape and size." While saying this he takes his hands, mimicking what he'll be doing during surgery; pinching my skin and lifting my right breast to higher and younger heights. "Do you have any questions?"

"Hmmm ... it sounds good to me and seems to make sense. Is this the procedure you'd perform on your own wife, if she had Jorge, that is?"

"Yes, this is the *exact* surgery I'd perform on my wife if she was in your predicament." *God, how I wish I wasn't in this "predicament."*

Looking to Ken, I ask his opinion. "What do you think, honey?"

"It makes sense to me," he replies with folded arms. And there you have it, we're all in agreement.

"You know, I'm really pleased with how everything has gone and I'm supposed to have an appointment next week with another Shape Shifter, but

I'd really like to get this over with. I'm going to let the Medicine Woman know you'll be doing my reconstructive surgery and get it scheduled. But please don't say anything to *my* Shape Shifter; I'd like to tell him myself. Again, he doesn't know I've scheduled these appointments. I think he feels obligated because we're such good friends."

"No worries, I won't say a word," he says, promising confidentiality. Silently making a mental note to myself, *tomorrow I'll contact the Medicine Woman and get this all scheduled.*

That afternoon I phone our Shape Shifter's office and inform Brianna about our recent appointment and intended direction. And more importantly, explained that our Shape Shifter is now off the hook. "Tell him thank you for everything."

No more than an hour later Brianna rings back. "Apryl, the Shape Shifter would like to discuss your plans in person. He wants to make sure he agrees with what THE Shape Shifter is recommending for you. Can you and Ken be here at 12:30 tomorrow?"

"Wow ... of course we can." I phone Ken, and once again he juggles his busy schedule to accommodate me.

Bringing the paperwork I was given by THE Shape Shifter, we watch as *our* Shape Shifter reviews it. Then unexpectedly he responds, "I don't agree with what he's recommending."

"Really?!" I thought for sure he'd be relieved he didn't have to perform this type of surgery.

"No. What he's proposing is reopening the scars in the crease of your breast. I get why he's suggesting that, but that would mean Jorge will be dragged through clean tissue. Nobody can predict what the fallout will be from that. It could leave behind residual cells and cause problems for you down the road.

"Second, he's suggesting a double breast lift, which concerns me because after chemo and radiation your left breast will change dramatically. There's no way to determine what size your breast will be after those treatments. Also, after radiation breasts with implants have a tendency to encapsulate."

Ken and I are both stunned, as if we just dodged another bullet. "But what about operating on radiated tissue; THE Shape Shifter said he doesn't like to do that."

"I'm not concerned about that. What I'm more concerned about is getting Jorge out of you—the sooner the better. Do you have a date set for the surgery?"

"No, we don't have anything scheduled yet. Would you be willing to do the surgery in tandem with the Medicine Woman and close me up?"

"I'd prefer you get through the surgery and all your treatments prior to having the reconstruction done. Plus, leaving the implants in during your treatments will help your breasts maintain their shape. You may be a little lopsided for a while, but no one will know any difference, other than you and Ken." He glances at Ken then back to me. "Apryl, Ken loves you. I'm sure he won't care if you're a bit lopsided for a while." Ken nods in agreement. "And *after* you've healed both physically *and* emotionally, that's when I propose we have the surgery."

Squirming a bit in my chair, I look to Ken for answers. "Apryl," the Shape Shifter says, "if you really want me at the surgery I'll be there for you. I care deeply for you and want only the best—whatever makes you most comfortable." Pausing, he then inquires, "What is it that *you* want?"

"I want Jorge the fuck out of me and all of this behind me." Feeling desperate I attempt to hold back tears and am embarrassed I used the "f word" in front of *our* Shape Shifter. Pausing, I inquire, "You really feel I don't need the reconstructive part until *after* the other treatments?"

"You know how I feel about you and Ken. I wouldn't lead you in the wrong direction. This is what I'd suggest for my mom or my own sister." He just said the magic words, and without a doubt, I know they honestly come from his heart.

Trusting our friend, I agree, "Okay, I'll wait on the reconstructive part and get the surgery scheduled."

"What I'd like to do, with your permission, is contact the Medicine Woman. I want to make sure she's the right surgeon and is on the same page as me. If not, I'll personally help you find someone I trust."

"Thank you so much, you have no idea how much this means to me." Standing to leave he gives me a big hug and one to Ken as well.

Reassuring me, he says, "Apryl, you're going to be fine. You're a strong woman and like I said before, this is just a little bump in the road for you." Words cannot express my appreciation for his confidence in me.

"Before you leave, give Brianna the Medicine Woman's phone number. I'll call you after I've spoken with her."

Later that afternoon he phones with his approval of the Medicine Woman. "I told her I wanted Jorge out as soon as possible and we've tentatively scheduled your appointment for August 26th. Make sure that works for both you and Ken, then contact her office and confirm the date. If you need anything, and I mean *anything* day or night, you have my mobile number, call me."

After ending the call I pick up the receiver and phone Ken at work. Finally, the date when Jorge and the Lymph-Along-Kid will be banished from my life is scheduled.

Life has come to a complete standstill while I attempt to fix this unexpected calamity. The pieces of my former self remain idly in my past, awaiting the day I am able to put them back together. As for the surgery, I feel that's going to be the easy part, relatively speaking. It's the anticipation I find difficult, making sure I have all the right doctors and procedures in place, while simultaneously dotting all my i's and crossing all my t's.

It's like being caught up in a windstorm that's haphazardly tossed you into a completely different country with no map, no form of transportation, nor any way to communicate. You're left to figure it out on your own. The reality is there is no guidebook with step-by-step instructions of what you're supposed to do.

As for the doctors, they're not much help when it comes to the reality of what you're going through. They'd rather pawn you off on their "nurse navigators" so they don't waste their precious time dealing with the human side of the disease. I wonder if they've become desensitized to it. After all, they do care for people who leave the world on a regular basis—it must be excruciatingly painful.

Up to this point, I think I'm doing pretty good. Still, I have friends voicing their concerns that I'm handling everything almost too well and wonder if I'm in denial. Sure, I've had a few minor *"I don't know if I can do this"* moments at night when Ken's had to literally pick me up and get me realigned. I truly don't know where I'd be right now without him.

It's important I acknowledge those individuals who selflessly give of themselves during a period such as this. Yes, those of us in a Tango are the ones going through all the treatments, but our loved ones have to stand by helplessly and watch. While they're not enduring the physical fallout we are, I know that the whole experience is as stressful on them—and in some cases more so—than it is for those of us actually going through it. They too have placed their lives on hold and are required to play so many roles that it's often overwhelming.

Take Ken for instance; since the arrival of Jorge, he's been pulled in every conceivable direction. He's had to be my caretaker, husband, friend, lover, parent, chef, chauffer, and psychiatrist. He's my . . . *everything!* And let's not forget the new addition to our family, Hugo, so you can add dog trainer and walker to the list as well. Of course it doesn't stop there. After all, he has his life as well and our business appears to be recovering from the economic downturn, requiring *more* of his attention.

Of course everyone has a breaking point. We were in our kitchen when his occurred. Ken had just made us lunch when Hugo had an accident, and at the same time he received a disconcerting business call. I of course had to chime in, "If you had let Hugo out he wouldn't have had the accident." No, I'm not kidding. I actually said that, and with complete disregard for his feelings. Why didn't I get up and let Hugo out?

It was as if our household were in chaos. Bracing himself against the kitchen sink, Ken took in a deep breath. Not making eye contact, he turned away from me and walked into the kitchen pantry, where he crumbled. His knees buckled as a torrent of tears streamed down his face. Over and over he sobbed, "I can't do this anymore. It's just too much. I don't know how much more I can . . ." I felt completely helpless and worst of all *numb*. I just sat there and watched him. I didn't move. I didn't console him. I just *watched*.

At some point, my compassion came back and I placed my arms lovingly around him. I clung to him as tears tumbled down my cheeks too. "I'm so sorry, honey. I know this is difficult for you too. I'm so very sorry I've been taking you for granted. I truly appreciate all you've done and are doing for me. I couldn't make it through this without you. *Please know that.*" And there we sat on the floor in the pantry of our kitchen. I love this man more than life itself! I would do *anything* for him.

12

Silent Strength
Apryl Allen

Be your own advocate. Prior to having surgery it's important to ask what the procedure entails. However, I must warn you—asking questions opens a floodgate of pre-op things to do. The most frustrating aspect? How are you supposed to know what questions to ask when you've never experienced anything like this before? And don't assume your doctor's office will handle the details—as challenging as it is, it's ultimately your responsibility to manage the entire process. Inevitably something will slip through the cracks, through no fault of your own.

For example . . . Imaging Center #2 called to confirm my needle localization—the pre-op appointment to insert the wire. Of course I took this opportunity to verify the exact details of the procedure. Why is it everyone seems taken aback when I ask questions?

"It's a guided insertion via mammogram or ultrasound. We only have your X-rays so it'll be up to the doctor performing the procedure," the voice said, sounding like a recording.

Perplexed, I anxiously inquire, "What do you mean you only have X-rays? I had both an MRI and mammogram completed by Imaging Center #1. Won't someone from your office be contacting the other Imaging Center to obtain those records?"

"I'm not sure. However, if they show up between now and two days prior to your surgery it would make the decision for the procedure a lot easier." She was all business and obviously not expecting an inquisition. *And, how, pray tell, exactly are they supposed to magically appear between now and then?*

Attempting to stay calm at the absurdity that no one has bothered to ask the obvious question, "Well, whose responsibility is it to get these records for you? I mean, my surgery is on Monday of next week, and if you require the MRI two days prior . . ." I silently did the math in my head, ". . . that would mean you'd need them on Friday, correct?"

"Actually, I'd recommend they be delivered no later than Thursday morning. And it would be the responsibility of your surgeon to get them to us."

Big breath, deep sigh . . . "Okay, I'll contact the Medicine Woman's office. In the meantime, can you please tell me exactly what this procedure will consist of?" You'd have thought I just asked her why the sky is blue.

Using a tone that implied I shouldn't inquire further she responds, "I'm not sure."

Why is this so difficult?! "Well . . . is there someone you can ask? I'm a bit apprehensive and would *really appreciate* it if you would clarify this for me. I like knowing *exactly* what to anticipate as I have a fear of needles."

Maybe I struck a nerve by explaining how apprehensive I was, or maybe she realized I wasn't going to hang up until I had all the details. Sighing, "It may take a while. If you don't mind holding, I'll attempt to find someone who knows the details." It's obvious this time she wouldn't be coming back with another "I don't know" response.

Keeping her word, I was on hold for quite a while when she returned, saying, "Okay, I spoke with one of the nurses and this is what she said you can anticipate . . ." describing the itinerary in detail:

12:45 PM	Check-In at Imaging Center #2
1:15 PM	Needle Localization:

    1. Follow the instructions given by your Medicine Woman prior to surgery *(I was told by Mabel I'd receive this via U.S. Mail later this week)*

    2. Wear a loose-fitting, button up the front blouse—no bra please

    3. The area of the procedure will then be numbed *(Now would also be a good time for me to take the entire bottle of Valium)*

    4. A needle, with a wire attached, will then be inserted via ultrasound or mammogram, at which time the wire will be guided to Jorge

> 5. The wire will then be attached to the titanium marker clipped to Jorge
> 6. The wire remaining outside my chest—YUCK—will be coiled up, covered with gauze, and taped to my décolletage
> 7. After the insertion, do not—*I repeat DO NOT*—raise your hands over your head
> 8. As quickly as Ken can get me to the hospital, please do so at this time!
>
> 3:15 PM   Out-patient surgery—lumpectomy & axillary lymph node dissection

"Thank you for this information. It's truly appreciated." I think even she was surprised to learn about the procedure.

After hanging up, I immediately dial the Medicine Woman's office. "Hi, Mabel, it's Apryl. I just got off the phone with Imaging Center #2 and found out the Center only has my X-rays, not my MRI or mammogram. Do you know if Imaging Center #1 has been contacted to send them over?"

"No. It would be the responsibility of Imaging Center #2 to obtain them." Okay, this isn't going *anywhere*.

Only because Mabel had talked me down from an OMG moment, I didn't feel right about pressing her for who actually was *responsible* for what—or maybe I'm just worn down from everything. Regardless, I wasn't interested in pissing anyone off, *especially* the Medicine Woman prior to surgery. It was obvious no one was going to go out of their way for me. So I contacted Imaging Center #1 myself.

"Hi, Iris! It's Apryl Allen . . . *again*. I'm sorry, but it appears Imaging Center #2 does not have the MRI or mammogram required for my needle localization procedure." In the back of my mind I'm thinking *this doesn't seem very professional on the Medicine Woman's part that I'm the one making this call*—I'm almost embarrassed. *But why should I be the one feeling uncomfortable? This only reflects on the Medicine Woman—but I chose her as my surgeon . . . stop it, Apryl, this isn't going to do anyone any good at this point.*

"No problem, we can have a copy made and have it delivered if you'd like," Iris offered. I was so relieved not to be having a conversation regarding whose responsibility it was to obtain them.

"My surgery's on Monday of next week and the Center needs them no later than Thursday morning of this week." Knowing Imaging Center #1 and #2 are literally across the street from one another, I then ask, "Do you think I should pick them up and deliver them to Imaging Center #2 myself or do you feel confident they'll get there by Thursday?"

"It's up to you. We can do either. We can have them held at the front desk for you or have them delivered." There was something in her voice that made me question whether this would actually get done.

"What would *you* do?"

Momentarily pausing, "If it were *my* surgery? I'd do it myself for the peace of mind and to ensure there are no mishaps." DONE!

"When will they be available for me to pick up?"

"Wednesday after 12:00."

Scrutinizing my schedule, "Okay, I'll be there at 2:30." Then as an afterthought, "Would it be possible to get a second copy for my own records?" It's just smart to have copies of past procedures. And, since I'm going to all this trouble, when I deliver them I'll inquire about what type of insertion will be done.

Later, I decided to call the Medicine Woman's office to verify I was given the correct times for Monday's itinerary. *Since no one appears to be looking out for my best interest — I will!*

"Hi, Mabel, it's Apryl again. I want to confirm the scheduling times I've been given by Imaging Center #2." Sounding frenzied on the phone, her response was jumbled.

"I can tell I'm catching you at a bad time. I'll get the details of the surgery when I drop off the order for the pathology report." Relieved she thanked me and we said our goodbyes.

It's strange. I find myself feeling scared, relieved, and a little insane. I mean for heaven's sake, if you think about it, I'm authorizing people to cut something out of me. I know it's a life or death situation, but it's just strange to think this is what we do. *Please God, help us find a cure.* I'm looking forward to having this unwanted and unexpected surgery behind me. And yes, Mom, I hear you . . . *Apryl D, you think way too much.*" She's right.

It's Wednesday, five days before surgery. Ken's at an out-of-town meeting in Las Vegas and I've planned to get some of my pre-surgery errands done. I had mentioned this to Adelaide and was elated when she offered to come with me. Honestly, I wasn't looking forward to doing this on my own.

We started with our High Priestess. Adelaide had graciously offered to share her appointment with me since I was unable to get in because she books out months in advance. Afterwards we'd have lunch then run my errands.

Who is this High Priestess? In a nutshell she helps keep my head on straight. But she also has a very special ability to connect with, well . . . loved ones who have departed planet earth. I know what you're thinking, *Great, Apryl's a Wind Chimer*—honestly I'm not! As a matter of fact, being Comanche I'm actually very leery of people like this.

My first appointment was in July of 2012 and I've only had a handful of appointments since then. During our initial meeting, I was completely taken aback. There are things I've told *no one*, not even Mr. Wonderful, and she inevitably worked them into the session, almost as if they were an afterthought.

Let's take, for instance, when you have a flash of a thought that's never voiced. *If my mom was here I'd ask her this . . . or, I wonder what the meaning of that is . . .* but nothing more comes of it. The question's never verbalized; it's just a fleeting thought that stays lingering in the ethereal world left unanswered because there's no earthly way to get the answer! At least that's what I thought.

With this in mind the High Priestess will, out of the blue, say, *"Oh, by the way, when you see X it's because of Y"* or *"Does this name, place or word mean anything to you?"* If you don't recognize the word or name, it will eventually surface, whether it's the next day or a few months later. Besides this uncanny ability, she's also a therapist who helps me put things back into perspective *without the use of drugs.*

Back to my shared session with Adelaide. After initial cordialities, we start the session and Adelaide takes center stage. At some point the High Priestess looks my direction and asks, "How are *you* doing, Apryl?"

Throwing caution to the wind I let go, "I don't *think* I can do this. I don't *want* to do this. As a matter of fact, I don't want to *be* here anymore." Tears fill my eyes and I glance at Adelaide, who appears to have had the wind knocked out of her, and I watch as her eyes widen with concern.

Calmly the High Priestess sits on her throne without movement, shrouding me in the warmth of her love. "Of course you can do this, Apryl." Her eyes are steady yet powerful, evoking the silent strength I'm so desperately seeking. "You're strong. Lesser people have been down this road before and they come out the other end just fine. Take me for instance . . ."

She then proceeds to tell us of her personal experiences with two very different cancers—not just once, but *twice* she's tangoed. She didn't take me into the details of her procedures, but instead discussed *my* feelings and *my* concerns and, yes, the depths of *my* despair. These are the same feelings she experienced herself firsthand.

Finally, the gray cloud that had been looming overhead began to dissipate. The claustrophobic, macabre tomb my world had become began to reshape and take on the vivid colors of my world and my future.

When we left, I couldn't thank Adelaide enough. However, I was a bit concerned with what was discussed in front of her. "Did I scare you with my candidness?" I inquired.

"Honestly, yes, but thank you for being so open and sharing." I could tell she was concerned about my mental state.

"Adelaide, please know I am not considering doing anything crazy. That's not who I am. But those were the only words that describe how I feel at this very moment. I don't want to be on this crazy roller coaster ride; I want off of it. But since I have no alternative I need help putting things back into perspective and the High Priestess has done that. She's truly amazing. I knew I needed to see her and am so appreciative you were kind enough to share your appointment. Truthfully, I can't thank you enough for spending the afternoon with me to run these errands. I wasn't looking forward to today."

"I know, and that's why I'm here." I am so fortunate to call Adelaide my friend, especially at this moment in my life. It's as if our paths have crossed at this *particular* juncture, for this *particular* reason. There's absolutely no question in my mind.

After lunch, we proceed to Imaging Center #1. I hadn't seen anyone here since I was diagnosed with Jorge. After being handed a package containing my records I inquired, "Would it be possible to say hello to Iris and the Breast Investigator?"

"Let me check for you." The receptionist buzzed back to their office, had a brief conversation, and I watch as a smile brightens her face. Cheerfully she informs me, "Absolutely. They'd love to see you! Do you remember how to get to their office?"

"Yes, thank you." A smile curled my lips as I proceeded down the infamous hallway.

Iris was the first to greet me and instantly gave me a huge hug. "Let me get the Breast Investigator; she'll be thrilled to see you!" I was then invited back to the Breast Investigator's office.

"How are you doing, Apryl?" the Breast Investigator inquired with a bright smile.

"Actually, things are going pretty well. My surgery's Monday. I feel a bit overwhelmed but am looking forward to having this all behind me." Then I briefly recounted what had transpired since I last saw them.

"I'm so happy to hear things are going well. You have the right attitude about this, which is going to take you *very* far. Your outlook is *everything*!" More than she'll ever know, I needed to hear these words.

"Breast Investigator, I want to thank you for saving my life . . ."

She was embarrassed and, with more humility than I've seen in a very long time, hastily interrupted my sincere impromptu speech on gratitude. "I was only doing my job."

"Yes, and because you did your job so well, I have a future to look forward to." My face lit up with heartfelt appreciation. Then, changing the subject, "I guess I don't need mammograms anymore since I have dense breast tissue and Jorge can't be seen on them."

With a shocked and worried look on her face the Breast Investigator stressed, "You couldn't be more wrong. Mammograms catch things other tests don't see."

"Really?!" This was something I wasn't expecting to hear. "Why not just have a sonogram or a MRI? I mean, the MRI does show everything, doesn't it?" Now I'm confused.

"Yes, they're good at detecting Jorge; however, MRIs often give false positives. If you had only MRIs, you'd constantly be in for unneeded biopsies. Honestly, if you told me I could only choose one of the three tests for the remainder of my life, I would choose a mammogram. But luckily we don't have to choose just one and therefore, in the future, every six months you'll be having something done. For instance, in December you'll have a sonogram and in June a mammogram."

Humph . . . the mammogram did detect the Lymph-Along-Kid. I left there thinking how lucky I am to have the Breast Investigator in my life. Thank heavens she pays close attention to her work. How many of us can say we do that? After thanking both of them again, they showed me the back way out of their office.

Adelaide was catching up on a few phone calls and quickly ended her current conversation when I reached the car. She couldn't believe what the Breast Investigator told me either.

From there, we drove across the street—literally—to Imaging Center #2. "Do you want to come in or wait?" I asked.

"There's a couple more phone calls I need to make," but then, as if an afterthought, "Unless of course you want me to come in?"

"Nah, I'm just dropping this off." Summertime in Phoenix is not the optimal time to be sitting in an idling car. "I'll be out in less than five minutes."

"Okay, I'll be here," she said, scrolling through her list of numbers.

Staying consistent with previous visits, upon entering the office no one greets you. Instead you're supposed to sign in, have a seat, and *wait* to be called, even if you're not there for an appointment. It kind of reminds me of the "Soup Nazi" on *Seinfeld*: 1) Sign in 2) Wait for your name to be called, and 3) Absolutely, under no circumstances, are you allowed questions!

Besides, after signing in, there's no one there for me to question. There are only two individuals working and they're both with patients. Taking a seat, I anxiously await my turn. I wait . . . and I wait . . . and I wait some more. I watched the secondhand tick away on my watch as the minute hand slowly swept from five to 10, then 15 minutes! I texted Adelaide *"You may want to come in, this is taking a lot longer than I thought."*

Of course no sooner did I send the text than my name was called. "Hi, I'm here to drop off these records for my procedure on Monday."

Hastily taking the package from me the clerk inquires, "Your name?" and I watch as she haphazardly punches it onto her keyboard. After misspelling my name several times she eventually gets it right and continues the interrogation. Satisfying her robust requirement for my personal facts, I then watch her rip open the huge manila envelope I delivered.

Plopping what is comparable to 100 pages of stapled reports on her desk, she reaches for her stapler remover. While yanking the staple from the first report, she messily takes its corner with it. Clearly, she hasn't been taught how to properly use a stapler remover. She then proceeds to scan each page of the report into an unbelievably inefficient scanner that's really only meant to scan a few pages of paper, insurance, and identification cards.

Due to the now torn pages, she has a difficult time feeding them into the scanner and attempts to bend each corner back into place prior to doing so. Agitated, I watch as she picks up the next set of stapled papers and begins this same process again, painstakingly feeding them through *one page at a time.*

Eventually the pile of pages got so high on the other side that the new ones being scanned through began to contort into various shapes, and worse, were sliding in between the other pages out of order. *Oh well, at least they're being scanned into the computer in the correct order,* I console myself. *Why isn't she picking up the scanned pages and placing them anywhere else on the vast empty desk she's sitting in front of?* I'm starting to lose patience, it's all I can do not to grab the staple remover, or the disheveled papers piling up, and organize them for her.

In efforts to divert my attention I ask, "Would it be possible to speak with someone about the type of procedure I'll be having?" If I'm going to be tortured and have to watch her scan all these pages, I might as well alleviate a concern. "I was told the exact procedure couldn't be determined until you received this information."

The clerk looks up from the scanner startled. Appearing to digest my request she crinkles her nose and apprises me, "I can't tell you about your procedure." *Duh.* "But if you're willing to wait I'll check to see if a nurse is available."

"Sure, I'll wait," and there I sat, thinking she'd eventually put the scanning project on hold and get a nurse.

Now I was glad I texted Adelaide; this is taking an inordinate amount of time. And yet she continues with the scanning. *Really?! Apryl, calm . . . find your Zen place!* And I wait while she scans all of the pages. Once finished she types a few things into her computer.

"Okay, let me see if I can find a nurse for you." Returning, "Please wait at the next desk. A nurse will be out shortly."

"Absolutely." *I'm getting good at waiting around here.*

It had to have been 20 minutes while I watched this dingbat clerk do one thing at a time. Realizing Adelaide may not have received my text, I decide to ring her.

"Hey, it's me! This is taking a lot longer than I thought—you may want to come up."

"Okay, I'll be right there."

Shortly after Adelaide arrives, a nurse appears. Luckily the nurse didn't take as long as the scanning did. "You have a question about your upcoming procedure?"

"Yes, I was told once you received the records I just delivered, someone would be able to tell me whether the needle localization I'll be having will be guided by ultrasound or MRI."

"I have no way of answering that. It'll be the doctor's decision on Monday." *Really?! Why is this so difficult?* So basically I just wasted an hour of my day. Well at least I know they received my records.

Without letting her see my frustration I smile. "Okay, thank you." Together, Adelaide and I leave Imaging Center #2, with no added peace of mind for my upcoming procedure.

Unlike me, Adelaide knew I required a female friend today. Truthfully, I haven't given much thought to what's physically going to happen to me. Her intuitive side told her I'd especially need her during this last errand to Lulu's Loot.

Lulu's Loot is basically a store within the, *ahem*, Center where I'll be having surgery. For whatever reason, I despise the name of the store—don't ask me why. Maybe they could have been a little more creative. Adelaide came up with a name that I feel best describes it, "Oh F#@%!!!!!!!"

I had no intention of coming here but, as an afterthought, in case they have something I might need, I decided to take a quick look. While perusing the merchandise a salesperson appeared. "Good afternoon ladies, may I help you find anything?"

My initial response is exactly what I say to all salespeople, "No, thank you, I'm just looking."

However, I *was* looking for something, a bra with no underwire. I don't know if you've ever attempted to purchase one, but they're virtually impossible to find. And rummaging through Lulu's racks of inventory proved the same. It was then I realized there were no bras anywhere. The only ones to be seen were out of reach, hanging on the display walls.

Pointing it out to Adelaide, I summon the salesperson. "Actually, you can help us. We want to see the types of bras you have, like those displayed on the wall up there." Motioning to a couple of fantastic looking sports bras, "Where are they?"

Inadvertently I got the full attention of both saleswomen in the store, each sporting pink medical-type poncho vests. As they approached, I noticed their smiles—warm deep gentle lines reflecting years of home baked cookies and sweetness that only grandmothers emanate. That's when I realized they were much *older* women.

"Oh . . ." one of them exclaimed, "we're volunteers. If you're interested in bras, then you'll need to see the *Sizer*."

Disappearing, she returns trailed by a woman who doesn't look at all happy. Her displeasure was obvious when she inquired, "Do you have an appointment?" *An appointment?!*

In unison both Adelaide and I reply, "No."

Instantaneously I feel this was a bad idea and, truth be told, I didn't *want* an appointment! What I *want* is to quietly walk around the shop and then inconspicuously make my purchase and LEAVE!!!!!!!!!!!!! I'm not sick, nor do I need someone telling me her story—*please let's not go there again*. I just want to be incognito and pretend I'm someone else, *anyone else*—the one *without* Jorge! Tears flood my eyes but I force myself to clear them.

I look to Adelaide and with a defeated tone said, "Let's just go . . ." I know she can see the terror in my eyes.

"Hold on a second . . ." and she actually turned her attention to this demon Sizer woman and began to speak with her.

"Adelaide . . . Let's go!!!" I said with a firmer, yet still defeated voice.

And what did Adelaide say to me? "Apryl, give me a second . . ." and I watch as she has the audacity to speak demon talk!

How dare Adelaide do this?! Does she not realize how difficult this is for me? Besides, nobody stands up to me when I put my foot down. Okay, maybe I've met my match, but what she doesn't realize is she's dealing with a Comanche!

Out came my war cry, "ADELAIDE . . . LET'S GO NOW!"

From behind I hear one of the volunteers exclaim, "Ooo . . . this is getting good now!"

The other one responds, "Mmm-hmmm!" And we all watch as Adelaide slowly turns in my direction.

Using a *"Don't mess with me"* tone, "We are NOT Leaving!" We then proceed to have a stare down. And would you believe this French seductress actually returned a *pleasant* gaze back to the Sizer, somehow winning over the demon woman's heart!

"Please, I'd love to have the two of you come back to the dressing room for a fitting," the Sizer kindly offered.

I was so upset. I didn't want to be here in the first place! This has been REALLY ROUGH on me! Adelaide, with tender caring eyes, flashed her dimpled smile my way. Warming my heart, I acquiesced, but not without a pout of protest while following both the Sizer and Adelaide back to the fitting room.

Once in her chamber, the Sizer produced all sorts of bras with hidden pockets awaiting prosthesis. While trying them on I found them to be quite chic. There was a bright red sports bra, then a black, white and cognac colored bra. I felt as if I were in a lingerie store choosing something wonderful for . . . well, Mr. Wonderful!

After reviewing my insurance, the Sizer informed me the bras wouldn't cost me anything because my plan covered them. "Consider yourself fortunate," she said, "Some plans only permit one bra per year." One bra? Who can wear one bra for an entire year? How do insurance companies get away with this?

Then she brought up the subject of the type of surgery I'd be having. "We have these really great vests that have pockets on the inside, so when you have your drain put in, it will conveniently hold the apparatus."

A huge lump formed in my throat. "I'll be needing that?" My eyes, betraying my heart, filled with tears.

"Yes, you will," the Sizer conveyed sympathetically. "Trust me on this. Get it; it will make your life a thousand times easier after surgery."

"Okay. May I see what it looks like?" At that moment Adelaide's phone rang.

"Sure . . ." The Sizer left to retrieve the vest and Adelaide joined her, not wanting to interrupt the fitting while she took her call. Feeling a bit deserted, I sat in the fitting room . . . alone . . . waiting.

Moments later the Sizer returned and, removing the vest from its plastic package, helped me try it on. To say the least, it was *ugly*. I stood and looked at this cream-colored unflattering vest and shuddered. The Sizer empathized, "Apryl, I've been where you are—actually worse, I had to have a double mastectomy, and look at me now! There is an end to this and you'll be *just* fine." Her softer side was calm and appeasing. "Apryl, I want to apologize for my initial abruptness. I was frustrated because doctors never tell their patients they're supposed to make an appointment for fittings."

"I'm sorry too, Sizer." In truth, we both owed each other an apology. "I didn't read the literature because I wasn't planning on coming here today. But now, I'm so thankful I came; I had no idea I'd need some of these items." I completely understood her frustration because the fitting took almost *two hours*.

Returning to the fitting room Adelaide asked the Sizer, "So do you have wigs we can try on?" My heart sank.

The Sizer directed us to a short hallway. Once through it we entered what looked like a make-up studio on a movie set, complete with rounded lights surrounding a mirror. Neatly aligning the dressing table were various kinds of brushes, along with samples of makeup, elixirs, potions and lotions. Mannequin heads, adorned with wigs, were displayed on several shelves showcasing an array of styles—short, long, curly, auburn, blonde and gray. There was even a baseball cap complete with a ponytail—you name it, they had it. Quite honestly it conjured up all sorts of fun surprises I could offer Ken when we dined out. He'd never know who he'd be meeting!

Adelaide pointed to a couple of wigs and plopped them on our heads. Flashing her gorgeous dimples, she struck a pose reminiscent of Jessica Rabbit. Sensually, she wiggled her curvaceous hips while making a sexy clicking sound with her mouth. "This is so much fun!" she exclaimed enthusiastically. While admiring herself in the mirror she giggled aloud, "Can I get one too?"

Not waiting for a response, Adelaide's attention turned to the baseball cap. Handing me a brunette one, she slid on its blonde twin. "Isn't this cool, Apryl? Look at the ponytail coming out the back!"

I turned my head to view the ponytail and reached up, letting the hair wrap around my left hand. "It looks just like my own hair when I wear a baseball cap." The realization of what could be left me grieving for the hair I still had.

"And that's exactly what it's supposed to look like—your *own* hair," the Sizer implored. "After your surgery, should you require chemo, you'll want to come in before your therapy starts. We'll have a fitting at that time."

"Will you be doing the fittings?" I inquired. I really like the Sizer now and feel completely comfortable with her.

"Yes, here's my card. I'll let you two play around here, but if you'll please excuse me, I need to order the items you'll be requiring after your surgery on Monday. We'll have them shipped here and everything should arrive on Friday. Although, I suggest you call tomorrow and verify they've been shipped; at the latest they'll be here on Saturday."

Playing briefly with the wigs, we then thanked everyone for their kindness and left the store. In my heart, I truly hope I won't be in need of a wig. But if I do . . . it's sure to be a fun fitting with Adelaide!!!

Leaving the store Adelaide asked if there was anything else she could do. "Would you like me at the hospital during your surgery?" I'm in awe of this woman and her generosity.

However, Ken and I had already discussed this and, since he's my loving control freak, he requested he be the only one present. *"I don't want to deal with anyone—I want my focus to be solely on you."*

"Thank you, Adelaide, but Ken said he can take care of everything at the hospital."

"How about dinner—can I bring over anything . . . chicken soup maybe?" *Seriously, she's offering to make us dinner—YES!*

"That would be incredibly nice!"

All in all, I'd say my errand day was pretty successful. And I'm so very thankful to have had a friend with me on this day—*thank you, Adelaide!*

13

I Believe

Apryl Allen

It's time to say goodbye. I know this morning is the only moment I'll have with no appointments or potential interruptions. My inner self, whom I've come to rely heavily upon during this period, is beckoning . . . *tell Jorge he's leaving.*

My heart's beating to an unknown drum, its rhythm urging me to gather my eagle feathers, a very special candle, medicine given to me by my Medicine Man, and a few other treasured items. I turn off all my phones and anything else that can possibly distract me during this moment. Carefully placing these sacred objects on my piano bench, I wrap my shawl around me and sit cross-legged on the floor, facing the window to a world filled with *life*. Meditating I reflect back on what was and what is to be.

Clearing my mind, I light sage, cedar and sweet grass. In a hypnotic trance I watch as the three types of smoke intertwine, performing a wraithlike dance before my eyes. Ancient smells immerse my senses and I drift to another place, or maybe another plane. Voices can be heard singing in the far-off distance. As they become more pronounced, I can feel the presence of my ancestors. Forming a circle, they begin a spiritual round-dance in my honor.

Gathering my eagle feathers, I begin fanning myself with the familiar smoke. Images of love, peace, and healing flash before me. In a meditative trance I sing to Jorge. Then, using spoken words, I tell him it is time for us to part. He's to leave my body—*forever*. I acknowledge his presence and thank him for the greater understanding I now have of life, but it's time for him to go. "On Monday, you are to leave and *never* return," I declare with conviction.

Quietly I sit and listen, surrendering my mind to the stillness of life. I can only describe what I felt as similar to a muscle twitch. It happened four times at the exact location where Jorge is in my left breast. He knows it's time to go . . . he's acknowledging his departure.

Filling my heart with reassurance and love, my ancestors quietly depart one by one, returning to their spiritual realm. And here I sit releasing tears, having cleansed my soul.

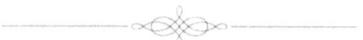

Earlier this week, I received a call from the surgery center wanting to schedule a pre-op phone call with one of its nurses. *What more could they possibly need to know after all the paperwork I've been required to complete?* I asked myself. Evidently they didn't believe what I put down in writing and want to verify the information in person. Gathering my Warrior Book and a pen, I plant myself in the kitchen awaiting the call. *I wonder if they're timely or if I'll be sitting here for a while?* I find myself questioning everything.

Promptly at 10:30 the phone rings. After greeting one another the pre-op nurse informs me, "We're required to go over a few items prior to your surgery on Monday. First, I'd like to verify the items you're allergic to. We have Percocet, morphine and medical tape—is this correct?"

Interestingly, the two items I'm allergic to turned into three—*where do they get their information?* "No, I'm not allergic to morphine."

"Okay . . ." and she types the change into her computer. "I now have three questions I need you to answer honestly." *That's an odd statement . . . why wouldn't I answer them truthfully?*

"Sure, I have no problem with that."

"Do you have a Living Will?"

Okay this is a strange question—not to mention quite personal. "Yes."

"It's not a requirement, but it would be a good idea to bring a copy with you on the day of your surgery should any unforeseen event occur. It'll make things much easier."

"Okay." *I didn't think it possible, but I'm beginning to feel more anxious about this surgery.*

"Are there any bruises or injuries caused by another individual we should be aware of or will see during surgery?"

"No." Although I'm answering these questions honestly, I'm now feeling panicky.

"After the surgery and upon your release, do you fear for your life or the safety of your well-being with any individual that will be at your place of recovery?"

Wow . . . really?! "No."

Seriously, they find it necessary to ask questions such as this? I could understand if the surgeon felt strongly there was a need for them but how strange to be asked them out of the blue. Ken was quite shocked too after relaying the questions to him.

On my list of "prior to surgery" errands I was to drop off, per the request of the Mad Scientist, the order for my pathology report. When I arrived Mabel appeared frazzled.

Taking a look at the order she seemed visibly upset. "This isn't the pathology report the Medicine Woman likes. She prefers a *different* report; besides, I've already sent the request in."

"Well, the Mad Scientist asked I drop this off to you. What should I do with it?"

"I'll shred it. There's no need for it." Handing it to her I watch as all traces of it disappear into her shredder.

Reaching for my Book of Life, I opened it to the list of questions I had compiled for pre- and post-surgery. I was in my *need to know now* mind-set. "I have a few questions I'd like to ask of the Medicine Woman. Is she available?"

"Let's see if I can answer any of them for you," she offered.

"Okay . . . How long will my surgery be?"

"I don't know, that will need to be addressed with the Medicine Woman."

"Okay. Do I need blood work done prior to surgery?"

"No." *Thank God!*

"How large of a margin will be taken around Jorge?"

"Another question for the Medicine Woman." This isn't going so well.

"Will margins be taken around the lymph nodes too?"

"No, she'll only be taking a sampling of your lymph nodes."

"I have a fear of needles; can I take a Valium prior to the needle localization? *Please say yes . . .*

"If you do, you'll need to inform the Medicine Woman *and* the doctor performing the needle localization."

"Would it be better if I didn't then?"

"I wouldn't necessarily say so, but to be on the safe side, I suggest you inform the doctors."

"I noticed some of the brochures mention lymphatic massage. Do I require this after surgery?"

"Another question for the Medicine Woman."

"Is there a list of items I should do pre- or post-surgery?"

"I mailed all that information to you earlier this week. You should have it no later than Friday."

"For the questions you were unable to answer, would it make it easier if I e-mailed them to the Medicine Woman?" I thought that she could look them over prior to phoning.

"We don't have e-mails." *Okay, this is very odd—not to mention a bit on the archaic side.*

"Why not?" I asked.

"The Medicine Woman feels she has enough to do and to add one more thing is overload."

After her response I wondered, *how proactive is the Medicine Woman when it comes to new techniques and technology?* However, I quickly dismissed it because the medical community—at least my small world of Dr. KnowItAll, the Breast Investigator and the Mad Scientist—all agree she's one of the *best*. Besides, she was on all of their lists of doctors to choose from.

At some point during our many phone conversations, I remember telling Mabel that I'd like to get my prescriptions filled *prior* to surgery. But I neglected to write it down, nor did I remember to ask her at this moment, when I had her full and undivided attention. We concluded with confirming my surgery-day itinerary.

In the end, Mabel said she'd have the Medicine Woman call regarding the remaining unanswered questions, but it never happened. When Friday's mail arrived in the afternoon, what I received was a single sheet of paper. It was a map with an access code for the surgery parking lot and nothing else. I attempted to call the office, but it was closed for the weekend.

For several years I've been seeing feathers everywhere! Some are amazingly beautiful and I've started a small collection. I know this is going to sound odd, but some of the feathers have been found in the most unpredictable locations. I wondered if they had a particular meaning and intended to ask an Elder of my tribe the next time I spoke with him.

Remember what I had mentioned about the High Priestess? How out of the blue she'll say something almost as if it were an afterthought? Well, that's how she won me over during our first session. Having not mentioned it to *anyone*, she ended with, "*Your mom wants me to tell you, when you see a feather that means she's with you.*" Again, this was NOT a question I asked nor did I mention *anything* to her about feathers.

There are many, many stories I can share of feathers miraculously materializing, but let's fast forward to Friday, August 23rd . . . While running my last few pre-surgery errands I asked my mom to give me a sign that she was with me. I normally question any and all signs I receive, but after you hear this one I think you'll even agree, it's time I stop questioning them!!!

At the request of the Mad Scientist, I scheduled an appointment with the Radiation Man prior to my surgery. Together the Mad Scientist and Radiation Man will decide the protocol for therapies post-surgery. I did have a bit of anxiety about the appointment, not as much as I did during the first appointment with the Mad Scientist, but it was close.

When we arrived I went directly to the front desk and signed in. While doing so, the receptionist asked if I'd completed the paperwork that was mailed to me.

"Yes, I'll get it." Ken, having heard the request, began rummaging through his briefcase for it. He was sitting maybe 10 feet from her desk and our chairs faced her direction. After retrieving the paperwork I return to her desk. "Here you go."

"Great, thanks," and she began glancing through the pages. "Actually, we'll need one more page completed," she said, handing me a single sheet of paper.

"Sure." And I seated myself next to Ken.

No sooner did I sit down than she informed me, "Apryl . . . I neglected to get your insurance card."

Fumbling for my wallet, I return to her desk and hand her the card. Once again seated next to Ken, I focused my attention on the blank lines requiring my personal information.

"Apryl?" calling my name again. "Sorry, I need to collect your co-pay."

During this period, no one has come in or out of their office. I should also add that Ken is one of those individuals who notices *everything*—nothing escapes him.

Returning once again with wallet in hand—what is this, the fourth time now?—I came to an abrupt stop two feet from her desk. She watched as I turned a pale shade of white and asked, "Are you okay?" Ken began to stand.

Had I taken one more step I would have walked on it. Instead there it was, resting peacefully on the floor, as if it had just floated down from an unknown opening in this four-story building—this office is located on the ground floor.

Slowly turning to Ken, "You're not going to believe this . . ." and I stepped aside, pointing to the floor in front of me to reveal a delicate four-inch white and gray *feather*! I was frozen!

Ken sat dumbfounded and shook his head in disbelief. "Your mom!"

The receptionist, curious at this point, stood peering over the counter above her desk. "Wow . . . how did that get there?!"

"I don't know, but I know who put it here!" I replied.

Looking a bit confused the receptionist offered, "Here's a tissue. I'll toss it."

Tenderly picking it up, I hand over the four-inch beauty. As she began to throw it away I came to my senses. "No wait. What am I thinking? I want it!"

"Really?!" She was puzzled, but handed it back to me. Only because there was no one else in the waiting room, I had to tell her why. After relaying its meaning she informed us, "I honestly can tell you we've *never* had a feather here in our office. And it's not raining outside so it couldn't have been tracked in."

I agreed but still can't fathom how we could have possibly missed it. Honestly, if you saw where it was, and the fact it was four inches *and* white, you'd agree too!

Now back to business . . . pulling a credit card from my wallet, I paid my $45 co-pay. While waiting to sign the receipt I silently thanked my mom.

Okay, Mom . . . I believe you're here! Humph—maybe that's the meaning of the license plate we saw PLSEBELVE. Thank you for being with me!!!

Feeling reassured from this other-worldly symbol, we waited to be called. At least I know there are no vampires around to take my blood. Then the door swung open and a cheerful woman stepped around it. "Apryl?" Both Ken and I stood and proceeded to follow her through the door.

First, we stopped at a scale and she noted my weight. Then, grasping some sort of vitals machine on wheels, we follow her into an examining room. Offering me a seat next to a counter with a computer on it, she introduced herself as Nina, the Radiation Man's medical assistant. She then proceeded to verify my personal information while typing it into the computer. Like others before her, I watched as she flipped back and forth between their form and my *"please see attached"* paperwork.

Chuckling aloud, she slaps her hand down on the countertop in jest and exclaims, "Oh, I love it! 'Medical Tape Loves Me!' This is the first time I've seen this. Why do you say it *loves* you?"

"Because when I attempt to take it off, it doesn't want to let go and often ends in a battle over who loves my skin more. I have battle scars from the last go-around!"

Making a note in the computer she then inquired, "And Percocet, what does that do to you?"

"Honestly, I've been told I'm not allergic to it, instead I have a very low tolerance for it. I get nauseous when I take it."

Turning to the next page she reads *"see attached"* again, and after quickly shuffling the papers, "Oh, I just *love* you! You have all your doctors listed with their contact information. You've even included your pharmacy! You just made my job that much easier."

Pulling over the vitals machine on wheels she asks, "Do you have a preference as to which arm I take your blood pressure from?"

Realizing I'm asked this question each time before blood draws, or when my blood pressure is taken, I find myself curious as to why and ask Nina to see if she can solve this mystery for me. "Why does everyone ask if I prefer a particular arm?"

"What side is your cancer on?"

Now that's a question I haven't been asked before. "My left side."

"Because it could cause *lymphedema*, especially after surgery. It occurs when the lymph channels are squeezed and that's what a blood pressure cuff does. After surgery you should be very protective of this arm and no longer have blood draws or your blood pressure taken from it."

"You've got to be kidding me? How come no one's told me this before?"

Taking my right arm she shrugs her shoulders. "I don't know . . . but you know now."

Just before inflating the cuff she looks at my feet. "Uncross your ankles, please."

Uncrossing them, I feel like a child asking, "Why?"

"Because when they're crossed it gives a false reading by raising your blood pressure." *This woman is so informative!* "Here, I'll prove it to you," and she took my blood pressure *twice*, once with my ankles crossed and the other with my feet side by side flat on the floor.

"Wow, I can't believe it went up that much."

"That's right! So next time, make sure you don't cross them." *Mental note: Don't cross ankles while blood pressure is taken.* "We're all finished; the doctor will be in shortly." Ken and I watch as Nina and the vitals machine leave the room together.

Making ourselves comfortable, Ken and I wonder how long we'd be waiting for *this* doctor. Happily, it wasn't long at all; less than five minutes later there was a light rap on the door. "Come in . . ."

Instead of the doctor, a polite young woman enters. "Hi Apryl, I'm Mimi, the Radiation Man's nurse practitioner." After introductions, she immediately starts asking the same questions Nina had, but then went a step further and inquired about Jorge and my upcoming surgery. When the Radiation Man joins us, I know he'll ask these same questions. Is this just to give the appearance we're actually doing something while waiting for the doctor?

Ending her interrogation, I watch as she pulls my favorite frock from a cupboard and lays it on the examining table. "Please change into this gown from the waist up with the opening in the front. The doctor will be in shortly," and she exists the room.

To our surprise, no sooner had I positioned myself on the examining table then another knock on the door. "Come in . . ."

The door opened and in walked a very serious-looking man followed by Mimi. After introductions we found ourselves discussing the very same information we went over previously with Nina and Mimi.

"I'd like to examine you now—please lie back on the table." After doing so he untied the pretty bow I had made on my gown. He then began to examine my left breast. YIKES . . . *his hands are cold!*

"You could have at least warmed your hands first," I teasingly said.

"Oh, sorry," he began rubbing his hands together and we all laughed.

Finishing the examination, "You can take a seat next to your husband if you prefer." *Yes, I do prefer!* As I seated myself I attempted to retie the bow in efforts not to flash everyone in the room—not that it mattered.

"I see your surgery will be this Monday."

"Yes."

"Until we have the results from your pathology we won't know exactly what the protocol of your therapy will be. What I can tell you is that radiation therapy comes *after* chemotherapy. And the norm for breast cancer with lymph node involvement means you'll be having radiation treatments five days a week for approximately one and a half months." No wonder my Shape Shifter said I need to make sure I'm comfortable with the doctor I choose.

"At the end of radiation therapy your left breast will have a tan, and besides being a bit on the tired side, there should be no other major symptoms. We'll be going over the exact procedure and potential side effects the next time we see you. Do you have any questions?"

"Yeah. Your medical assistant told us about something called *lymphedema*. No one's ever mentioned this before. Is this something I need to be concerned about?" *And why didn't my doctors tell me about this? Instead I get to hear it from their assistants.*

"Yes, there is the possibility of lymphedema, but with diligent care of your arm, you shouldn't have any problems."

"Okay. I don't have any other questions." I turned to Ken. "Do you?"

"No," he replied simultaneously, shaking his head.

"Good luck with your surgery and if you have any questions in the meantime, please feel free to call."

As we were leaving we noticed a different receptionist, the one with the beautiful smile, sitting up front. "Hi, Malaika! We were unaware we'd be coming to this same office for radiation treatments."

"Yes! And we look forward to having you back!" This girl was absolutely charming, not to mention genuine. These appointments will definitely be easier when I'm greeted by that smile!

As we left the facility I felt a reassuring calmness come over me. I let out a long breath, grabbed Ken's hand and gave it a warm squeeze. With him by my side and the kind individuals at this facility, I feel I'll actually make it through these appointments.

After returning home I researched *lymphedema*. Below is a brief description from the notes I took:

> **Lymphedema** *is swelling that occurs in an arm or leg most commonly caused by the removal of or damage to lymph nodes as a part of cancer treatment. Although lymphedema tends to affect just one arm or leg, sometimes both arms or legs may swell. Lymphedema is caused by a blockage in the lymphatic system, an important part of the immune and circulatory systems. The blockage prevents lymph fluid from draining well, and as the fluid builds up, the swelling continues. There's no cure for lymphedema, but it can be controlled by diligent care of the affected limb.*

During this same research, I also read somewhere that it was an old wives' tale. I figured I'd get to the bottom of it by making inquiries to my league of extraordinary doctors. It was then I remembered the feather from earlier that day safely nestled within my purse. Carefully unwrapping it from the tissue, I placed it on a paper towel on the kitchen counter and began admiring its beauty. I wondered if there was significance to its gray and white colors. Of course I had to research them:

> **White** *is associated with light, goodness, innocence and purity. It is considered the color of perfection. It can represent a successful beginning.*
>
> **Gray** *is the color of sorrow. It is also the symbol for security, maturity and dependability. It signifies responsibility and practicality*

I feel the surgery is going to be relatively easy for the most part. Although I must admit I am a little nervous about the lymph node dissection. Mostly, I'm anxious to hear the results regarding Jorge.

In preparation for the surgery I've painted my toes a light blue that has an iridescent light purple tinge to it. It was the color of my wedding dress and the color I painted my toes on that day. My fingernails have no polish, as instructed for the surgery. With nothing else left to do I decided to look up the meanings of the combined two colors of my polish:

> **Light Blue** is associated with health, healing, tranquility, understanding, and softness
>
> **Light Purple** evokes romantic and nostalgic feelings. It also has short wavelengths, thus, it's high in energy

I still have my smile but these past few nights have been excruciating, requiring the assistance of my little friend, Mr. Valium. Thursday night was a bit bumpy for us as anxiety got the better of me; it seems I don't take Mr. V until I've crashed and burned. Looking back, I really should have taken him when I went to bed. Honestly, I thought I could do without, which I did, but really I should have taken him. More so for Ken's peace of mind and, in the end, *mine too*. I did take one last night and will again tonight. I'm not sure if I'll need to take one prior to the 12:45 Monday needle localization appointment. However, if I feel the slightest bit of an OMG moment coming on, I won't hesitate.

Climbing into bed I snuggled up to Ken and buried my face in his chest. "I wish I could crawl into your body and return to mine after all these procedures are done and over with." Breathing him in, my eyes filled with tears.

"I know, honey. I wish I could do that for you," he said with a wounded voice while wrapping his arms protectively around me. Before drifting off to sleep, I silently prayed *please help me with creating low levels in Jorge*. I then left it in the hands of the greater deity to determine my ultimate fate.

14
It's Too Late
Sabrina Malheiros

The morning of the dreaded surgery has arrived. I'm feeling a bit groggy from my little pal Mr. Valium that I took last night. While fulfilling my, shall we say, morning duties after my eight-hour slumber, I turned a little too quickly and smacked the left side of my upper lip against the doorway to our toilet room. *Ouch!*

While assessing the damage in a mirror the voice of the pre-op nurse starkly echoed, *"Are there any bruises or injuries caused by another individual we should be aware of or will see during surgery?"* And my next thought was, *oh great—they're going to think my husband beats me!*

Walking into the kitchen Ken's gaze immediately spotted the lump on my lip that felt the size of Mount Kilimanjaro. I quickly grabbed an ice pack to deter the swelling and any potential bruising, which in the end went unnoticed. *Thank goodness!*

In my mind the most terrifying part of the surgery will be the needle localization. I was feeling pretty calm after I took care of my lip and decided not to take Mr. Valium, primarily because each medical person I spoke with told me if I did take the little yellow pill, I would have to let my doctor know. Feeling it could cause a potential problem, I opted not to take it. Besides, I didn't need another mishap, especially after my run-in with the wall.

It turns out the waiting before the needle localization was worse than the procedure itself—the reception area was cluttered with people. Having only five minutes to spare *prior* to the actual procedure, "Apryl?" rang throughout the waiting room. Feeling a bit unstable, I stood and walked towards the not-so-happy-looking in-take Nazi Clerk. There are six desks, but only three are manned, with one clerk currently at lunch.

Once seated in front of this Nazi Clerk, she asked in her much expected strict tone, "Name?"

"Apryl Allen." No witty quips; clearly she's not the joking type.

"Date of birth?" And we continued in this manner until her voracious appetite for my personal information was satisfied.

Then came the kicker. She handed me three pages of paperwork that needed to be completed. Knowing the drill, I quickly scanned them for the required information I had pre-printed. To my dismay, I realized the three pages were actually *six* with questions on both sides.

To add insult to injury, the Nazi Clerk was impatiently watching me. I frantically began filling in the blank lines while simultaneously motioning for Ken to bring my pre-printed materials. The clerk was not at all amused by my ability to multitask.

Closing in on the fourth page of questions, my *I've got this under control* attitude crumbled. I stared blankly at words that literally made no sense. They were clearly medical in nature and after reading them a second time, I assumed they were actually meant for the doctor.

Looking to the Nazi Clerk, "I don't understand how I'm supposed to answer these questions?" pointing to the blank lines.

The Nazi Clerk, appalled I questioned something, peered over her spectacles at me and pursed her lips. Not looking at the paperwork, she folded her arms and glared at me, silently criticizing, *I can't help your stupidity*. Finally, she broke eye contact and read the questions.

"Leave it blank," she replied in a single drone.

While attempting to speedily complete the last two pages, a nurse arrived looking extremely agitated. "Where's Apryl Allen? We're ready to start her procedure."

As if I wasn't present the Nazi Clerk motioned with her head in my direction, "She's still working on the paperwork," as if it were *my* fault!

I know what you're thinking ... *Duh, give the paperwork to the patients when they arrive*. Obviously there'll be questions on the form, but that's when they should offer, *if you don't understand a question leave it blank and we'll go over it when your name's called*. Okay, so no one asked for my opinion and I should just sit quietly with my arms folded and mouth shut. Which is exactly what I did after the frenzied rush. I took a seat *again*.

But seriously, did I really need this added stress prior to surgery? And what about the nurse who came looking for me? I could only deduce she must have found something better to do.

While seated, the butterflies in my stomach quickly turned to hornets attempting to get out. Then I heard, "Apryl Allen?"

As I began to stand Ken reminded me, "Honey, give me your jewelry."

Since I was diagnosed with Jorge I've been wearing my mom's dog tag from her service in the Women's Army Corps during WWII. After kissing it, I carefully lifted the chain over my head and lovingly handed it to Ken. I then removed my wedding rings and watched as my thoughtful husband carefully added the rings onto the chain. After doing so he then placed them around his neck and kissed me tenderly as I stood to leave him for the first step of the surgery. He didn't let me see his heartbreak or fear but I knew, as he helplessly watched me leave the waiting room, tears followed.

Once through the door, the attendant asked me to follow her to the changing room. "Please change into this gown with the opening in the front." Having complied with her request, I slid open the curtain and stepped out. The attendant then instructed, "You may place your clothes in one of the lockers here." After I turned the lock and pinned the key to my gown, the attendant returned. "Please have a seat; someone will be with you shortly," and she motioned to another waiting area.

I can't bring myself to sit anymore. Luckily for me there are windows in this room facing the mountains to the east—the view is stunning. Storm clouds can be seen gathering over the distant mountains and I allow myself to drift away. This waiting room is about the same size as the one where I left Ken. There are maybe six women waiting and I hope their appointments are for anything other than a serious illness. I'm sure it was only a few moments, but it seemed like forever before a nurse appeared calling my name.

Still not knowing what type of procedure I would have, I was incredibly relieved to be taken into a room with an ultrasound machine. Curious I asked, "Can you tell me which doctor will be performing the procedure?" I had previously researched the doctors at this facility and had narrowed it down to three.

"The head doctor in this division."

When he arrived, he introduced himself and that's when I wished I'd taken the entire bottle of Valium because my nerves began a trapeze act.

Mentioning this to him he inquired, "How did you do with your biopsy?"

"I only punched the doctor once!" He and the nurse looked at one another and burst out laughing.

"Yeah, well, I'm a great punching bag!" I was thrilled he had a sense of humor.

He then began the inevitable, "I'm now going to numb you just as the Breast Investigator did." I immediately put myself in the same mind-set as I did for that procedure. I told myself I was having electrolysis done. Funny how pain in the name of vanity is tolerable. "And here's the little prick" *dang . . . that so doesn't sound right!*

Honestly, it wasn't bad at all. Then, with no pain whatsoever, he went deeper with the numbing shot and soon he announced, "Okay, you're all done!" I was shocked! It literally took five minutes—if that long—for the entire procedure!

The doctor wished me well and left for his next victim; then the nurse took over and proceeded to bandage me. Remembering my previous battles with the medical tape I told her, "Medical tape loves me . . . could you possibly use a small amount?"

"Sure, not a problem. But I don't want to use too little because the wire could get pulled and end up tearing your skin."

Quickly addressing her concern, "Whatever you think necessary is fine." To my relief she did not wrap me as I had been previously.

After she finished the bandaging she instructed, "Let's take it slow; carefully stand up." She helped me return to a vertical position and once she felt I had my balance asked, "Are you doing okay?"

"Yes, I'm doing fine." *Wow!!! I feel my mom's strength coming through!!!!*

The nurse opened the door to the treatment room and pointed to a chair just outside of it. "Please have a seat and someone will be with you shortly."

"What for?" Another small detail I wasn't told about.

"A mammogram. Please have a seat."

Great . . . another mammogram. A few minutes passed when a tech appeared, informing me, "I'll be taking a few images." Once we entered her room, complete with mammo machine, she requested, "Place your arm up here and hold onto this bar." *But wait, I was told not to raise my arms!* Once she was satisfied with the images, "You may relax now." I watched as she began typing on her keyboard.

"Would it be possible to see the mammogram?" I mean it is Jorge we're talking about here.

"Sure . . ." and she turned the monitor for my viewing pleasure.

Hmmm . . . not bad! "But the wire isn't hooked to Jorge . . ."

"We only place the wire *next* to him," she informed me.

"Thank God!" I chortled aloud. "I was wondering how they were going to achieve that feat!" Remembering back to when I was first told they'd be clipping the wire to the titanium marker and questioned *what if they missed—what then? See what I mean? My mind works in mischievous ways!*

"Okay, we're all finished. You can return to the changing room across the hall and change back into your clothing. After doing so, please take a seat in the waiting room and someone will be out to get you." I happily obliged and quickly changed into my button-down denim shirt. I returned to the beautiful view in the waiting room. The storm clouds were closer now . . . and I drifted off once again to another place in time.

About five or so minutes later a man appeared with a wheelchair. *Surely that's not for me!* "Apryl Allen?"

Cringing, I approach the man, "I'm really fine. I can walk on my own."

"We don't want any mishaps and use the wheelchair to avoid having your wire shift."

Sounds very logical to me—I will happily sit in your wheelchair! And I seated myself as he so kindly asked me to do in the first place. With a smile on his face now, "Okay, let's get you down to the shuttle bus! Here's the mammogram you just had taken; give it to your surgeon when you see her."

"Of course, but I don't require a shuttle bus. My husband's here waiting to drive me." And this is another perfectly good reason why I'm thankful I didn't take Mr. V this morning. I have my wits about me!

He seemed surprised to hear this. "Oh . . . okay, let's go find your husband." *Do people not have others helping them during something like this? I can't imagine going through this alone!*

Ken, seeing me in a wheelchair, asked with alarm, "Is everything okay?"

Calmly I replied, "Yes, they don't want the wire shifting."

"Oh right . . . I'll go get the truck," and he immediately went down the stairs to get our SUV and the Wheelchair Man and I proceeded down the elevator to meet him.

The truck and my beautiful husband were waiting for me when we arrived at the patient pick-up area. I thanked the young man for his kindness and quickly hopped aboard the carriage with my prince charming and off we went to the Surgery Center.

Surgery . . . oh the ill-fated surgery! *Interesting fact*—it's been two months since this whole crazy adventure began, when the Lymph-Along-Kid was biopsied on June 26th, to this exact day of my surgery—August 26th.

As I mentioned before, we were mailed a sheet of paper from Mabel with a special code to get into the parking lot next to the surgery center. After pulling through the gate, we were pleased to see there were ample spaces close to the main entrance. Ken pulled under the front portico. "Honey, I can walk—" but stopped mid-sentence. "Oh I forgot . . ."

"The wire," Ken said, finishing my sentence as he pulled up to the front door. "Stay in the truck . . . I'll get the door for you." The quintessential gentleman, of course. Cautiously, he helped me out. "Find us some good seats after you check-in—preferably ones that aren't near any TVs or people." I couldn't have agreed more.

As I entered the building I was greeted by an empty reception desk cluttered with plants. Upon closer inspection I noticed a sign-in sheet. I thought it was strange that no one was here to greet me, although I guess at this point they assume patients know the routine. I sign in and stake out a couple of chairs incognito as Ken requested.

Everything about me has gone numb and I feel as if I'm in a bad dream on the verge of waking. We sit patiently awaiting my fate. After about 10 minutes a check-in clerk appears. "Apryl?"

Standing, I find my knees to be workable but extremely wobbly. "I'm here."

We follow her around a short bend in the hallway and she motions for us to have a seat at her desk. I look around and there's absolutely no one else in the facility, other than the fellow patients and their loved ones we left in the waiting area. Again, same questions, different facility. I was expecting her to hand me the notorious forms needing to be completed, but instead she just continued asking questions and typed my answers into her computer. "Okay, last question. Is English your primary language?"

"Sí," I replied, laughing nervously from my belly with everyone joining in on the joke.

After signing my John Hancock on a few papers, she then handed me my copies. "Okay, we're finished here. You may have a seat in the waiting area again and someone will be with you shortly." Hands down, this is the shortest check-in I've had since this dreadful Tango started.

Once again, Ken and I seat ourselves in the waiting area. You can't help but look around the room and wonder what the other individuals are here for. I'm by far the youngest, at least on this day.

I'm sure you've heard it said before, people love to hear their name spoken, but that doesn't apply to me, at least not today. "Apryl Allen?"

Standing, I slowly turn to face my grim reaper. Instead, it was none other than—*I swear*—Jane Lynch in the flesh! On exceptionally unstable legs I hear myself answer, "That's me!" and with a cheerful voice!

She looked at me, pretending to size me up and down. "I have only one question for you—Prada or Gucci?" She then bit the end of her pencil in anticipation of my answer.

Are you serious??? Laughing, because obviously I didn't hear her correctly, "I'm sorry?!"

"Well, your gown of course," she replied. It's a very important detail!!!"

"Oh, hmmm . . ." I began thoughtfully, "that's such a difficult question. I guess Prada. What the heck!" I could feel a small amount of tension dissipate.

Jane then looked to Ken. "If you wouldn't mind, we need you to wait here until we get Apryl into *bed*." Then changing to a juicy voice with a titillating tease, "I'll return for you l-a-t-e-r!" simultaneously strutting backwards while provocatively wiggling her pencil at him. Whirling around, she led me down the remainder of the corridor, all the while leaving Ken breathless! *I LOVE IT!!!* This woman is *exactly* the type of person I love in life!

Once we entered the prep area she handed me a package of purple apparel, minus the Prada logo of course, all of which was wrapped in plastic. "Here's your new wardrobe. Remove everything but your panties. Once you've changed, place all your personal belongings in this plastic bag." She then handed me a clear plastic bag with a draw string attached.

Pointing to a pair of white stockings atop the bundled package, "The white knee-highs have holes in them that are meant to be placed at the balls of your feet. Put those stockings on first. The fuzzy purple socks go over them."

Upon closer examination of the warm fuzzy socks, I realized they had paw prints all over them—*how did they know I have dogs? And how thoughtful . . . they want to make sure my feet stay warm.*

While attempting to throw together this unique ensemble, I hear the Medicine Woman arrive. Not using the cheeriest of tones she inquires, "Is she about finished?"

I replied from behind the curtain, "These couture outfits are difficult to put on!"

I could hear the Medicine Woman's puzzlement through the curtain and Jane quickly appeared to assist.

"You look great!" she said, astonished to find I donned my new attire perfectly. "It appears you're ready for your debut!" As she pulled the curtain back, I made my entrance.

I guess I was expecting my Medicine Woman to greet me, but she was all business and didn't appear to be in the best of moods. As she stood making notes in my chart, I became a bit worried. She's going to operate on me and I want a smile on her face. So, using my most pleasant tone, of course, "Are you happy?"

With a deadpan look and *"I don't have time for this"* tone the Medicine Woman replied, "What?"

"Are you happy today? I want to know you're in a good place," I asked energetically. You would have thought I had tried to hug the Queen of England or made some other faux pas. The staff stood frozen; holding their breath.

Realizing I was serious, her attitude immediately changed. After all, I am the one who hired the Medicine Woman and I want her in good spirits while working on me.

"Oh . . . Yes, I'm happy." Her response could have used a little more energy, but it was acceptable.

"Great . . . I guess we're ready then!"

Jane asked I follow her to an area with curtained-off surgery tables. "This one here's your beauty. Go ahead and climb aboard." While pulling over a tray on wheels, she informed me, "I'll be putting your IV in."

"Okay, but just so you know, I have small rolling veins."

"Piece of cake," and with nothing more than a pinch it was in.

While waiting for the inevitable, I decided to ask the names of everyone who would be working on me. Of course there was Jane, whom we already know. Then Missy, the assisting nurse who looked to be 20-something, arrived and asked me a bunch of questions I don't remember as Marsha typed my responses into a computer.

The Medicine Woman then started toward me. Not making eye contact, she approached with caution, staring at the sheets covering my chest. As she lowered them, "Just to verify, I show your surgery is going to be on your left breast. Is this correct?"

"Yes, I replied and wondered whether I should be nervous by her question.

"Okay, I'm going to mark it with an X," using a *purple* sharpie pen, of course.

Marsha then asked a few questions and ended with, "We appreciate you asking all our names, but you're not going to remember them." Everyone chimed in their assent.

What they didn't know is I have my mom's memory. I can pretty much remember most things with accuracy—in fact, I remembered everyone's names! Okay, I forgot the anesthesiologist's name but that doesn't count because he was administering a liquid memory loss potion at the time I asked.

Not noticing Jane had slipped away, she reappeared with none other than Mr. Wonderful by her side. I don't remember what we spoke about. What I do remember is feeling the softness of his touch and his pleading, loving eyes looking into mine.

Before long Jane returned. "Sorry to break up this party, but it's time for your hubby to leave."

Having his hands full with all the items we brought, he stood juggling them before leaning over. With tears running down his beautiful face he whispered in a low voice for my ears alone to hear, "I love you more than life, honey. Please know I'll be with you throughout this entire surgery." This man *really* loves and adores me ... *boy, this is difficult to write!* He then kissed me. "I'll see you soon, love ..." and he gracefully disappeared behind the curtain.

That's when I wanted to jump off the table and grab his hand and run as fast and far as we could away from *everything*—to *anywhere* but this room, with these people. But it's too late and I keep my composure. The next thing I remember is waking up with the night nurse.

Agnus was buzzing around talking to various people. Suddenly she appeared by my side. "On a scale of one to 10, 10 being the worst, how's your pain?"

I don't remember my reply. She returned to her buzzing. My mind was fuzzy ... "Would you please tell my mom to come back?" I remember asking a woman standing at the head of my bed. She looked lovingly into my eyes and I remember feeling a softness emanating from her, yet no words were exchanged. She then looked towards Agnus—I assume with hopes she would do something about my request. Quite honestly, I don't think Agnus even knew she was there. Then I watched as this unknown woman left my bedside and walked out the door. She never returned.

A group of about eight nurses appear, with one taking center stage. "I just wanted to say goodnight to everyone."

All attention was then focused on her. "Happy Birthday! Have a wonderful time tonight!" Everyone chimed in with their own adulations.

Someone then inquired, "Where are you going for dinner?" and that's when stomach-churning chatter about their favorite foods filled the room. I felt my stomach do a somersault as nausea began to take over. I could hear someone calling for Agnus' assistance, and then realized I was beckoning her.

Not wanting to leave her cohorts, she eventually broke herself away from the crowd. "How are you feeling?" she inquired, not at all happy with me.

"I'm feeling nauseous and in a little bit of pain." She walked away and reappeared with a shot needle. As if I were a rag doll, she turned me over and stuck it into my left buttocks. I remember thinking *Yikes!* But I didn't feel anything and drifted off again.

Agnus reappeared. "Apryl . . . Apryl . . . on a scale from one to 10 how is your pain?"

"About a two," I replied.

"The same as you felt before?"

"Did I say two before?" I was confused and didn't remember my first response. Besides, I thought I'd told her I was at a five or six. *Oh well*, I thought to myself, *at least the nausea has subsided.*

More buzzing around. When she finally came back over I told her I was thirsty.

Once again she disappeared and returned with a cup of ice and proceeded to spoon-feed me. I couldn't believe how parched I was, and thrilled to find the ice was the small, easy to chew kind, unlike the medium hard cubes given to me after my hysterectomy that I tried to refuse but couldn't because every time I opened my mouth to tell them I didn't want anymore, more was shoved in.

Agnus set down the cup. *But wait, I'm still thirsty! Rats* . . . she left again. I watched as she buzzed around the room. When she returned, I admitted, "I'm a little scared. Will you stay here and talk with me a bit?"

"Don't be afraid." Then, as an afterthought, "Pretend you're in Turks and Caicos walking on the beach."

"Oh . . . have you been to Turks and Caicos?" I inquire.

"No." Then using an almost accusatory tone, as if I'd been caught doing something I shouldn't have, she asks, "Have you?"

"Yes, my husband took me there for my 40th birthday." Remembering the trip well, I told her about the hotel we stayed at and then, being proud of the fact, inform her how my husband designs hotels, and *blah, blah, blah* . . .

"Where do you live?" Not waiting for my answer, she pessimistically quipped, "You must have a *nice* house."

Suddenly, she leaned in real close and, just shy of a whisper, asked another question. This time I felt a warning from deep within that alerted me she was asking something way too personal and that I shouldn't answer. I don't remember the question, but it didn't matter because she disappeared again. I wasn't impressed with her, and with much clarity and certainty, can definitively say the feeling was mutual. *Note to self: If ever I or anyone I love* requires surgery, request to be by their side as soon as they're out of surgery. Preferably before they wake.

Soon, she was by my side once again. "Agnus, will you stay with me or get my husband, because I'm starting to feel scared again."

She then proceeded to feed me ice, all the while repeating, "Apryl . . . wake up. Apryl . . . wake up." Disappearing *again*, she returned with some sort of contraption. She handed me what felt like a milk carton jug and stuffed something or another into my mouth. It was a rubbery pliable mouthpiece that I thought she had said I was to blow into. *Yuck!*

Firmly she reprimanded me, "No . . . you're supposed to take a deep breath while it's in your mouth. And try to get this little ball to the yellow marker." She walked away again. When she returned: "Apryl . . . wake up. Apryl . . . wake up!" Over and over she kept saying this. *Please, someone stop her, I can't stand being treated like an idiot!* I drifted off again. When I opened my eyes I was still holding the contraption in my right hand and had the dreaded something or other in my mouth.

I could hear another woman in the bed to my right jabbering away. She asked a different nurse, "Will you stay and talk with me? If you won't, can I talk to the lady in the bed next to me?" *She was referring to me!*

Suddenly Agnus reappeared. Using my tongue, I pushed the rubbery thing from my mouth and let it fall onto my chest. I had to remove it quickly because I was unsure how long she would be around before she buzzed off again.

"Agnus, why is that woman so much more awake than me?"

"Could be many reasons, but you need to wake up!" She left again and reappeared saying, "I have your scripts here," and wrote something down on a clipboard.

My what? Oh dang, my prescriptions—I forgot to get them filled prior to surgery! "Agnus, will you please fax them to my pharmacy?"

"NO. We can't fax narcotics!" In my heart I knew this wasn't true. I'm prescribed Tylenol with Codeine due to my low tolerance to pain medications which *can* be faxed but I just didn't care anymore. I did my best to listen as she proceeded to go over the checklist with me. "You're supposed to do your exercises twice a day," flipping through the pages attached to the clipboard, she inquired, "Did the Medicine Woman give you the page with your exercises before your surgery?"

"No . . . I don't think so." My head was reeling.

"Hmmm . . . okay." Shrugging her shoulders, she disappeared again.

She must have left to get Ken, because he arrived at some point after my conversation with her. I was so tired I just wanted to sleep. I know he arrived after I asked Agnus to fax my prescriptions; otherwise, I'm sure Ken would have insisted she do it. Lovingly I feel Ken squeeze my hand.

Agnus appeared again. "Two to three times a day you'll need to empty Apryl's lymphatic drain." She pulled out from under the sheet what looked like a clear soft rubbery hand grenade at the end of a long clear tube.

Yuck! That's attached to me? I thought. Unease masked Ken's face as he listened intently to the instructions that ensued. In my groggy state I attempted to pay close attention as well, just in case Ken missed something.

"I'll show you how to do it." Agnus then positioned herself next to Ken. "First, you're going to uncap the *grenade*." (*Sorry, I don't know what else to call it.*) Ken and I both observed closely as she removed the cap. "Next, you'll need to clear out the tube like this." She then pinched the top end of the tube closest to my underarm with her thumb and index finger. Using her other hand in a similar fashion, we watched as she pinched the tube just below where she was holding it. Then sliding her fingers down the length of the tube, she squeezed a reddish colored liquid into the gadget.

"You'll want to make sure you've squeezed whatever drainage is in the tube down into the grenade *before* you remove it. After doing this, whatever's in the grenade will need to be emptied out." We watched as she squeezed its contents into a measuring cup. "Once you've emptied it, you'll need to clean the end of the tube and the cap with an alcohol pad." She began cleaning both of them.

"Where do we get those?" Ken asked, referring to the pads.

"Any pharmacy carries them," she replied, pausing from her instructions. "Before you replace the cap, squeeze the grenade like so," and we watched as she emptied the majority of the air from it. "While it's deflated you'll place the cap back on—and that's it."

"Would it be possible to get enough pads from you to get us through a couple of days?" Ken inquired. "I'm not sure when I'll be able to get to a pharmacy to purchase them."

"Sure," and she left with the measuring cup in hand; we assumed to get the pads. Returning several minutes later, the measuring cup and pads were a thing of the past.

"It's time for you to take a walk to the restroom." Looking around the room Agnus signaled for a woman to assist me.

A very nice woman with a Russian accent appeared and helped me out of bed. She steadily held my arm while assuring my drain was not compromised as we walked to the restroom. *Why couldn't she have been by my side when I first woke up?* I thought. She likes to talk and was extremely nice, which I really appreciated.

When we came out of the restroom she and Agnus together seated me in a very comfortable Barcalounger and, with Ken's help, they proceeded to change my clothes. I watched as the plastic drawstring bag slowly emptied of my personal belongings. When he got to the bottom, the last item remaining were my flip-flops.

"I don't want to wear those," I told Ken. "I want to leave my socks on," because my feet were perfectly comfy cozy!

"Okay, she's ready to go home," Agnus announced. "If you want to pull your car around we'll meet you in the patient pick-up area."

It seemed to take only seconds from the time they rolled me out in the Barcalounger—yes, it had wheels—to our SUV that miraculously appeared at the sliding glass door exit. My prince charming rushed to assist me as I stood readying myself to climb into our vehicle. Yes, I was ready for home sweet home.

It was storming on the drive home. A huge lightning bolt sliced through the darkened sky and thunderous drums answered its electric display. Ken and I were in awe of its beauty and reveled in the rain that ensued. What a relief it was to be headed home. Then I remembered where I was and why we were out this evening.

Suddenly I became very G-R-O-U-C-H-Y! I knew the night nurse could have faxed the prescriptions. Silently I berate myself for neglecting to have this done prior to surgery. *How could I forget?* Worse, I proceeded to tell Ken how to drive home . . . excuse me, to the local pharmacy.

"Ken, I don't want to be alone. Please don't go into the pharmacy. Can we go to one that has a drive-thru?" Then a little later, "I just want to go home. I don't want to wait for the prescription to be filled."

"What do you propose we do then?" he asked, attempting to stay calm.

"Clíona offered to help. If we drop it off, I bet she'd pick it up for us."

"Okay, get her on the phone for me." Both Clíona and Adelaide made sure Ken had their numbers prior to my surgery and told him, if we needed anything at all, to call them. I found her name, dialed her number for Ken and handed him the phone as it began ringing.

"Hi Clíona, it's Ken. I guess we are in need of help. We didn't get Apryl's prescriptions filled and she doesn't want me to leave her alone. If we drop them off, could you possibly pick them up for us?"

"Absolutely! Is there anything else I can do?"

"Thank you, no," and I listened as he told her which pharmacy. They spoke a bit more about how the surgery went, and Ken ended the call expressing his appreciation for her help.

As we drove up to the pharmacy's drive-thru window, Ken told the young pharmacist I just had surgery. "Could you possibly fill it quickly for us?"

No special privileges here. "Sure, give us 10 minutes." It was around 8:00 at night, and the pharmacy didn't seem all that busy. "Please wait in the parking lot," she directed Ken.

"What do you think, honey?" Ken asked. "Shall we wait or do you want to go home?"

"I can wait 10 minutes." I wasn't in any pain; I just wanted to be at home in bed.

He quickly phoned Clíona. "Hi, Clíona, we're terribly sorry to impose on your time, so I checked with the pharmacy and they can fill it immediately for us. Thank you, but we won't need you to pick it up."

"Okay, if you need anything at all . . ." Ken thanked her again and ended the call.

At 10 minutes exactly we drove back up to the window and, with prescriptions in hand, we're finally on our way home. Again, I started to feel unsettled. *Ken is normally so organized. What's wrong with him???* Obviously the more appropriate question is *what's wrong with me?*

Before I knew it, I was home in bed and Ken was serving me the chicken soup Adelaide had lovingly prepared on a tray with crackers. I was ravenous! When my stomach reminded me numerous times throughout the day I was hungry, I appeased its relentless demands with the thought of this soup.

My mouth was watering as I blew on the soup to cool it, but I didn't need to worry about its temperature. It was *spicy* hot and burned my throat as it went down. I was so upset . . . *why would Adelaide have put jalapeños in it?*

"Ken, it's spicy hot!"

"What?!" He himself took a cautious taste of the soup. "Wow! That is spicy . . . Honey, I'm so sorry. Let me go see if we have a can of chicken soup."

What?! I'm relegated to eating chicken soup from a can? I cried and whined to Ken. "I was so looking forward to her soup . . . I'm so upset . . ." and *blah, blah, blah! Poor Ken.*

Unfortunately, while I was eating my canned nourishment, Adelaide phoned. While Ken was speaking with her I of course demanded to talk, half wanting to hear my friend's voice and the other to whine! With a bit of reluctance, he handed me the phone.

"Hey, how ya' doing?" she sweetly asked.

"Ken always has everything so together but tonight it's just a mess. And, why did you put jalapeños in the soup?"

"What?! I didn't . . . I put white pepper in it. It shouldn't be that spicy—but I thought you liked spicy foods, so that's why I added it."

Crossly I replied, "I do . . . but this tastes like it has jalapeños in it and I can't eat it! Now I have to eat chicken soup from a can . . ." and lord only knows how long I went on like this. *Poor Adelaide.*

Needless to say, the torturous conversation did finally end. We hung up and, pouting like a five-year-old who didn't get her way, I ate my penance of canned soup and fell fast asleep with the tray on my lap.

15

Erased

Annie Lennox

My eyes are closed. Gradually I become aware of my surroundings. I attempt to move. Yesterday's activity registers disapprovingly. My left arm wants nothing to do with the effort. I enlist Ken's help and he places his hands under my back to help me sit up, positioning me somewhat vertically, I then swing my legs over the edge of the bed. Blood rushes to the areas where Jorge and the Lymph-Along-Kid have vacated. A harsh throbbing ache explodes; involuntarily I take in a sharp breath. Slowly I rise to welcome the new day, without *him*.

We begin the first of our two to three times a day routine of empting my drain. I don't know how Ken can stand it. I personally can't watch him do it; it makes me ill to my stomach. There's absolutely no physical pain, only mental anguish on my part. No sooner does Ken get me settled than the phone urgently rings. It's the surgery center checking in on me.

"I'm doing fine. Thank you."

"And how was your overall experience with our facility?" the voice questioned.

"You'll need to speak with my husband," I replied, handing the phone to Ken.

I listened as Ken informed the caller "the night nurse neglected to give us the items required for emptying her drain."

Whoever this woman was told Ken, "It's not a big deal. Just use the lines on the hand grenade to record the number each time you empty it."

"What?! We're supposed to be recording the drainage? No one said anything about that!" Ken was agitated. After ending the call, he suggested I ring Mabel.

"They said what?!" Mabel was as shocked as we were. "That is absolutely incorrect! They should have provided you with a measuring cup to record the precise amount of drainage in cc's. You should've also received a chart to record the date, time, amount in cc's and color of drainage. Was that given to you?"

"No, they didn't give us anything," I replied dismayed, wondering how a facility in the business of healing could neglect to give such vital paraphernalia.

"I'm sorry, but you'll need to go back to the surgery center and get those items, along with the form."

After hanging up with Mabel, Ken and I examined the grenade. Its measurements only reflected 25, 50, 75, and 100 increments. There was no way we could accurately measure the drainage using it. Angry and exasperated, my faithful husband left to retrieve the necessary paraphernalia from the surgery center the morning *after* my surgery.

While awaiting his return, I remembered my conversation with Adelaide. Utterly embarrassed, I cringed at the thought that I dared complain about something someone did from their heart. *I'm sure she'll never speak with me again. And to think she went to all the trouble to make me soup from scratch—and I complained about it?! I don't even know what to say for myself!* I called to apologize, fully expecting Adelaide to say, "Please don't call again."

Instead, her response was, "I'm so sorry. I'm making a new batch as we speak with *no spices.*"

"You still love me?" I asked, fearful of the answer she'd give.

"Of course . . . you were under the effects of anesthesia. Everyone's strange with that in their system."

I was stupefied. No one has ever . . . I mean, Ken puts up with me but he has to—right?! But someone who has known me for less than a year, *and* after being spoken to in that fashion? She's an angel!

"I'll bring the new batch over tomorrow," she said with an upbeat attitude.

With a much lighter heart, I reveled in my surgery being a thing of the past and spending the day with my husband. Surprisingly, I found I didn't want to be in bed. Instead, I was up and around—*not doing much of course*. But still, both Ken and I were amazed at how good I felt.

"Since you're doing so well, would you mind if I went to the office tomorrow?" He's been sacrificing most of his urgently needed time at the office for me, and during a crucial time for our business. Our company is finally at a turning point with new projects on the horizon and Ken is desperately needed. Besides, he knew Adelaide was coming over and I wouldn't be alone. He added, "I'll only spend half a day."

"You can stay the whole day if you need to." I was feeling energized. Maybe it was because the dreaded surgery was finally over. Or maybe because I knew Ken loved me and I had friends to support me. Who knows? All I know is I feel happy and content.

Wednesday morning, Ken headed to the office, and I spent the morning doing a couple of light loads of laundry and watering houseplants. Adelaide stopped by for lunch and, as promised, brought a new batch of chicken soup.

She arrived with her dimpled smile carrying a basket that contained the pot of soup, all the accoutrements needed for this homemade nourishment and flowers! As we talked over lunch, I modeled the vest we got from Lulu's Loot. I showed her the conveniently placed pockets inside that kept the grenade out of sight and harm's reach and, more importantly, far from my mind's imagination.

While discussing the chicken soup saga, we realized I'd had a tube down my throat, which was probably the culprit for feeling the first batch was so spicy. But *really* . . . who would go to all the trouble to make a second batch of homemade soup? *Am I as good of a friend as she has shown to me?* I silently wondered.

After Adelaide left I took the opportunity to sit and ponder everything that had transpired up to this day—probably not the best choice of things to do. Looking back at all the faux pas prior to surgery was disheartening. But was I the one to blame? The surgery was scheduled so quickly that I never gave it a second thought that the only time we met with the Medicine Woman was at our initial consultation. Wasn't there supposed to be a pre-op appointment? I guess it was because I'd had so much interaction with Mabel at her office, it felt as if I was dealing with the Medicine Woman herself. I had considered that meeting an interview for the position and for some reason thought there would be another appointment prior to the actual surgery. At minimum I was sure I'd be speaking with the Medicine Woman again *but it never happened.*

Feeling anxiety starting to build and wanting to ease my worry I asked myself, *do I feel comfortable having the Medicine Woman as my surgeon?* Absolutely YES! I feel strongly she was and is the correct choice and, based on what I see in the mirror, find myself very pleased with the outcome. Plus, every doctor I've spoken with says she's one of the best, especially because she focuses solely on *breasts*. *I guess it's better than focusing on e-mails.*

In the end, it was only due to my naïveté that some things slipped through the proverbial crack. Honestly, I'm beginning to feel a bit neurotic. But then again . . . this is not a normal part of my life. However, *it is for my surgeon.* She should have prepared me to the best of her ability. As the saying goes, "It isn't her first rodeo!"

Based on my experience, I suggest if you ever require surgery, schedule it for first thing in the morning. The reasons are many: The doctors are at the start of their day, you won't end up having to fast all day and moreover, you don't end up with the night shift. I did attempt to change the appointment to an earlier time, but the first one available was on September 17th and I didn't want to prolong the surgery any more than I had to.

But that is nothing compared to the foremost mistake I made on my surgery date. The absolute most important item at the top of every list is to get your prescriptions filled *PRIOR* to having surgery! If you forget, have someone else fill them for you while you're in surgery. And don't let any nurse tell you he or she can't fax your prescription to a pharmacy. As long as it's not narcotics, they absolutely can! *Apryl . . . change your frame of mind! It does no one any good to dwell on this, especially you!*

In an effort to avert my attention from the *"should haves, could haves, would haves,"* I started busying myself around the house again when the Medicine Woman called. Remember when I'd mentioned to Ken that if she didn't get all the margins I would have to go in for *another* surgery? But he had corrected me, saying I misunderstood, and they test the margins *at the time* of the surgery? Well, evidently I had rolled the dice and didn't realize I was gambling.

"Good afternoon . . ." I greeted the caller on the phone, not recognizing the number on our caller ID.

"Good afternoon, Apryl, this is the Medicine Woman. I'm calling to let you know all the margins were clear around Jorge and as suspected, only one out of the nine lymph nodes taken was angry. The other eight were all healthy!"

"Okay, let me get this straight . . . had the margins not come back clear I would have required another surgery, but because they're all clear I don't need to?" I wanted to make sure I understood *exactly* what she was saying.

"That is correct."

"That's fantastic news!!!" *Jorge and friends are officially gone!* "Since I have you on the phone I do have a couple of questions. Are there any exercises I'm supposed to be doing? I wasn't given anything after my surgery."

"Yes, raise your hands over your head twice a day and hold them there for five seconds."

"Is there anything else?"

"Nope." She's definitely not a woman of many words.

Realizing it was 10 business days until my pathology results would be received, I then inquired, "Is there any reason why I need to keep my appointment with the Mad Scientist for this Friday, especially since we won't have the results from my pathology report?"

"No, I'd call and change it. He won't have the results for, at minimum, 10 days from the surgery." *Done!*

"I notice my left arm and fingers appear to be a little swollen."

"That's normal and should go away over the next week or so." *Thank God!*

"I also have a massive headache, is this normal?"

"I doubt it has anything to do with the surgery; I recommend you take whatever it is you take for headaches." *But wouldn't the Tylenol with codeine take care of this?* Feeling a bit like a hypochondriac I dropped the subject.

"Okay, thanks for the call and good news." *How about that, a phone call I wasn't even anticipating and it was GREAT News!*

Quickly phoning Ken, I told him about the call and the possibility I could have required another surgery, but thankfully the surgery was successful! The only thing we could figure was this information about the surgery must have taken place while he had stepped out during the appointment.

Note to self: Make sure someone else is present when meeting with a doctor so you both can take notes about an upcoming surgery, unless you're recording the conversation on your smart phone. It's imperative you have a second set of ears present.

Had I known the Medicine Woman didn't test the margins at the time of the surgery, I would have definitely obtained a second opinion from another surgeon. Surely technology has advanced to the point this can be done. I could be mistaken, but I recall hearing about this somewhere. Again, this is what's so particularly frustrating to me. How are you supposed to know what questions to ask when you've never experienced anything like this?

Hanging up with Ken, I then called the Mad Scientist's office and spoke with his medical assistant, Deadra. After explaining the dilemma, "So we'll need to reschedule my appointment."

I could hear her typing on her keyboard, "Ten days from your surgery would put it on Monday, September 9th, and the Mad Scientist will be on vacation."

"Okay, what's his first available appointment when he returns?" Mind you, this is only *THE* most important appointment of all, the final piece to my puzzle and the one that tells me literally what my life will consist of over the next six months!

"Hold on, let me check." While on hold, I silently pray she can get me in on the first day of his return. "Okay, we can get you in on Thursday, September 12th at 2:15."

I was absolutely elated. "Thank you, Deadra; this means the world to me!"

Hanging up I make a mental note to call her back the day before the appointment to verify the office received the results of the pathology report. Heaven knows we've already been down that road before. There's no reason to go and have my blood drawn and wait for 40 minutes to simply smile at the Mad Scientist—*right?!*

Later that afternoon, I sent an e-mail to The Inquisitive Minds:

> *From:*   *Apryl*
> *Sent:*   *Wednesday, August 28, 2013 5:55 PM*
> *To:*   *The Inquisitive Minds*
> *Subject:*   *ADA Update – Surgery Results!!!*

FANTASTIC NEWS!!! Surgery went great ... I'm feeling Great and the best news of all, ALL the margins were clean around Jorge and as suspected only 1 out of the 9 lymph nodes taken had cancer. The other 8 little lymph nodes were as healthy as could be! I just now received the phone call from my Medicine Woman!

SOOOO YIPIEE!!!!!! Jorge has been officially ERASED! I'm just thrilled! Thank you all for your prayers, thoughts and love! Hope you all have a wonderful holiday weekend if I don't speak with you in person.

Next stop will be with the Mad Scientist on September 12th when we receive the results as to the stage and level Jorge is at.

Again . . . Jorge has left my sanctuary and I am a VERY Happy Girl!

Big Hug & HUGE Kiss to everyone!!!

After pressing the send button, I immediately start my twice a day exercise and attempt to lift my hands over my head. *Yikes!* It's horrifically painful and I can't get my left arm to completely straighten—it appears to be stuck at 60 degrees of my normal range of motion. It absolutely does not want to comply with my efforts to raise it over my head.

Throughout the week I persevered through the pain and faithfully completed my *twice a day* morning and evening exercises. Some days, when I was feeling really motivated, I did it at noon too! Then, I decided to add noon to each day, furthering my efforts for a complete recovery. Eventually I included everyday house chores as exercise too, using my *left* arm to place clothing and dishes in upper cabinets.

Rewind back to when I picked up my bag of goodies from Lulu's Loot . . . not only were the anticipated bras and vest in the bag but a pink heart pillow about eight inches in diameter had been included with my treasures. *Okay, I'm starting to get sick of the color pink and now hearts too,* I thought to myself. And dismissed the heart as yet more paraphernalia you receive when encountering Jorge.

Now back to my chores. It was time for our monthly bills. While organizing I came across the little heart pillow that somehow ended up on my desk in the office. When I picked it up I noticed a tag was attached to it that displayed the logo and name *"Breast Cancer Comfort Hearts"* and in fine print under the logo it read:

> *This heart has been made just for you with love and support from your friends at Breast Cancer Comfort Hearts. This heart pillow is designed to assist in your recovery. Put it under your arm on the side(s) that you've had surgery and it will bring you comfort and well wishes for a speedy recovery.*

After reading this I realized when I've been sitting with Ken watching television my underarm, where the Lymph-Along-Kid was, began to have a deep dull ache to it. The only way I could alleviate the ache was to put my left arm up on the back of the couch, but then my shoulder would start hurting and my arm turned ice cold.

That night I thought I'd give the heart a try. I couldn't believe it—the pillow did *wonders* for me! Looking back, I wish I'd spent more time in the store perusing its many items. Who knows what else I would have found there. Evidently, the Sizer knew what I would need and included it as a gift for me. One day I'll have to call and thank her for her kindness.

Cliona stopped by Thursday afternoon and brought with her lunch, a book and welcomed conversation. Earlier that morning I had seen a snake on our back patio and filled her in on all the details. Of course, I just knew there was some greater purpose to the appearance of our recent guest and, prior to Cliona's arrival, had researched what it means when a snake comes calling . . .

> **The Snake**: *When a snake presents itself you can expect death and rebirth to occur in some area of your life. (Jorge.) Change and healing will soon follow. (My current status.) Snakes have speed and agility. (Ken and*

I personally witnessed this.) When a snake comes into your life you will find changes and shifts occur quickly and are recognized and defined easily. Also, look for rebirth into new powers of creativity and wisdom. (I look forward to it!) Using their tongues, snakes have a keen sense of smell, which is why it flicks in and out so much. People with this talisman will find themselves extremely sensitive to smells and fragrances. (I've been complaining to Ken about unfamiliar smells, maybe it's because I'm only able to take sponge baths, but he claims he can't smell anything—that's my prince!)

After Clíona left, I was exhausted, probably from all the excitement of Mr. Snake! So I decided to lay down on our living room sofa for an afternoon respite. However, my nap took an unexpected turn while I drifted in and out of consciousness. Feeling cold I thought, *the air conditioner is blowing on me—I should move.* But I was so fatigued I couldn't get myself to lift a finger and continued on with my slumber. Around 4:30, when I finally did wake, my chest was all tight and I knew a cold was coming on. Phoning Ken at the office I found myself feeling frustrated at the fact I required yet more of his time when I informed him I wasn't feeling so well.

"Can you please pick up a humidifier for me at the store on the way home? And more apple juice please!" Friday I slept all day and felt horrible. Saturday I felt better and continued lounging around the house. Sunday I felt as if I took a step back and Monday was the same. Needless to say the surgery and chest cold were starting to take a toll on me.

That afternoon my 92-year-old *pia* phoned. *Pia* means mother in Comanche. In our culture, if your mother passes away, it's our custom her sister takes her place.

"I'm so sorry I haven't phoned. I couldn't remember whether your surgery was last Monday or today."

It was wonderful to hear her voice, which sounded so much like my mom's! Overwhelming emotions took over and I began to cry. "Oh, *Pia*— I'm so sad!" I sobbed, "I've come down with a cold and between this and my surgery I'm beginning to wear down."

We talked for a bit more. Then with my mom's authority and her wise insightfulness, my *pia* said, "You need to get the attitude back you had when we spoke before your surgery. *Happiness* is the best medicine when you're sick!" She was right and after hanging up I set my heart on changing my state of mind!

What would make me feel better? I asked myself. I'd just *love* to take a shower and was sick of the only article of clothing I was able to wear during this past week—the cream-colored vest I got at Lulu's Loot. Truly, it wasn't the most appealing article of clothing—I felt like a cream puff wearing it—but it did save me a lot of grief. The pockets it had on the inside held the apparatus for my lymphatic drain perfectly—*thank you again Sizer Woman*.

What I wanted was to feel comfy cozy and this vest just wasn't doing the trick. My arms have a tendency to get cold and when I'm sick that's the last thing I want. Not to mention I found myself wanting to feel feminine and look pretty—I mean *really* ... there's no need to wear something unappealing.

I went into my closet and began perusing my wardrobe for something I could convert into a similar style. *Something* I could alter with ease, though I knew this would be difficult since any article of clothing would require pockets on the inside. Sorting through the clothing on hangers, my mind came to life with what I wanted it to feel like—mid-thigh length, something I wouldn't mind lounging around the house in, and definitely something easy to wash in case of an unexpected spill.

And there it was, in the back of my closet hanging amidst my bathrobes—my gray mid-thigh length, long-sleeved, zipper-up-the-front house jacket. It would be easy to convert and the pockets on the outside of the jacket were at just the right length. All I have to do is cut a slit into the pockets from the inside of the jacket, then sew them so the material won't fray. It worked like a charm and quite frankly ... I was impressed with my ingenuity and thankful to my mother for teaching me to sew.

Now for my sponge bath *in the shower*; I'd have to be extra careful not to get this dang drain contraption wet. Using much caution, I enjoyed my half body wash and upper half sponge bath. After drying off I slipped into my new but old house coat. It felt delectable! I felt like a whole new person, and even better, I actually felt *Happy* again! *Thank you Pia!*

When Ken came home that evening I recruited his help to wash my hair. He prepared the counter in our laundry room for the blessed occasion by laying down towels to lessen the hard surface of the countertop for me.

My husband is always so thoughtful! Then, using our step ladder, I climbed its steps and lay down—it was *perfect!*

He began washing my hair in the sink; it felt amazing! Of course, because I couldn't raise my arm over my head, Ken had to blow-dry my hair for me. He did a pretty good job, although he should definitely keep his day job. Now I was ready for a night on the town—*well almost!*

Tuesday, one week after my surgery, was the follow-up appointment with my Medicine Woman. Upon my arrival, Mabel requested yet again I don the infamous gown with the opening in the front. After doing so, the Medicine Woman came in wheeling her laptop computer on the rolling table. While she was punching in information I inquired, "How much of a margin did you take around Jorge?"

"Let me see . . ." Adjusting her glasses to view the screen better, she said, "One centimeter-plus."

Hmmm . . . okay. At this point I have no complaints, at least from what I can see, that is. After the surgery she had placed clear bandages, approximately 3 x 5 inches in size, over each of the incisions. I didn't dare look at how the drain tube was attached for fear of fainting.

She then asked, "Did you bring your report with the details of your drainage?"

"Yes," Ken replied as he reached into his briefcase to retrieve it. I was hovering around 28-ish and knew the tube wouldn't come out until we got down to 24 ccs.

The Medicine Woman then added the previous day's amounts. "Eight plus 19 equals 27. Okay, it can come out."

Wait . . . what?! Did I just hear her say it was coming out? Yippee, I get the tube out! But then I realized, *Oh shit . . . she's gonna take the tube out!*

I looked to Ken with fear and trepidation written all over my face. Without hesitation he said, "Honey, look at me, not at the Medicine Woman."

The Medicine Woman stood up from her chair. "Okay, place your hand on my right shoulder," and as asked I placed my left arm—the side on which I had the surgery—gently on her shoulder. She then fiddled with the tube a bit. "Hmmm . . . we're going to have to take the bandage off first because the tube isn't budging."

When I heard this, what should have been butterflies fluttering inside my stomach felt more like a buffalo stampede. With great distress I clamored, "I have to be honest: I'm a little scared."

Without any hesitation whatsoever, the Medicine Woman replied, "Well, I'm not!" and *R-I-P!!!* As quick as lightening she had it off. Truthfully, it wasn't as bad as being waxed down you know where!

"Now, there might be a little burning after the tube is taken out," and, without giving me a chance to think about what she just said, out it came. Luckily I felt *nothing*! Whew . . . I can't tell you how RELIEVED I am that it's over!

I let out a ginormous breath and the Medicine Woman exclaimed, "Ah . . . so you do know how to breathe!" She then began cleaning the previously bandaged area and after finishing said in jest, "Now get out of here. I need to tend to patients who are sick!"

We all laughed, although mine was more of a *thank God it's over* chuckle. I then looked my Medicine Woman in the eyes and in a half-whispered, yet heartfelt, voice uttered the words "Thank You!" My eyes filled with tears that began tumbling down my cheeks.

Grasping for control of my emotions, and before she could leave the room, I voiced a worry. "I do have one concern I'd like to inquire about. My left bicep is *really* sore; it feels as if it had the workout of a lifetime."

"That's probably due to the fact your arm was at a 45-degree angle during the surgery."

"Okay, but the inside of my left arm, my underarm, part of my shoulder and back leading all the way to my shoulder blade, are completely numb. Is this normal?"

She went back to her computer and looked at her records. "That's because it took a lot for me to pull your muscles apart to get to the Lymph-Along-Kid. He didn't want to budge so I literally had to pry him out!"

And that's when I realized, my angry little guy was probably upset because I neglected to say goodbye to him. Yes, I had said my goodbyes to Jorge, but not the Lymph-Along-Kid, and he was the one that saved my life!

She then gave me approval to shower!!!! Oh . . . how I can't wait to feel that warm water streaming down my body. I readily began making plans to rid myself of this house coat and into clothing from my former life!

Before the Medicine Woman left the room, she said, "Get with Mabel before you leave. Let her know I don't need to see you again until January." *Really?! How WONDERFUL!*

The moment she closed the door Ken stood and clasped both of my hands within his. Instead of placing his arms around me, fearful of causing pain, he leaned towards me, allowing our foreheads to touch. Together we watched as our tears tumbled to the ground. Honestly, this has been so *very* difficult for both of us!

Later, as we were riding down the elevator, I realized the Medicine Woman *must* have e-mail because she brings her laptop that's connected to the Internet via Wi-Fi to each appointment. Maybe the truth is she doesn't want to *deal* with e-mails from patients—nor does Mabel. At this point I really could care less. Now onwards and upwards . . . it's time for healing!

The next stop will be with my Mad Scientist, when we receive the results of the pathology report. I'll learn all of Jorge's intimate details—the stage, level and risk factor of my naughty boy. *Oh please God . . . let the news be the best it can be* I silently pray.

Ken had to get back to the office when we returned home. He made sure I was comfortable, and knowing me so very well implored, "I don't want you looking at yourself until I return home tonight. We'll look together, okay?" Satisfied I was in a good place, he left.

And that's when my curiosity took hold . . . what *did* my scars look like? I couldn't wait, I had to see them. The Medicine Woman had placed a Band-Aid over the hole where the tube was and said we could remove it the next night. But I had to see what the two scars looked like from the surgery.

Walking into our bathroom I turned on the vanity lights over my mirror. I then looked deep into my eyes and asked myself, "Are you sure you want to do this, Apryl?" The answer was obviously *yes* as I began unzipping my house jacket.

However, before I opened the jacket I once again looked deep into my eyes. "Are you sure you want to do this?" I again questioned myself aloud, pausing this time for several moments. Then, with much clarity, "Yes!" I opened the jacket and undid my sports bra that hooked in the front.

The scar where Jorge used to reside was a three-inch long thin black line. It didn't look bad at all. There were no divots or crevasses or even visible stitches. As a matter of fact, without the thin line, you'd never know I had surgery. Then I looked to the place where the Lymph-Along-Kid had been. *Oh my God . . .* my skin looked like it had been rolled into a three-inch-long No. 2 pencil. And, holding it together were black stitches sewn with a rope stitch.

Leaning against my bathroom counter, it felt as if my breath had been knocked out of me. I needed to hold onto something to stabilize myself. I stared deep into my eyes. *Oh, Apryl . . . what has happened to you?* I just stood there in disbelief. I was expecting my breast to look like it had been through hell, but not my underarm. This was unexpected—*why didn't anyone warn me about this? I mean, I understand the breast, but my underarm? No one had said a thing to me about this other than I was having a lymph node dissection. No wonder my arm was giving me such pain.* I stood in front of the mirror staring at myself until finally coming to my senses.

Of course I called Ken to tell him. "Hi, honey . . ." I said in a childlike voice.

"You looked at yourself in the mirror, didn't you?" *How did he know? Does he have a camera hidden somewhere or am I that transparent?*

"Yes . . ."

"And . . ."

"Well, my breast looks really good, but I wasn't expecting my underarm to look like this." My words were jagged, attempting to convey what the mirror reflected.

"Honey . . . it will heal. More importantly, I love you. We got rid of Jorge which means I get you for that much longer."

"I'm going to call the Medicine Woman's office. I want to make sure this is going to flatten out. I don't want a big old raggedy scar here."

"Remember what our Shape Shifter said, Apryl. He can fix it, so don't get all worked up over it."

"Yeah, you're right, but I don't plan on having another surgery for a while. I want to make sure in the meantime I'm not going to look like Frankenstein . . . *although* Halloween is just around the corner," I cackled, ending the call on a laughable note.

As I waited for Mabel to answer the phone my thoughts reflected back to my mom; she had gone through this by *herself.* It was heart wrenching to think she did this *all by herself*. Yeah, my siblings were there to help out to some extent, but none of us really understood fully what she was going through. And she *never once* complained about pain. My heart wrenched just thinking about her.

"This is Mabel," the distinct voice greeted.

"Hi, Mabel! It's Apryl Allen. I know I was just in, but I have another question. I just looked at my scars . . . my breast looks fine, but I wasn't expecting my underarm to look like this. Is this normal?"

I could hear Mabel's mind working. "I'm not sure what it looks like so you'll need to speak with the Medicine Woman, hold on . . ." I was placed on a brief hold.

"Twice in one day, Apryl . . . how can I help you?" the Medicine Woman chided.

Voicing my worry, "Where the lymph nodes were removed my skin is all rolled up and stitched. Is this normal? Will it flatten out eventually?" Silently I wished I had the courage to ask, *why didn't you tell me this part would be worse than the breast surgery?*

"Yes." Again with the one-worded response.

"So it will eventually flatten out." *Did she not hear the concern in my voice?*

"Yes, it will flatten out." *Gee, thanks for adding a few more words.*

"Okay, well . . . I just wasn't expecting this. I appreciate you taking my call."

Satisfied it would ultimately diminish, I sent Ken an e-mail to ease any concern he might have as well. Then I contemplated, *maybe I should have taken the Shape Shifter up on his offer and had him close me after surgery. Well, what's done is done and he did say he could fix it,* I consoled myself.

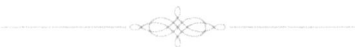

Jorge was sent in for testing to a company called Agendia. As the Medicine Woman said, "It will take approximately 10 working days to get the results." Since this report will reveal everything about Jorge, I wanted to know exactly what Agendia was and rummaged through the paperwork I was given. Of course I searched online as well.

I learned Agendia created a genomic test that studies the genes and behavior of a cancerous tumor to predict the risk factor of its return by uncovering the hidden biology. Another test will further identify its subtype, which will provide additional information about what therapy the tumor will respond to best. Below are their two types of tests:

- ***MammaPrint** studies 70 prognostic genes that determine the risk of recurrence. The test results will be one of two: Low Risk (10% chance) or High Risk (29% chance) of the cancer returning within the next 10 years. Results are given based on what would happen if the patient had no treatment at all (neither hormonal nor chemotherapy[1])*

- ***BluePrint** investigates 80 genes that identify the functional molecular subtype of a tumor, of which there are four: 1) HER2 (also called ERBB2); 2) Basal or triple negative; 3) Luminal A; and 4) Luminal B. Each of these subtypes respond differently to various therapies. This test will allow the patient and physician to determine the most effective treatment[2]*

Ultimately, these findings will help me and my Mad Scientist design a personalized treatment plan aimed at decreasing the risk of Jorge returning. The nice thing about this test is there are no intermediate results. It will be either high or low, chemo or no chemo, to be or not to be—it's a definitive answer!!

Speaking of answers . . . this waiting for results is excruciating. I'm praying we receive them in time for our next appointment with the Mad Scientist. Honestly, the waiting alone is making me insane!

It's now Wednesday, the day we're allowed to remove the final bandage, a simple Band-Aid that was placed over the hole that held the tube for my drainage. The aversion I have to medical tape once again rears its ugly head. My skin is raw and I'm finding it hard to stomach.

---

[1] Buyse M, et al, J Nat Cancer Institute. 2006; 98:17; 1183-92

[2] Gluck S, et al Breast Cancer Res Treat. 2013 Jun; 139(3):759-67

Around 7:30 that evening Ken finally addresses the elephant in the room. "Come on, let's take the Band-Aid off and go to bed early." He knows I'm filled with anxiety about removing the bandage.

Many of my friends and acquaintances have been saying over and over how strong I am. I have to admit, I do feel I've finally reached the pinnacle of inner strength my mother attained. It's something I've always strived for. However, a few friends have voiced their concern that I've been burying my feelings. On the contrary, I have taken this *very seriously* and feel it wouldn't help anyone, especially Ken, if I were a constant blubbering mess. Instead, I've attempted to match this terror with strength. Until tonight, that is . . .

Ken was incredibly gentle as he lovingly and carefully removed the last bandage. Once it was completely off . . . that's when I crumbled. "I don't have the strength to be strong anymore," I said to him and he held me as I literally fell apart in his arms. A flood of tears drenched the T-shirt he was wearing. This has been one of the most difficult things I've had to face in my life!

That moment, while Ken was holding me, has never stopped. It continues to be felt throughout time. His love—the love we share—is what's getting me through this. *Thank you kamakʉna (Comanche meaning beloved), thank you!*

Pain—each time I think about complaining the thought that *this could have been so very worse* comes to mind, and I close my mouth. My left arm is the only thing that's really sore at this point. The Tylenol with codeine does help, but I'd rather not take it. With each passing day the use of my arm is returning. I'd say my range of motion, lifting my arm out to my side then straight up over my head with no pain, is about 80 percent of its normal capacity.

However, parts of my left arm, both the bicep and triceps, hurt when they're touched. Even a gently placed fingertip that ever so softly runs along these areas is *painful*. It's especially tender just to the left of my underarm. Along with the pain is the lack of sensation. The Medicine Woman said the feeling should come back within eight months and I know it will only be a brief period of time before the pain subsides too.

Once again I enlist my Inquisitive Minds to assist me in creating the best outcome possible for this unwanted Tango:

From: *Apryl*
Sent: *Friday, September 06, 2013 1:44 PM*
To: *The Inquisitive Minds*
Subject: *ADA Update – Special Request!*

I'm proud to report the smile has returned to my face completely . . . now I'm awaiting my next marching orders! Once again I'd appreciate it immensely if you would keep me in your prayers, hearts and thoughts that my risk factor for future cancer comes back LOW — less than 10 percent would make me extremely happy!

With all my heart and love, I continue to remain . . .
Apryl.

16

El Tango (de Roxanne)
Jose Feliciano, Ewan McGregor & Jacek Koman

Waiting. It's enough to make a person go insane. The appointment—when I'm to learn of the results from my pathology report—was initially scheduled for Friday, August 30th, four days *after* my surgery. Since we wouldn't have the results at that time, it was only logical I question the need for it. It speaks volumes of the decisions doctors make (or not) and their communications with one another.

On September 11th, the day before my highly anticipated appointment, I phoned to verify the Mad Scientist had indeed received the results.

"His staff is at our other facility today, but you're welcome to leave a voicemail," the operator offered.

The few times I've left voicemails for Deadra, she's returned my call either at the end of the day or first thing the next morning, so I had no problem leaving a message. However, just to cover all the bases, I decided to verify with Mabel as well. Initially, they go to the Medicine Woman, who then forwards them on to the Mad Scientist. *Dang . . . voicemail.* I leave a message for Mabel too.

That afternoon Deadra returned my call. "Yes, we received your results."

"Wonderful! You wouldn't by chance be able to give them to me over the phone? Or is someone there that can?"

"No, we can't," Deadra snickered. *Humph . . . am I starting to break the ice with her or is that a mocking sneer?*

"Rats! Well I've waited this long, what's one more day? I'll see you tomorrow afternoon!" Ending the call a bit disappointed, not to mention frustrated, I reassured myself, *it's only one more day, Apryl.*

At the house my mobile phone doesn't always work due to bad reception. Hence on Thursday morning the sound indicating I had a voicemail chimed and I listened to the message. It was Mabel. "Yes, we received the results last week and I sent it to the Mad Scientist's office using two different methods." *They've had my results for a week? I'm on pins and needles and no one gives it a second thought to call me?*

Truly, I don't understand why patients are kept in suspense with regard to their own test results. Don't medical professionals realize this is your future at stake? And let's not forget about sanity. I mean ... why couldn't the Medicine Woman have told me the results? Or why couldn't Patience call with them? I paid for it! *Give me the damn results!* But no, you're required to come into the doctor's office, at the physician's convenience, to discuss your options. I guess if you didn't come in for an office visit the doctor wouldn't get paid.

Ken arrives at 1:50 and together we drive to the appointment in silence, both of us contemplating what our future will hold. We arrive. I'm now on the lookout for any sign from my mom. I want to know she's with me. None yet, but in my heart I know she's only a whisper away. We arrive at 2:20 and proceed with the normal routine—sign in, pay my co-pay, and complete the redundant paperwork.

"Apryl Allen?" We're escorted back to waiting room #2. Staying consistent with office protocol, I'm taken to have my blood drawn by the vampires. This poking and prodding is really getting old. Finally, I've satisfied their thirst and I'm allowed to rejoin Ken in the waiting area. My name is called at 2:35 and we follow Ramona into the examination room. Ken and I are both praying it won't be the normal 40-minute waiting period.

Ramona takes my vitals. "Everything looks good," she says, placing the equipment back in their resting spots. Then, nonchalantly before leaving the room, she says, "You'll be meeting with either Patience or Mirage today since the Mad Scientist is on vacation."

Flabbergasted, we respond in unison, "What?!" *Did she just say the Mad Scientist is on VACATION????*

"Yeah, he gets back tomorrow," and without waiting for our response, she closes the door behind her. Ken and I are in disbelief; saying I'm distressed would be a vast understatement.

"How could this have happened? I told Deadra I wanted his first available appointment when he *returned*." My mind was reeling. "They better be able to give me my results . . . and I'm asking for my co-pay to be refunded. This is absurd!" I then added, "But only after we get the results will I demand the refund."

Ken, exacerbated, nods his head and asks the inevitable, "What are we supposed to do with the information once the *nurse practitioner* gives it to us? I most certainly do not want her telling us our game plan. She's not the doctor. This is ludicrous!!!"

"They could have called me with the information if that's all this appointment is about." Then an even worse scenario occurred to me. "What if it's not Patience, and instead Mirage, whom we've never met?" All the answers were the same. *I don't know.* Deep dark blackness was all we felt.

"How can they treat their patients like this? Surely they know the severity and torment of what we're going through?!" I asked as my heart wildly thumped, fearing the unknown.

The room always seems to be slightly warm, but today I actually feel the walls closing in around me. The air, thick and foreboding, makes it difficult to breath. *I wonder if this is what a jail cell feels like,* I ask myself, unsure of how much more I can take.

And we wait . . . it feels as if time is literally at a standstill. Twenty-five minutes have now passed and no nurse practitioner.

"Ken, I'll give it another 10 minutes—until 3:15. If no one show's up I'm going to get someone."

"No, *I* will get someone," he said, disgusted. It felt as if we were captives awaiting our fate in this macabre cell while eternity passed. And the room continued to grow warmer.

It's 3:15. Ken, determined to bring this atrocity to someone's attention, exits the room, leaving the door slightly ajar. I hear him speaking to someone—his impatient yet assertive words are barely audible: "Who's in charge here?" A response is given, but I can't quite make out the words.

Then, without warning, an ill-tempered shriek erupts, "Do NOT raise your voice at me!"

No . . . No . . . she didn't just say that to my husband, who's put his life on hold for me! Ken says something in response but it's hard to discern.

Offering no consideration to our mismanaged situation, this impetuous creature then foully screeches, "GET OUT OF MY FACE!"

Now my Comanche blood is heightened and I'm on the warpath! I fling the door open, and realize I've yanked it from Ken's hand that was resting on the knob. I look from him to about four feet away, where I lock eyes on what appears, to my dismay, to be a soulless Native American imp! How can this woman be Native American? I'm thrown but only for a nanosecond. I walk past Ken and up to this beastly imp-worm and plant myself directly in front of her.

"Don't you dare speak to my husband like that! If you want to know what it's like to have someone *actually* in your *face* . . . HERE I AM!"

I stand locked in a stare down; her eyes, a black *emptiness*, a being without a soul. How can someone with this temperament, and clearly no compassion, be working in a facility such as this?

Breaking her stance, she raises her hand up IN MY FACE and spinelessly attempts to slither away though an open door. *How dare she do this!* Enraged I follow the pathetic creature into an office, where Patience, and I assume Mirage, are typing away on computers. Everything at this point has gone a little fuzzy. It takes all my willpower not to grab this cowardly imp by the neck and throw her across the room.

I'm feeling dizzy and no longer in pain—adrenaline has taken over and the room begins slowly spinning. Trailing close behind this soulless-imp-worm I, with no fear whatsoever, get within an inch of her face!

With clinched fists out comes my war cry. "You do NOT treat me or my husband this way!" Patience and Mirage are in disbelief, frozen in place with mouths gaping.

Up comes the imp's right hand, *again IN MY FACE*, and using my left hand—the side I had surgery on—I grab it and easily take it down.

"You have no idea how much I want to punch you right now!" It takes every ounce of my being to contain the seething rage.

The cowardly creature flinches and pulls away. Both Patience and Mirage are now half up out of their seats, not quite knowing what to do!

Patience finds her voice first. "What's going on?"

My eyes break from this spineless creature and I look to Patience. "Is this how you treat your patients? This is the *cruelest* thing I've ever experienced." Tears fill my eyes and I hear myself loudly recounting the steps I took, the phone calls with Deadra, all to ensure a meeting with the Mad Scientist.

I don't know who said it, but someone pointed to the creature. "That's Deadra."

Are you serious?! This is Deadra? Whom I've painstakingly attempted to form some sort of relationship with over the phone? This is the insipid voice that I finally got a snicker from yesterday?!

All eyes went to her as she incredulously said, "You never *asked* if the Mad Scientist was here."

Are you kidding me? This is her response? "You're right, I didn't ask that yesterday. I did *two weeks ago* when I called to reschedule the appointment."

With a lilt in her voice, as any selfish child has who gets caught in a lie, "No, you didn't."

My right hand slams down hard on Patience's desk and I explode. "I am a *fucking* CFO of a multimillion-dollar company. I'm methodical in EVERYTHING I do! How dare you insinuate otherwise?"

Then out of nowhere a dark, hefty, short-cropped, curly-haired woman enters wearing hot-pink and royal blue eye shadow. This menace of a woman, dressed in scrubs, steps in between me and the soulless-worm. "Back off and keep your hands off my staff!" she bellows, throwing her hefty weight around.

Are you fucking kidding me??? How did I become the villain here? And yet she continued in her repugnant manner. "We have people on their way to handle you!" She was actually saying this to *me*!

Ken wasn't absent from this explosive moment. He tried a few times to calm me down by gently reaching for me. However, each time he did, I'd turn to him with a raised index finger and, speaking through gritted teeth, countered, "Give me a moment here!" Knowing I was still in pain from the surgery, and not wanting to hurt me, he quickly abandoned his attempts.

Disgusted with this torturous persecution, I turn to leave but my exit's thwarted by two women blocking the doorway. I immediately recognize the Nightmare Navigator. Both women appear a bit fearful while cautiously attempting to assess the situation. Recognition slowly emerges within the Nightmare Navigator's eyes. Looking aghast, she uses a somewhat shaky voice and shudders, "Apryl . . . what's going on?"

Looking from the Nightmare Navigator to Ken, I give up, *broken*. Words of despair escape my lips. "I can't do this anymore." I attempt to find my way down the endless hall, back to the jail cell to collect my things, and leave this hell-hole of a place!

Ken trails behind with a shattered heart, attempting to console the fragments that are left of my sanity. The unknown woman calls to Ken, pointing to the door we came through earlier. Ken delicately grasps my arm and leads me back down the hall to where the imp-worm had slithered from, back into the wretched cell. Patience, Mirage, the Nightmare Navigator and the unknown woman all enter the jail cell too. Words of concern spew from their lips. Wildly, tears stream down my face.

"Can we at least get the results from Apryl's pathology report?" I hear Ken ask.

"Of course . . ." and Mirage quickly disappears to get the results.

"What happened?" Patience asked. Ken told of his encounter with the soulless creature.

Finding my voice again, I use the unknown woman as a human example. I put my hand in her face as Deadra did to me. "What's the first reaction you have to this? Move my hand from your face, right?!" All three women were mortified. I then asked, "Are you all that desensitized towards your patients? I mean, no disrespect, I know you're dealing with people who have cancer, and sadly, some don't make it, but how we were treated today is unconscionable!"

The unknown woman takes this moment to introduce herself. "I'm Storm, a nurse navigator . . ."

> *No longer hearing her words, I find myself standing in an empty room facing a worn-out dance floor. Unexpectedly an electrical thunk is heard and a shaft of light spews down from the ceiling. A woman with dark hair wearing a red dress is seen sitting on a chair. The light cascades down her body, threatening to reveal her innermost secrets. She stares down at the broken wooden floor beneath her. She remains unmoving, presumably broken herself.*
>
> *Forbidding seductive notes from a flamenco guitar waft through the air, drawing me deeper into her world. A yearning to let go engulfs my spirit, as my soul recognizes the music to an all too deranged movement. As if it were my own heartbeat, I feel the rhythm emerge from a*

> *shadowed guitarist as the heel of his hand beats heavily between notes upon his aging guitar.*
>
> *Captivated, I stand idly by and watch as this woman begins her ill-fated dance. Sadly, she appears to be worn down and ragged. I realize at this moment I am looking at myself.*

Muted voices can be heard. "Apryl, we are so very sorry for the treatment you received by Deadra. It is unacceptable what she did. The Mad Scientist will be *mortified* when he finds out tomorrow."

> *The words echo from afar, like water dripping deep within a dark dank cave. The voices have no beginning or end; they just bounce off the walls into muted nothingness. I'm spent and don't care anymore—about anything. I just stand here alone in a trance— hypnotized by . . . El Tango!*

As the Tango ensues another voice echoes within this hellhole, "What can we do to make things right?"

> *A faceless man, muscular in stature and full of strength, crosses the dance floor. Anger can be felt seething within his body as he grabs the arm I had surgery on, spinning me around. With no care or concern for me, he brutally ravages my body and wantonly pulls me towards him.*

"I don't know. I'm so disheartened . . ." and *blah, blah, blah* I hear myself sob.

> *The room begins spinning again, as tears once more fall and disappear into the broken, dried wood of the dance floor. Another man appears in this morbid Tango and I'm thrust into his arms.*

"Oh Ken . . . I'm so sorry!" Ken physically envelops me as I place my hands over my face and cry into his chest.

The second man lifts me into the air and spins around, then hurls me like a rag doll into the waiting arms of yet another beastly man. The music continues its chilling strain as this new evildoer maliciously twists and turns me at his whim, dipping me within an inch of the broken floor.

Sobbing, unable to contain my emotions, I utter, "I don't understand how anyone can treat someone so dispassionately."

Violently I'm winched from the tortuous dip and flung back into the arms of the first devil-dancer. "I would never treat anyone this way!" I say to the faceless brute.

The door opens to my cell. Mirage has returned with the news of Jorge. In a somewhat happy yet compassionate voice, she says, "Well . . . we have good news for you, your cancer level came back *LOW*!" Then using a little more excitement, because she saw my mind was still reeling, exclaimed, "Apryl, this is *GREAT NEWS!* It means if you did absolutely *nothing* from this day forward you have less than a 10 percent chance of Jorge returning!"

Yet the wretched Tango continues on the broken floor.
I'm now being flung from madman to madman.

Everything appears to be in slow motion as the words tumble through the air . . . *Jorge's level is Low*. All this waiting, and what should have been a celebration has turned into this?!

"How about if we get you in to see the Mad Scientist as his first appointment of the morning? Can you be here at 9:00?" someone asked.

Numbly I respond, "I don't know . . . okay, fine." I felt depleted and completely beaten down. These past months I worked so hard to be upbeat and happy. It seems no matter what you do in life that's positive, there's always someone waiting, lurking in the shadows, ready to crack you over the head in efforts to drag you down to their level.

Ken's as emotionally upset as I am. I notice his distress as he continuously raises his hand to the collar of his shirt to straighten it. It's a habit of his I'd seen before.

Patience looks anxiously to Ken. "You're not having a heart attack, are you?" We all let out broken chortles. "No, seriously. I trained as a cardiologist nurse and that's one of the signs I was taught to look for. Are you feeling okay, Ken?"

Grimly he responds, "Yes, I'm fine. I'm more concerned about Apryl. She's going to be in a lot of pain later. She's still healing from surgery and this was not a good thing to have happen to her." I felt a lump form in my throat . . . this man always puts others before him, looking out for those he loves.

Everyone then looked to me. "Are you okay?"

"Yes, I just want to go home but I need a moment to compose myself before I leave. And I refuse to pay for this appointment."

> *The Tango slows. One by one the devil-dancers brutally shove past me while exiting the dance floor, leaving me desolate, depleted and powerless to face this alternate world on my own. Back where this wretched Tango began—in the chair looking down at the broken wooden floor beneath me. The lights fade to black. The dance ends the same as it began.*

That's when I feel the soft caress of my husband's hand. I'm not alone! Everyone in the room appears to understand my request and begins to file out. As each one passes, they again apologize. Both Patience and the Nightmare Navigator give me a welcomed, yet painful hug.

After the door closes, I seat myself in a chair within the wretched cell. Deprived of the victory from several months of a forced Tango, tears again stream down my face while I attempt to gain control over this relentless display of torment. I glance in Ken's direction; he too has broken down. To be treated like this during a time when you're supposed to be *healing* is hideous and immoral!

Composing ourselves we quietly leave the jail cell. The soulless imp-worm is back at her desk, snickering repulsively with her cohorts. As we walk by her station I silently ask myself, *why and how could this have happened?*

In silence Ken and I ride the elevator down to the first floor. As we approach the doors to leave the building I look down. There on the carpet peacefully lays a gray and white feather. My mother was with us and witnessed this repulsive and disgusting debacle in its entirety. The glass doors release and numbly I walk through them.

"I know it hasn't sunk in yet, baby, but you just dodged the biggest bullet of your life! Let's go celebrate this victory!" Ken said, attempting to sound triumphant and change our mood.

"I don't know, Ken . . ."

"You don't have a choice; we're celebrating! I'm taking you out for a martini."

Finding our way to the end of the bar, we seat ourselves where we knew there wouldn't be many people. As we began sipping our first martini (yes, first) a beautiful woman walked in the room and sits one barstool away from me. Her presence is magnificent and her energy mesmerizing. After a few moments she's flanked by two friends, each emanating her own beauty and presence.

Not wanting to appear as if I'm gawking, I turn my chair and full attention to Ken. As if by magic, subtle soothing harmonies can be heard wafting in the air, beckoning me to enter their beautiful realm. Enchanting and alluring, each carefully placed note captivates my heart, stirring my soul. I can hardly believe my ears; these three *Angels* are joyfully humming rhythmic melodies together.

While my second beverage of the afternoon begins shaking in its icy container, I turn to the Angel seated next to me. "Excuse me, but before I have my second martini and am unable to speak intelligibly, I want to tell all three of you how lovely you are! I just love the energy you all exude!" I then proceed to share with the Angels why Ken and I are here celebrating. "My risk factor for another *Tango* came back *Low!*" Of course I leave the ill-fated debacle out of the re-telling.

My second martini is frostily placed within my grasp. As I reach for it, all three Angels pick up their glasses as well and begin toasting me. I watch as my drink sloshes on the counter in front of them. Not caring, they all laugh and join my revelry. At last, it's beginning to feel like the celebration I've so desperately longed for.

> *Snowflakes gracefully begin falling from heaven, blanketing the fears of what could have been—erasing them from my world and my future.*

The Angel sitting next to me turns my direction and begins singing the song "Wind Beneath my Wings." Resonating within my soul, tears once again begin to fall. Harmonies follow suit and, much sooner than I cared for, the song is over. A gift from my mother—*this was no happenstance!*

All three Angels then introduce themselves, each giving me a much needed hug and kiss. Later, after returning my attention back to Ken, I overhear them toasting the Angel that arrived first. "Happy Birthday!"

I quickly apologize for stealing her thunder. "Are you kidding me, honey . . . not at all!"

Before I could stop myself I hear myself say, "I'd love to sing 'Happy Birthday' to you," and proceeded to do so with a weakened and battle-torn voice.

"Thank you!" she said, and reciprocated with a sweet kiss on my lips followed by another hug. Since my head was still reeling from *El Tango*, I did not realize to whom I had just sung "Happy Birthday." Of course she was a famous singer. Truly these women are ANGELS!!!! I wonder if they'll ever know how they lifted my spirits this afternoon.

17

Black & White
Apryl Allen

I canceled the 9:00 meeting with the Mad Scientist on Friday the 13th. The thought of returning to that jail cell today after *El Tango* is sheer torment. Right now I should be reveling in the wonderful news of Jorge. Instead I'm literally spent, both physically and emotionally. I've phoned the Nightmare Navigator, only because the operator supposedly can't find any of the other three women we met with yesterday; she was my last choice.

When she picked up I inform her, "Instead of the appointment at your office I would rather speak to the Mad Scientist on the phone." This made perfect sense to me; he has the time set aside for me anyway.

"Okay, he could possibly do it after 2:00 but I need to verify this with the Mad Scientist and will get back with you around noon." *What happened to my 9:00 appointment? Screw it, I'm too drained to argue.*

Around 12:30 the phone rings. "The Mad Scientist will do his best to call you, but he's stacked with appointments today, and being that it's Yom Kippur he has to be home before sundown. So he may not get back with you until Monday."

Once again I feel dejected and tormented. If the Mad Scientist considers himself religious, what could be more virtuous than giving someone long-awaited news about a life-threatening disease. After all, he took the Hippocratic Oath, which requires a physician to swear he or she will uphold a number of professional and ethical standards. One specifically emphasizes "... *warmth, sympathy and understanding* ..." I guess it's easier to turn a deaf ear and blind eye to a horrid situation. All I'm asking for is peace of mind. Sadly, this seems to be the norm for most people—me first, then you.

As I lay despondently on the couch I keep replaying yesterday over and over in my mind. Then I begin wondering, "What does *Low Risk* actually mean?" Does it mean a lesser form of chemo, a pill, or no chemo at all? What about the stage of my cancer? I was supposed to learn *all* of the results from my pathology report yesterday. But the only information I was given is that Jorge is *Low Risk*.

Feeling I can't make it another day without knowing the particulars, I phone Ken. "I guess I get to wait until Monday to learn about all the details of Jorge."

"What? Why?" Ken's concern is once again heightened.

"Because when I spoke with the Nightmare Navigator she said the Mad Scientist is leaving early because it's a Jewish holiday this weekend and probably won't have time to call today because of his busy schedule." I felt like a child whining to her parent.

"Text me the Mad Scientist's phone number," was all he said. Moments after texting him, Ken phoned back, "You *will* receive a phone call from the Mad Scientist today before 5:00."

After we hung up my phone began ringing. Concerned friends were inquiring of my test results. After hearing of the debacle they offer the only thing they can—more loving support. My mom must be hard at work in efforts to find my smile, although I didn't know it because I was a blubbering train wreck.

The phone rang one last time; it was Clíona. "You don't have a choice. I'm stopping by to say hello in an hour." Without giving me the opportunity to decline, she ended the call.

I really don't want any visitors. What I want is to sulk in self-pity and drown myself in my sorrows with no interruptions—something I've purposefully abstained from since the news of Jorge.

But isn't it interesting how life is? Everything is cyclical. It starts at a particular point and ends almost in the same exact place. The news of Jorge all began while I was with Clíona, and now here she is by my side when the phone rings its urgent peal at 3:45 . . . it's the Mad Scientist calling.

"Okay, Apryl, BIG breath and let it out . . . I'm here with you! And don't bring up what happened with his assistant. We're only interested in Jorge!" *God . . . she has no idea how powerful those words are to me and the fact that she's here with me at this very moment in time . . . how can this be?* Truthfully, I don't think I could have taken this phone call alone.

I do exactly as she suggests . . . I take a deep breath in and let it out, then answer the phone. "Hello?" My voice sounds depleted.

Using an insipid, forlorn and nasal tone, the Mad Scientist is barely audible in his reply. "Hello." Dead air . . . absolutely *nothing! And I wait . . . still nothing. What kind of game is he playing?*

"Hi, Mad Scientist, how are you?" I ask, breaking the muted silence. *This is no game—this is my life! And this is whom I've entrusted my future with—not to mention my well-being?!*

"I'm good and you?" his heart wasn't in the question. He could care less.

"Faring well, thank you," I reply.

"What can I do for you?" he asks with an indignant tone. *What can you do for me? Is he serious?*

"Well . . ." I attempt to swallow over a lump that has formed in my throat. "I was given the news yesterday I'm at *Low Risk*, but I know there are other parts to the diagnosis. For instance, can you tell me what stage Jorge was?"

His response is unnervingly slow . . . almost as if he's bored. It's evident by his demeanor that he doesn't want to be speaking to me. "Jorge is Stage 2. I'll let you Google its definition yourself." *He'll let me Google it . . . fantastic. How much am I paying this man?*

"Okay . . ." I scribbled *Stage 2* on a piece of paper as Clíona attempts to decipher it.

"You're ER and PR Positive, which means your body will react to hormonal therapy, meaning you *may* not need traditional chemo. But I want to verify this with a fellow oncologist before I say for certain."

I felt my breath catch from within and asked again, just to verify I heard him correctly, "So I may not need to have chemo?" Clíona, standing next to me, does a quick little jig.

I don't know if it was because he could hear my distress from the past months melt away over the phone, or the fact he was pleased I didn't take him to task about the soulless imp-worm. All I can say is he finally came to life. The jovial voice of my Mad Scientist, the one I've entrusted my life to, the one I knew from his office, finally resurfaced.

He proceeds to give me all the information I've so desperately been awaiting. "You're considered Low Risk Luminal A. If you had been B you would have required chemo—but I'll explain that in more depth when I see you again. When's your next appointment with me?"

"I don't have one."

"Okay, I'll have *Ramona* call you to schedule it. Who's your radiation oncologist?" *God—do doctors not remember anything about their patients? Shouldn't they have tickler notes or something in their files to remind them what's been discussed?*

"Who you referred me to—The Radiation Man," I remind him.

"Okay, you need to get an appointment scheduled with him as well."

"All right. Thank you for your time; I greatly appreciate it. And have a good holiday weekend." *I can't help but be myself.*

"Thank you ... goodbye." When the phone clicked off I took in a huge breath while using the kitchen counter for support, since my legs are wobbly from all this anxiety.

Before my raw emotions had the opportunity to seize the moment, hurling me back into the mind-numbing months that preceded it, Clíona averts my attention. She unexpectedly breaks into an animated Irish jig, tapping her toes and kicking her heels, attempting to recreate an unpracticed *River Dance!* She then starts singing notes we all sang as little children with no rhyme or reason, no definitive tune other than the thrill of life and pride in being part of this spectacular moment in time!

After the fascinating display of joy and elation, Clíona then proceeds to wrap her arms around me, squeezing me as if I've just won the lottery! Exuberant laughter and hugs are exchanged, followed by numerous, numerous kisses all over my face! I'm sure our several high fives could be heard echoing throughout our community! She's MAGNIFICENT to be with when receiving news such as this! Honestly, in all my life, I don't think I've ever had another woman offer such a beautiful display of emotion towards me.

She then exclaims, reflecting back, "And to think we were together in the beginning when you received your diagnosis and now we're together again when you received your results!" WOW ... *isn't life amazingly stunning?!*

After Clíona left, returning to her world, I phoned Ken with the wonderful news. "I'll be home shortly, honey ... I can't tell you how relieved I am to hear this news." Then his voice cracked. "I love you!"

Only because I'm too tired from stress and having been up all night until 4:00 this morning, I'm now ready to celebrate the grand news—*tomorrow!* Okay, maybe a little tonight with my husband!!!

Retreating to our living room, I peer through our picturesque window—out into a world filled with *life*! I thank every form of life around me. I thank my beautiful husband. I thank my friends. I thank the Inquisitive Minds. I thank my mother, my father, and my ancestors. I thank the Universe and God! I am so very thankful . . . to be *me*!

Coming down from the wonderful high, I sit and contemplate what my future now holds. I'm not sure if I want to continue with the Mad Scientist; after all, Deadra is his assistant. She can make my life extremely difficult from this point forward if she so chooses. Not to mention she has full access to all my personal information. The Nightmare Navigator assured me the debacle would be addressed with the Mad Scientist. The only outcome I feel would be appropriate is to fire Deadra.

I find myself drifting back to our initial consultation with the Mad Scientist, when he asked my nationality and I proudly responded *"I'm Comanche."* It was then, with a chuckle, he told us he had a difficult hot-headed Native American working for him. What he neglected to tell us was that *she* was his assistant.

When Ken returned home, after greeting Maddy and Hugo first, of course, he gives me the most beautiful hug and kiss. "I love you. I am so thrilled to hear that more than likely you will not require chemo. I can't even begin to tell you what a huge relief it is," he said, kissing me again. Releasing our embrace, he inquires, "So did the Mad Scientist apologize?"

"No," I reply glumly.

"After all that and he didn't apologize?" Ken's beside himself.

Questions consumed our conversations throughout the evening— WOW . . . *He didn't apologize?! Why didn't he? What about Patience's comment, "When the Mad Scientist hears about this he'll be mortified?" What about the Hippocratic Oath?*

In the end, Ken and I surmised this obviously wasn't the first time Deadra has done this. Primarily due to everyone's reaction in the end to the debacle, she knew she could get away with it. It's only apparent to us, unless she's fired, she'll continue with her evil doings. I hope the Mad Scientist realizes this and takes appropriate action. No one—*and I mean no one*— should *ever* be subjected to what we were! No matter your state of health.

In the end, we decided to keep the next appointment with the Mad Scientist only because we want to hear his thoughts on treatment. If he doesn't address the debacle personally with us at that time we'll more than likely leave his office, never to return.

Besides the scars from surgery I now have emotional ones, ironically from the people who are supposed to help me heal. They say it's *"The Fight Against Cancer,"* but there is no *fight*. I did nothing more than everything I was told to do. *Fighting* cancer is purely an effort to rid it from your body — and mind. Finding the *cure* and *healing* is what we as people should aspire to. Sadly, looking back, I find the *fight* is with our healthcare system: doctors, their office staff, the facilities, insurance . . . and the list goes on. Let me say it once more — healthcare and those involved in any aspect of it are expected to promote *healing*!

The next morning the news of Jorge is still reverberating throughout every fiber of my being. I review the detailed list I created about Jorge after my phone call with the Mad Scientist. I was disgusted over the fact I had to research a few of them on my own. Opening my laptop, I begin scouring the various cancer websites and took down the following notes:

- **Low Risk** – *means I have a 10% or less chance of recurrence if I did absolutely nothing for the next 10 years.*
- **Grade 2** – *a tumor grade is a way of classifying tumors based on certain features of their cells. The tumor grade is directly linked to prognosis. Using a microscope, a pathologist studies the tumor tissue removed during a biopsy to check: 1) How much the cancer cells look like normal cells (the more the cancer cells look like normal cells, the lower the tumor grade tends to be) and 2) How many of the cancer cells are in the process of dividing (the fewer cancer cells that are in the process of dividing, the more likely it is that the tumor is slow-growing, and the lower the tumor grade tends to be). Together, these two factors determine the tumor grade.*

These grades are usually classified as:
- *Grade 1: The tumor cells look the most like normal tissue and are slow-growing (well-differentiated).*
- *Grade 2: The tumor cells fall somewhere in between grade 1 and grade 3 (moderately-differentiated).*
- *Grade 3: The tumor cells look very abnormal and are fast-growing (poorly-differentiated).*

- **Stage 2 AT** (*stage 1 and 2 breast cancer is often called early breast cancer*):
  - *Stage 2A: The cancer is smaller than 2cm and has spread to the lymph nodes in the armpit OR is bigger than 2cm and has not spread to the lymph nodes OR it can't be found in the breast but is in the lymph nodes.*
  - *Stage 2B: The cancer is smaller than 5cm and has spread to the lymph nodes in the armpit OR is bigger than 5cm but has not spread to the lymph nodes.*
- **ER and PR Positive** *which means my receptor status will respond to hormonal therapy.*
- **Luminal A Molecular Subtype** *(had it been Luminal B, I would have required chemo). "Researchers are studying how molecular subtypes of breast cancer may be useful in planning treatment and developing new therapies," one of the websites indicated. Another stipulated, "Most studies divide breast cancer into four major molecular subtypes. At this time, molecular subtypes are used mostly in research settings. Prognosis and treatment decisions are still guided by tumor stage, and tumor characteristics."*

Once again I find myself waiting for the Mad Scientist, this time to confirm his interpretation next week with a fellow oncologist. One reasoning is there are smaller subtypes within Luminal A that respond differently to various therapies. The other reason, he wants to corroborate his rationale because I'm so young. Ultimately, he feels confident my protocol will be radiation followed by hormonal therapy via a pill I will take daily for the next 10 years.

The only downside to all this is I'm still reeling over how I received this news. It came with a horrendous moment and at a huge expense to me both emotionally and physically. The range of motion in my left arm went from 80 percent and feeling good, down to 45 percent and in a lot of pain. Although it had been two weeks since my surgery, I can definitely say I lost one week's worth of healing as a result of the debacle.

Throughout the rest of the weekend I find myself constantly pondering *El Tango*, wondering how and why it happened. It's now on a continuous loop in my mind, incessantly playing over, and over.

"Apryl, you need to stop," Ken said, interrupting my spiraling thoughts.

"Honey ... I just don't understand why it happened. How can people be so cruel? Do they not understand the mental anguish I'm already going through?"

Ken chuckled to himself, "You seem to think life is black and white and there's an answer for everything. But there's not. Instead of looking for the answer to how and why, think about the fact that you just dodged a bullet. What could have been an unbearable experience has just been lessened. You continue to get good news. Focus on *that* instead. Now is your time for healing. Please sweetheart, concentrate your energies on healing!" Ken pleaded.

I realize it isn't just me affected by *El Tango*; Ken has been too. It's killing him to see me in such agony. It takes everything in me to turn the never-ending loop off. I catch myself watching it, more precisely reliving it occasionally, and have to force myself to focus on the good news that eventually followed.

Ultimately the debacle faded and was replaced by the Inquisitive Minds and their part in my healing process. I truly believe with all my heart the reason I continue to receive good news about Jorge is because of them! They kept me in their prayers, thoughts and hearts, and some of them even enlisted leagues of people within their place of worship. *I'm in awe!* Though I do not consider myself a religious person, I do consider myself spiritual. Unequivocally, without any doubt whatsoever, I believe the reason I have been spared from what could have been a very different outcome is clearly because of the Inquisitive Minds. I was and continue to be protected!

The Mad Scientist phoned unexpectedly. Luckily for me, I've been living by my phone in anticipation of any and all news pertaining to Jorge and the Lymph-Along-Kid.

"Hi, Apryl, this is Ramona from the Mad Scientist's office. He would like to speak with you if you have a moment."

"Yes, I'm available."

"Hello, Apryl . . ." he began, sounding a bit more animated than the deadpan voice he used during the previous phone call. "As we discussed last week I gave the results of your pathology report to two fellow oncologists, who separately researched the same information. Due to your *one* lymph node involvement, we all came to the same conclusion. You will *not* require chemo! Instead we'll put you on hormonal therapy; a pill you'll be taking once a day."

"That's fantastic news and a HUGE relief. Thank you. What's the name of the drug I'll be taking?" I wanted to know so I could research it.

"Tamoxifen." I asked him to spell it.

"Have you scheduled your appointment with the Radiation Man yet?"

"Yes, I'll be seeing him on Thursday."

"Good. I'll get with him and inform him of our findings. In the meantime, let me get Ramona back on the phone to schedule our next appointment." When I finished the call we had scheduled it for Friday, September 19th. I couldn't help but wonder if the Imp-Worm was still working there, but quickly ushered the thought from my mind. I had more important things requiring my full attention than that dismal creature. After pouring myself a tall glass of sparkling water, I begin my research on the drug called Tamoxifen . . .

18
Nowhere to Run
Michael McDonald

The phone peals unexpectedly. The voice on the other end of the line claims she's the patient benefits representative for the Radiation Man. From her title, it sounds as if she represents the patient but, in fact, she wants to discuss an invoice related to my PET/CT scan that ACME Insurance hasn't paid. It didn't take long for me to surmise she's in accounts receivables; more than likely my deductible hasn't been met and she wants to collect the payment. *And to think, Ken and I are attempting to digest everything that's happening to our world, yet bills do not wait!*

"I'd like to verify what payments have been made towards my medical bills first. If indeed my deductible has not been met, I'll pay it when I come in on Thursday." *Note to self: Time to review my medical bills.* I've been attempting to ignore the mounting pile of papers but I knew the time would come when I had to face them. I find them to be daunting, and worse, the majority of them remain *unopened*.

"Fine. Just to let you know, there's another outstanding bill from the Mad Scientist's office as well. Your insurance company has informed us it will cover your blood work, but not the blood draws."

"Really?! So how do they propose we get blood out of me?" A logical question, I thought.

"Exactly; we don't have an answer for that one yet. Also, I noticed you were given a $45 co-pay credit and wasn't quite sure why. Do you know what it's for?"

"Yes." I knew *exactly* what it was for—*El Tango! So they did credit me for that appointment*, I silently thought to myself, *or was it just the co-pay?* Not wanting to relive the debacle, I inevitably found myself recounting the appointment with her in brief.

"I can't believe that happened!" she exclaimed. Then, using the exact same words Patience, Mirage, Storm and the Nightmare Navigator did, "The Mad Scientist is going to be mortified when he hears what happened."

"That's what I thought too, but he has a funny way of showing mortification since he didn't offer an apology during our two recent phone calls."

"He will . . . I'm sure of it." I believed her. He probably just wants to do it in person.

"So that's what the credit is for."

"Do you want me to apply the credit to any of these invoices?" She was attempting to sound helpful but I knew it was really about collecting money.

"Let me verify my records first and I'll let you know on Thursday." She seemed pleased with that suggestion.

After we hung up, I went back to researching Tamoxifen. Satisfying my curiosity, I had compiled a list of questions in my Book of Life for the Mad Scientist. And then the inevitable—I turned all my attention to the pile of medical bills that seemed ready to topple.

Sifting through the unopened envelopes, I start by creating two piles: one for medical bills and another for insurance. I found the majority of the envelopes to be from ACME Insurance and decided to start there. After opening them I find they primarily consist of EOBs. The terminology "EOB" is often used in lieu of *Explanation of Benefits*; these statements are sent from your insurance provider. They basically detail the breakdown of what will and will not be covered.

As for the medical bills, it was minutia in comparison to the EOBs received, only four in total. While reviewing the EOBs, I'm taken aback, I didn't realize how many people were involved with my Tango, and I have yet to receive their bills. Without their invoices, going solely off the EOBs will be difficult as they're based primarily on codes, and I'm not familiar with the medical jargon. Then I remembered an Excel spreadsheet I had cleverly concocted from a past surgery and decided to implement the matrix in an attempt to reconcile what's been billed, what's been paid for by insurance and ultimately, what I owe.

Among the four unopened medical bills is a purple envelope from the Medicine Woman. I knew this was the report I had requested from

Mabel summarizing my surgery. Might as well open it and start a file for these reports too. However, when I picked up the purple envelope it was extremely light. *That's odd. I'd have thought the report would have been several pages*, I mused.

Clasping my letter opener in one hand and the envelope in the other, I slit it open. As I unfold the single sheet of paper that's the sole content of the envelope, I stand aghast. Within the purple casing dated September 9th—thrown haphazardly into my pile of bills—is a one-page report from a company called Agendia, detailing Jorge.

My heart sank deep into my belly. If I had only been prudent and opened all of these envelopes as they came in and organized them like I usually do, I would have known what my future held! And *El Tango* . . . it probably wouldn't have happened. At least I wouldn't have been so out of my mind. *Oh dear God . . . how could I have done this?*

After the initial shock was over, I continued to organize the rest of the paperwork. However, it was extremely difficult since I hadn't received the majority of invoices from my doctors or the medical facilities to compare against the EOBs. I did attempt to decipher the EOBs and found if it had a date that coincided with an appointment in my calendar I could deduce what it was for, but if not . . . let's just say it was inordinately frustrating.

I then attempted to enter the EOBs into the Excel spreadsheet, but gave up on that idea too and decided to finish it after I've received *all* of the invoices. Once I have everything it'll be easier to reconcile.

In the end I entered into the spreadsheet whatever payments I had personally made to date, and matched them to the few invoices I had received. I then found their matching counterparts in the mound of EOBs. Once finished I determined my deductible had not yet been met and I did owe the $500 plus balance due for the PET/CT scan.

Afterwards, I returned to Agendia's report and picked up the phone, dialing Ken's office number. "You won't believe what I just found . . ."

My appointment was scheduled for 4:30 Thursday afternoon with the Radiation Man. However, I received a phone call from Nina, his medical assistant, that morning inquiring if it could be moved up to 3:15.

"We want to get your alignment set up on the radiation machine for your upcoming treatments and all the techs leave at 4:00. Can you possibly come earlier?"

"Let me check with my husband. I think we can, although we may be a few minutes late."

"That won't be a problem," she assured me.

Once again Ken found himself rearranging his schedule and we arrive at 3:20. The receptionist at the front desk with the beautiful smile greets us as I sign in.

"Our patient benefit rep has asked to see you first," we were told. Boy, they don't mess around with the bills. I thought I'd see her *after* the appointment. Oh well, what did it matter, I needed to pay and might as well get it over with.

This office is completely different from upstairs where I had appointments with the Mad Scientist. It's not the architecture or interiors that's different, but rather the attitude of the people. Everyone here is actually *happy* and they make me feel like a *person* when I walk in the door, not someone in the middle of a *Tango*.

After greeting the patient benefit rep I inform her that I haven't met my deductible. As I hand her my credit card, she asked, "So how are you doing since *El Tango?*"

"I'm back to 70 percent range of motion in my left arm and am feeling more like my old self again!"

"I'm sure happy to hear that. When are you scheduled to see the Mad Scientist again?" she inquired.

"Tomorrow afternoon . . ."

"Well, I'm sure he's addressed the situation and everything will go smoothly from this point forward so don't give it a second thought." I agreed, but silently thought to myself, *it sure would have been nice if he had offered some sort of apology during our phone conversations.*

A cheerful voice greeted me from behind; it was Nina. Leading us down the hallway into an examining room, she proceeded with taking my vitals. "Everything is well within the normal range," she informed me, smiling as she removed all the gadgets.

Mimi, the nurse practitioner, arrived and we chatted while Nina finished logging my vitals into the computer. After she left, Mimi explained what the protocol would be and what I could anticipate from my upcoming radiation treatments. "Today we're going to be taking measurements to align you on the machine."

It was around this time the Radiation Man walked in. Joining in the conversation he explained what my treatments would consist of and reiterated what Mimi told us regarding potential side effects.

"For this procedure, you'll be lying on your back and the radiation waves will be aimed horizontally across your body." Interestingly, he also tells us, as many doctors have in the past, "Of course, nothing is definitive; all treatments and side effects are different for everyone."

"Can you please explain *exactly* what the treatments will consist of?" I didn't want any surprises. Lord knows I've had my share of them.

"Sure," the Radiation Man complied. "Radiation beams will be emitted through your left breast horizontally as you lay on your back, skimming your chest cavity. Because you'll be on your back, it should not hit any vital organs, such as your lungs or heart." *God forbid!* "However, there's always a chance it could as nothing is 100 percent guaranteed. These treatments will be five days a week and will last for approximately five to five and a half weeks. At the end of this period, we'll be adding an additional week focused at the front of your underarm, where the Lymph-Along-Kid was, to irradiate that area as well."

Mimi then handed the Radiation Man a couple sheets of paper. "These two pages are identical; they're a list of the potential side effects that could possibly occur from radiation treatments. We'll need you to sign both, one for your records and the other for ours." It was a form they not only wanted, but *expected* me to sign prior to treatment, releasing them from any and all liabilities.

How safe are these treatments? I thought to myself as Ken and I quickly perused the list. Then we noticed an asterisk on one of the rare side effects—*Death!* As if reading my mind, the Radiation Man interjected, "The asterisked side effect has never occurred in all my years of practice."

Whew! "Believe me . . . I won't be your first!" I informed him.

Now, I had planned on bragging to all of my friends how I don't have tattoos; instead, I have three endearing new scars: The removal of Jorge, the removal of the Lymph-Along-Kid and one I hadn't anticipated, a scar from the drain. The drain was placed just below my underarm and is exactly where the circumference of my bra wraps around me.

But then I was told by Mimi—*drum roll please*—"You're going to be tattooed."

"What?!" Yep . . . that's right, I heard her correctly.

"No, we don't do hearts, stars or smiley faces. These tattoos will look like, shall we say . . . freckles." She smiled coyly and continued with the explanation. "This will enable us to align the machine perfectly each time you come in for radiation treatments."

"Wow . . . Really?!" This was the last thing I expected.

"Do you have religious beliefs that requires you forgo them?" she inquired, obviously reading the concern on my face.

"No. I just didn't realize I'd be getting tattooed." *Gulp.*

"Yes, they'll be three of them." Again a placid smile. And then, as if she had just informed me what the weather was going to be, she continued with, "Also, during these treatments, please do not wear deodorant or put lotions on prior to the appointment," completely diverting my attention from any questions or concerns I had about the tattoos.

"I can wear deodorant during this period, right?" *Argh . . . I'd hate to lose any friends.*

The Radiation Man interjected, "Afterwards you're welcome to, but you may be tender and it could cause some irritation. It's basically up to you."

Mimi then reached into a cabinet and placed my favorite style of gown on the table. "Please undress from the waist up and change into this gown with the opening in the front. Benny will be in shortly for your alignment."

"The same Benny who did my PET/CT scan?" I inquired.

"Yes," and she stepped out the door, closing it behind her.

"Oh, good, Benny! He's the happy young man who made me feel extremely comfortable during my PET/CT scan," I reminded Ken.

Benny arrived with his smiling face and charming personality. This time Ken stayed behind in the examining room as he was anxious to answer some very important e-mails. Benny offered to leave the door open so he wouldn't feel confined to the room.

As I followed Benny down the hall, he explained, "We use the same PET/CT scan machine to align your treatments. We'll then perform a quick scan of your upper region for the Radiation Man to confirm we have you positioned correctly." Arriving at the VLM, "Apryl, you remember Thomas? He'll be one of three techs you'll be seeing during your radiation treatments." Since I know I'll be nervous for all my appointments, it was reassuring, because Thomas is as pleasant and comforting as Benny.

Remember how I said the bed for the PET/CT scan machine was comfortable? Well, this time it wasn't. Yes, the triangular pillow was placed under my knees, but there were no other comfy cushions. Instead, in place of the pillow was a deep blue 2 x 3-foot inflated air cushion. Once on board, I felt as if I were laying on a hard table or countertop. Underneath the air cushion was a half cylinder-type holder that would keep both my head and neck straight, at the same time ensuring my head was maintained at a certain level.

Thomas instructed, "Place your arms above your head on the cushion." Once I did he added, "Make sure you're comfortable. You'll be in this position for 10 to 15 minutes each time you come for treatments." Luckily for me my arms didn't need to be straight. I'm still in a bit of pain from the surgery.

He then began to open my gown. "Please be careful ... my left nipple is *extremely* sensitive," I cautioned, not knowing exactly what he would be doing. "I can barely stand to have shower water touch it." With sympathetic eyes he proceeded mindfully.

"Are you in a comfortable position?" he asked, confirming I was indeed relaxed.

"Yes."

"Okay, turn your head slightly to the right and lift your chin a bit." He then began to release the air out of the pillow. "You're going to feel the pillow flatten out as I remove the air. This will leave an imprint of exactly how you're lying on the machine."

Lasers were then projected onto me while Benny stood off to my left taking photos. Using the lasers, they pinpointed three separate locations for aligning the machine. They then marked me with an "X" using a black Sharpie pen at each spot the lasers pointed at. Where the beams were coming from exactly, I haven't a clue. They then covered the newly marked Xs with clear half-inch circular stickers. The first "X marks the spot" is located on my left breast between the 9 and 10 o'clock position, if you were facing me. The other two are both mid-range on the left and right sides of my rib cage, the left being a half inch higher and a little more forward than the right.

"These are where the tattoos will be placed. When you shower don't scrub this area. If a sticker falls off, try to put it back on; you shouldn't have any problems with them," Thomas informed me.

Benny then asked something, but I can't remember what, because when I looked at him to answer, he quickly chided, "Don't move! You need to keep your head and arms in the exact position we've placed you." Abandoning his question, he continued, "We're now going to do a short scan of your upper body." As I had done before, I closed my eyes, primarily because I felt a twinge of claustrophobia setting in. And just as he said, the scan was maybe three minutes start to finish. *Thank heavens!*

Then it was over. They both greeted me as the bed slid out from within the scanner. Knowing I was still sore from surgery, they gently helped me sit up. Thomas again reminded me, "Please don't take the stickers off; we'll do that at the time we mark you with tattoos."

"What does the radiation machine look like?" I had to know. I'm at the point my imagination is running amok and I can't take anymore *"just wait to find out"* scenarios.

"We'll take you on a quick tour if you'd like," Benny eagerly offered. "While you're changing we'll make sure no one's in the room. I'll come and get you in a moment."

After I changed, Benny escorted Ken and I back down the hall, where we joined Thomas and started the tour. "When you arrive for each appointment you'll sign in. After your name is called you'll then come to this changing room and place a gown on with the opening in the *back* so it can be easily removed during your procedure. You'll place all your personal items in one of these lockers and hold on to the key."

We then proceeded down the hall to the infamous room containing another VLM. It too was quite futuristic looking with cameras inside, no windows and a large thick door. The door reminded me of something you'd see in a recording studio, except this one is marked with hazard signs.

Stepping out of the treatment room, Thomas indicated "During your treatments the techs will sit here." The desk was about eight feet from the ominous door and the chairs faced in the opposite direction. "They'll be monitoring you from these four computers. During treatments, should you need anything, just ask out loud as there are microphones in the room. All we ask, no matter what, is don't move from your position. We can respond back via the speakers in the room." Hmmm . . . sounding more and more like a recording studio—I sure wish it was. "Oh, and music will be playing in the room too."

Thanking them for the tour Ken and I left, with me feeling much more at ease. Now the only question that remains is what will the treatments *feel* like?

The next time I'm here in this office I will be permanently marked. Not quite how I envisioned my first tattoo, that is, if I ever wanted one. On the upside of things, I'll be finished with radiation treatments just in time for the holidays! Ho, ho, ho!!! What a crazy unexpected ride this has been!

A friend of mine invited me for lunch one afternoon. I learned some very interesting facts from her that I think we can all benefit from. Her brother is the doctor who researched and linked deficiencies in Vitamin D3 as being a contributing factor for breast and colon cancer. But before I go on, I'd like to give you a little background about my life since 2010.

2010 and 2011 had been HIGHLY stressful years for me. Not only had the economy gone bust, but our administrative staff turned over, leaving me as the sole party to hire and train new personnel.

On the upside of things, my album *Shape Shifter* was nominated for four NAMMYs, winning the Best Pop category and, adding to the excitement, qualified for seven GRAMMYs! I was also in the middle of writing a Latin-American album with a classical flamenco guitarist from San Miguel de Allende, Mexico. This same year I was asked to sing with the Phoenix Symphony. After my performance, I was approached by two individuals wanting to know if I knew of anyone that could write a Native American Musical. My response: *"Yes . . . me!"* So during this year, I was in the middle of research for this project too. All of which were placed on an indefinite hold until I could get our office realigned. To say I was stressed is an understatement.

Another friend commented how she couldn't believe I could juggle so many projects. Although she did warn me, *"Be careful . . . you look really stressed and that's not good for your body."* Then one morning I awoke with the most excruciating sore throat I think I've ever had. I pleaded with Ken, *"Please call Dr. KnowItAll."* Then realizing it was Sunday, *"Maybe we* should go to the ER or one of those urgent care centers. I've never felt this horrible before!"

Ken decided to try Dr. KnowItAll first, and left a message with his after-hours answering service. I don't recall ever contacting Dr. KnowItAll after hours; did he even have an answering service? To our surprise—more so mine—he returned our call and told Ken he would phone in whatever it is he recommends when you have the flu. I took the prescription faithfully.

However, after the required seven days of taking it, I didn't feel any better. So I called Dr. KnowItAll's office and was told I needed to come in for an appointment. I would have preferred not to leave the house and wasn't feeling well enough to drive. So Ken drove me.

During the appointment Dr. KnowItAll drew blood and checked for Valley Fever, the Nile Virus and whatever else he thought I could possibly have come down with. They all came back negative. *"You just have the flu and need to let it run its course"* he gave as a prognosis. So I waited.

After being on and off sick for almost a year, a friend said, *"It sounds like your immune system is run down. Try taking some vitamin C."* Why not, I've tried everything else. After one day of vitamin C I felt so much better. I thanked my friend for her recommendation, wherein she suggested I find a good naturopath.

After doing so, the naturopath found I was considerably deficient in Vitamin D and was testing positive for the Epstein-Barr virus. *"It appears you recently had mono and it's not clearing your system."* How did I get mono?!

Armed with this new information, she placed me—and another not so willing participant, Ken—on a vitamin regime. Going from nothing to taking I don't remember how many pills is painstakingly . . . well, painful. It's like counting calories or points on a diet. Who wants to do that? I even acquiesced to vitamin IVs (and you know how I loathe needles), which I did three or four times for a period of about a month. Finally, I was out of the woods and back in the saddle of life.

Of course, Dr. KnowItAll in the past preached he'd read an article about deficiencies in Vitamin D being a contributing factor to breast cancer. But if he believed this, then why didn't he run blood work to see if I was deficient in this area? *Absolutely* I would have taken it had I known this.

The reason I turned a deaf ear to the idea was because Dr. KnowItAll touted my mother's breast cancer as the reason I should be taking Vitamin D every day. Well . . . sadly, I didn't take it to heart, solely because my mom's Tango was from estrogen being administered to a woman for the first time when she was 77, causing all sorts of health issues for her.

Now I'm not saying my stress or deficiencies in vitamins are what led to my tango with Jorge. But I can't help but wonder if I'd been taking vitamins all along would I have attracted him? Now back to my friend's brother . . .

After lunch, I went home and researched her brother's background. I read a few articles and, more specifically, read an interview in which he discussed our need and requirements for vitamins *and* minerals. When asked more specifically about them, he used the term micronutrients and explained that every person's needs are different.

Vitamin D3 is now a daily regimen of mine. In fact, testing for it is incredibly simple and your doctor can run this test during your annual exam. I'll be forever grateful to my friend for sharing this information with me. After I'm through all my treatments, I'll be revisiting what vitamins I specifically need to be taking for my health and future.

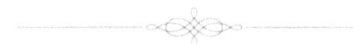

We arrived for our appointment with the Mad Scientist exactly on time. Nothing seemed to have changed, and I followed the normal protocol —sign in and pay co-pay, complete paperwork, wait for name to be called, head back for a two-vial blood draw, and wait in second waiting room with Ken for my name to be announced *again*.

Surprisingly our name is called by someone other than Ramona. This nameless face asks us to follow her to a jail cell. In doing so, we have to walk past the Imp-Worm's desk. I couldn't believe my eyes; there she sat with her back to us. *How is she still working here?* I could feel my Comanche blood start to simmer.

Once in the jail cell this new face, who didn't introduce herself, took my vitals. Only this time my blood pressure is a bit elevated . . . *hmmm, I wonder why!*

"The Mad Scientist will be with you shortly," was all she said to us prior to exiting the room. That's when Ken and I both take note as to the time on our watches . . . let the waiting begin.

While waiting, I became a little perturbed with Ken because I wanted to address *El Tango*. However, he insisted, "Do not go there. We need to focus on you right now." Once again, I find myself silencing my voice—*and the bad guy wins.*

Surprisingly, instead of the normal 40-minute wait, the Mad Scientist walked through the door within 10 minutes.

"You don't hate me do you?" he asked of me, then looked to Ken. *This is the first thing he asks after how I was treated?*

Unenthusiastically I respond, "No, I don't hate you."

After seating himself, he reiterated his findings. "As I said during our last phone conversation, you will not require chemotherapy. I've verified this with two of my fellow oncologists and they all concur that *no chemo is required!* So basically you got three opinions, *plus research,* for the price of one!" he added gleefully.

"That's really terrific news," Ken said, looking to me in an attempt to make amends for our previous conversation.

"That is great news . . ." I agreed matter-of-factly and opened my little green Book of Life. "I have several questions for you, a few specifically concerning the drug Tamoxifen . . ." I was in disbelief of its side effects. We've all heard the commercials for various drugs on television; this one is no different. *Why would anyone in their right mind agree to take this pill?*

When I was younger I attempted to go on birth control a few times. However, each time I did I became Jekyll and Hyde. My mood swings were off the chart and this was while taking the *lowest* form of birth control. As Ken can attest, I do not do well on drugs. If I get a headache, it has to be really horrible before I take something for it. I don't know why I'm this way; it could be because my mom did not push drugs on us. Instead she would comfort me with love or attempt to get my mind off of it by playing games or teaching me something new. It always appeared to work! Oh, back to the Mad Scientist . . .

My first question is, "Can we start radiation therapy on October 7th? Ken wants to take me away for five days prior to starting treatments."

"Where are you going?" the inquisitive jovial Mad Scientist was back in full form.

Being that I was a bit agitated with Ken from our private conversation I replied—*but please know I absolutely do not feel this way whatsoever*—"he's taking me to California where we got married and where we'll probably get our divorce!" I glared at Ken.

Ken just sat there deadpan and, well, the Mad Scientist didn't quite know what to say. His back was to me at the time, but I saw him and Ken exchange a look that translated to *I've got one of those at home too — they can be brutal! Sigh!!!*

"I don't have a problem with it, but you'll need to get the approval of the Radiation Man. Next question?" No one in the room was going to tread on my now staked out ground.

"I'm getting conflicting responses from doctors. The Radiation Man said I shouldn't have blood draws or blood pressure taken from the arm I had my lymph node dissection on because it could cause lymphedema. When I questioned the Medicine Woman about it, she informed me it was an old wives tale. What are your thoughts?"

"I'm going to defer to the Medicine Woman for that response." *Great . . . thanks — keep it noncommittal.* "Next?" he inquired.

"Speaking of the Medicine Woman . . . the stiches on my left breast are starting to poke through my skin. They're getting longer with each passing day and now they're starting to catch on my clothes." I opened the examining gown revealing my new scar.

"Let me take a look—" and he opens my gown completely. "Hmmm . . . they look fine," prodding them. He then said, "If they continue to be bothersome you may want to call the Medicine Woman."

While closing my frock I inquired, "When do you propose I start taking Tamoxifen?"

"After you've completed your radiation treatments." There was absolutely no hesitation or considerate thought before his response.

"Okay, but I noticed one of the potential side effects could be blood clots. My mother got them in her legs when she was put on estrogen and three of my siblings have deep vein thrombosis. If I have it, does that mean I'm unable to go on this particular drug?" *This is maddening. Why is he not catching these potential concerns? Did he even look at my family history form?*

I continued on with my findings. "Also, all of my brothers have heart problems, one of which is heart arrhythmia; my mother had this as well. And one of the more concerning side effects for me personally is mood swings. I truly don't want the next 10 years of mine and Ken's lives to end up being bouts with Jekyll and Hyde."

"As for the deep vein thrombosis, that is an issue. We'll need to have additional blood work done to see if you have it. When was your last period?"

Again ... do doctors not remember *anything* about their patients? "March of 2003 when I had my *hysterectomy*."

"That's great news. There are a couple of other pills I can put you on; however, they're for post-menopausal women ... but since you've had a hysterectomy you don't need to worry about it. Let's get you back to the lab for more blood work."

"What? More blood work? But they just did it ..."

"If you don't want to do it now, you can schedule another appointment and have it done at a later time."

Sigh ... "No, now is as fine a time as any. When will we get the results? Today?"

"No. It won't be until the end of next week."

"How will we learn of the results? Will you call me?" *God ... how I hate the waiting game.*

"No, but you can call the office at the end of the week and speak to Ramona about the results. And I'd like to see you again at the end of October." We then follow him out to the soulless Imp-Worm's desk. Thank goodness she wasn't there and we watch as he flounders, looking for someone to help him.

Out of nowhere a vampire materialized. "Is there something you need, Mad Scientist?"

"Yes, I need more blood work completed on Apryl. Here's her file." We said our goodbyes and once again I found myself sitting in one of my least favorite chairs. Another poke and *nine more vials later—I'm really getting tired of this.*

Relieved to have left that hell-hole of a place, I realized I neglected to write down the other two drugs the Mad Scientist proposed in lieu of Tamoxifen. So I phoned his office and asked the operator to put me through to Ramona, or whoever could give me the names of the drugs.

I was placed on hold for a brief moment and then was transferred to the person in charge of all prescriptions for the Mad Scientist. After consulting the Mad Scientist, the additional drugs he proposed were Arimidex and Femara. Of course I had to ask her to spell them. Why are names of drugs so difficult to pronounce, let alone spell? This would now become my number one priority for tomorrow—researching these additional two drugs.

Speaking of the next day, it was so strange ... those pokey stiches that morning had miraculously disappeared. It was so bizarre; one day they're hugely bothersome, then simply they're gone—*nothing*. To say the least, I was relieved, both that they were gone and I didn't need to schedule another doctor's appointment.

I started the next day with a cup of coffee, my laptop computer and Google. By around 2:00 in the afternoon I found the two new drugs the Mad Scientist was suggesting to be no better than Tamoxifen. And they all shared the same side effects, night sweats, mood swings and bone pain. Basically, these Jorge-fighting pills will put me into early menopause.

The more I thought about it I realized, *I'm at Low Risk with a less than 10 percent chance of having Jorge return. Does that mean in this particular breast? Or is it throughout my entire body?* Radiation would take my risk down by 35 percent, which would mean if I were at 10 percent—my pathology report states *"less than 10 percent"*—but let's just say I were at 10 percent, radiation treatments would take me down to 6.5 percent. *Okay, maybe radiation is worth it since it is a contaminated area.* Then after further delving into the Jorge-fighting drugs, statistics showed taking it would reduce my risk in *half*—that would bring it down to 3.25 percent.

What?! Is it worth it to take a drug to lower my risk by only 3 percent? I mean, if my risk was at 80 percent and taking it would bring my risk factor down to 40 percent, okay, how soon can I take my first pill? But I'm at 3 percent ... AND *there's no guarantee!*

From this point forward, my number one priority for my health will be my biannual ultrasounds and mammograms. I won't miss one! And *if*—this is a big *IF* because I'm absolutely confident my body is clear of any and all future Tangos—Jorge mysteriously returns, I know what to do and at that point will seriously contemplate the Double M.

Still more thinking and mulling what to do. Then the thought occurred, it's time to enlist the advice of my gynecologist. I'd like to get his take on this. He called me back around 5:30 that evening. I love my gynecologist; he sincerely cares and exudes compassion. He *listened* to everything I had to say just as if I were in his office.

I ended with the drugs the Mad Scientist felt I should go on, including Tamoxifen. My gynecologist explained, "The other drugs, Arimidex and Femara, can be used on pre-menopausal women. They're currently used to treat endometriosis, so you needn't worry about them. And of the three, I suggest you take Femara. The chief complaint I hear from women, besides the mood swings and night sweats, is they have pain during sex. The pain can be treated with vaginal estrogen, but it's *another* drug with *other* side effects. I'm sure it wouldn't be a problem to take it in conjunction with Femara, but we'd need to verify that with your Mad Scientist prior to prescribing."

He concluded with, "Apryl, what you're talking about is *quality of life*. If indeed it drops your risk only by 3 percent, I have to agree with you, the side effects aren't worth it. Please make sure this is the case, though. I also agree with you to go ahead with radiation, but I'd like you to research that as well prior to having those treatments. You did an inordinate amount of work to come to this conclusion and I feel confident you will do the same with radiation. If you need anything at all I'm here until the end of the week, then I'm going on vacation. Otherwise I return in mid-October."

"Thank you, Dr. Gyno. Unless I come across something by the end of the week I feel confident about what we've discussed. Besides, we have until the end of November to make a firm decision on hormonal therapy." After I hung up, I felt confident and content with the decision I made *not* to take the prescription drug.

That was until I called the Mad Scientist to confirm my assumption. "Yes, it's less than 10 percent but *only* in the current location. Jorge could come back *anywhere* in your body." *But doesn't everyone have this potential risk?*

"Okay, but unless you tell me I'm *absolutely* out of my mind I think I'll forego hormonal therapy."

"Apryl, you're *absolutely* out of your mind. If you were my sister you'd be taking it!" I wasn't expecting the Mad Scientist to sound so agitated.

"Seriously?!"

"Yes, you asked me to tell you and I am!" Now it was clear he was upset.

"Thank you, Mad Scientist, for your time. I'll see you at the end of October. Goodbye."

My heart's in turmoil—*I DON'T KNOW WHAT TO THINK or WHAT TO DO!!!* It's sheer torment. There's nowhere to run, let alone hide! I truly don't want to take these drugs and risk crazy side effects to my body, my mental health and most of all, wreak havoc on the love of my life and heart, Ken! The stress is horrifically maddening with no definitive black or white answer; instead, everything's gray! And the doctors. *"You have this, ergo, you do that even though there's no 100 percent guarantee of anything."*

I totally get why my beautiful mother, upon hearing her Tango had returned two years later, got up off the table and said, *"No . . . no more—I'm done."* I will find the silver lining though. I always do!

19

A Million Miles Away

Lenny Kravitz

Tattoos. I've never really contemplated having one. However, this week I will be permanently marked with three of them. I'm actually a little nervous about being *inked*, imagining what we've all seen on TV, and dare I say what many of you may have experienced; the oversized machine gun-type applicator which will leave a dot the size of a freckle. At least it will be small.

When I was initially told about this appointment I thought it was for tattoos only. How silly of me; of course they need to take a few X-rays. When I arrive they ask me to change into the lovely gown, with the opening in the back—a welcome change. Then Thomas and three twenty-something female techs escort me into the radiation room. I'm asked to lie on the table, where the inevitable will eventually happen—radiation treatments. That sounds so final . . . doesn't it?

Positioned at the head of the table is the blue foam form Thomas had previously molded to my upper body. I'm asked to climb aboard and take my position. They then proceed to remove the upper portion of my gown and lay it on my belly; I am now nude from the waist up—*argh!* They then ask me to place my arms in the mold so they can confirm my position is indeed correct. Without any warning, as if they've been told I have the plague, everyone suddenly takes two steps back. And the radiation machine comes to *life*.

Three or four round and square paddles swing around me as I lay horizontally on the table. The largest of the paddles is round and comes to a complete stop looming above me. Staring up at the paddle I can see my reflection in its glass plate. That's when I notice on my left breast a ruler of light can be seen on my skin. Using this ruler and red lasers, the techs align the black Xs to the machine.

Satisfied with the alignment, a tech began to remove the round stickers over the Xs. "Holy cow you're right, adhesive really does love you!" she said, confounded by its hold. Eventually she did get them off, but I have to admit, it was a little on the painful side. Especially on my left breast which seems to be on sensitivity overload!

To ease my apprehension of the inevitable she adds, "The tattoos are nothing compared to taking these stickers off." *Oh . . . I hope so!*

Now you might assume the elder of the group, Thomas, would be inking the tattoos. Nope, it was one of the young girls. *Oh my . . . I really hope she's had ample experience working the machine!* To my relief, and somewhat dismay—I mean, if I'm going to get a tattoo it should be worthy to talk about—she pulls out a small shot needle, if you can even call it that, pre-filled with black ink.

Starting with my right rib cage she begins . . . I feel nothing—*absolutely nothing!* Then to the 10 o'clock location on my left breast; this one, however, is on the tender side and interestingly, so is the left rib cage. But I felt nothing more than a quick pin prick. The tattooing was officially over.

Returning to the changing room I attempt to see what the tattoos look like in the mirror hanging on the wall. Initially all I see are red marks. *Is that a freckle, mole or is that the tattoo?! Nada . . . inconsequential!* Yippee, now I'm ready for radiation therapy. I'm as excited as a deflated ball attempting to bounce.

After leaving the facility, I feel a little dazed as I climb into my car and start the engine. The soft sweet notes of Amos Lee immediately fill my senses. I've finally made it to the last song on his album. Storm clouds can be seen brewing to the east as I start to drive. And as if they were speaking to my soul his lyrics drift from the speakers: *"Facing winds that break the strongest of chains . . . We all know that the storm is coming. Everybody wants to know which way to go . . ."* and I wonder . . . which way I will go?

I've been extremely lethargic since my surgery. Often, I find myself taking naps during the day—it's quite frustrating. It seems all I'm able to do is one or two minor activities; then, when I return home, I end up sleeping for a few hours. And that's after eight to 10 hours of sleep at night.

During our mini-vacation all I seemed to do was stare at the ocean and sleep. Well, it was relaxing and that's what we went for. Spending half a day in the city of Carmel walking around proved to be too much as I became physically spent. I felt bad for Ken because in the past we've had such wonderful memories here and now he's relegated to watching me sleep.

I have to admit I did freak out a couple of times, solely due to the anxiety over my upcoming radiation treatments. I know what you're thinking—*talk* to someone about *their* experience. Sadly, the wretched patient advocate and Nightmare Navigator have instilled such fear in me that I honestly can't bear to hear another horror story!

A sharp searing pain on my bottom lip rouses me awake. When I completely come to I realize I've bitten my lip hard enough to draw blood. Not knowing what these treatments or their aftermath are going to be like is terrifying. *Fear of the unknown,* I think, climbing out of bed. Peering into the bathroom mirror, I assess the damage; it's not pretty. My lip is black and blue. After tending to the wound I begin my morning routine, remembering to skip the deodorant until *after* the ill-famed appointment.

Needless to say radiation treatments aren't difficult; they're very similar to X-rays and I feel nothing. (Although, that could be because I'm still numb in this area.) When I first arrive, I change into the lovely gown and proceed down the hall. Turning the corner, one of the techs is usually seated in front of the monitors, while the others are in preparing the room. Thomas is usually the first to greet me. He escorts me through the large thick door brandishing brightly colored hazard signs, then down a short corridor to the notorious machine.

It's *almost* like a five-star hotel experience since everyone's lined up waiting to greet me with a smile. Protruding from the machine, a bed has been set to my exact specifications, with a hard foam pillow meticulously placed at one end. The courteous techs are willing to do whatever it takes to make my 15-minute stay all the more palatable. Sadly, there's no comfortable cushion awaiting me, just the hard cold surface of a table with a single sheet covering it, attempting to disguise the reality of why I'm here.

Forgetting to open the back of the gown prior to lying down, I quickly realize *you can't remove it if you're lying on it!* My first appointments went something like this . . . after laying down I immediately place my arms in the casted form, only to be politely reminded, "Please take your arms out of the gown." Complying with their request, they fold the top part of the gown down over my chest, thankfully revealing nothing. It only took me a week and a half to get the routine down.

While lying on the hard surface, I'm flanked by two techs. As the lights dim they lift the sides of my gown and place them on top of my torso, revealing my rib cage tattoos. They then align the tattoos by positioning me, using the sheet underneath to some projected light.

"Don't move; *we'll* use the sheet to move you." *Easier said than done!*

After aligning my rib cage tattoos, they then lower the gown over my left breast. It's then I realize the largest of the paddles has been looming overhead and within its reflection a ruler of light can be seen projecting onto my breast.

"98.9," one tech chirps.

"98.9 . . . okay, ready," another replies in response.

Gently placing his hand on my knee Thomas soothingly coos, "Just relax; we'll see you in a moment." All the techs then file out of the room and the lights slowly return to their original brightness. Rather than silence, I'm now keenly aware of the radio station that's been playing in the background. This is when the machine comes to life.

A paddle appears to my right and aligns vertically with my upper body, then another on my left, all moving with efficient grace and knowingness. Suddenly the entire machine itself turns, but curiously the bed stays in the same position. When it stops, the large round paddle from the beginning reappears at my right. Through its glass case, small thin steel rods can be seen, reminiscent of steel keys in a music box, only these are smaller in width and very close together. The keys slide into their intended positions, taking on a one-dimensional shape of my breast. The arm attached to the paddle then angles itself to my upper right, obviously aimed at the location Jorge recently vacated.

Lying on my back for this mechanical spectacle, I have no choice but to stare up at the ceiling. Thankfully, this facility was kind enough to install one of those faux light fixtures that, when illuminated, simulates landscape scenery, in this instance a bougainvillea swinging lazily beneath a cloudy blue sky. *Hmmm . . . anyone for lemonade?* And because I'm lying here with nothing else to do, I allow myself to enter its artificial world and watch as the clouds actually begin to drift!

Around this time the bed jerks and moves slightly, returning me to reality. Once again I'm aware of the music playing in the background. Thomas and two of the techs now enter and return my gown to its proper and modest location, then assist me in sitting up.

Since my appointment is from 11:40 to 12:00 noon, which includes the time it takes to change into the gown, we end each session inquiring about lunch. Then someone kindly walks me out the corridor and we all say our goodbyes and I return to the dressing room to change. My deodorant has now become a permanent fixture within my purse and I put it on prior to leaving. I haven't noticed any stinging or rashes from using it. As a matter of fact, I feel nothing at all because my underarm is still numb from the removal of the Lymph-Along-Kid.

The only thing I've really noticed during this first week of treatments is I'm *extraordinarily* fatigued. Ken and I think, and the Radiation Man agrees, it's due to all the stress from the surgery and fear of the unknown. I've had to cancel a few things simply because I've been too drained. However, it does appear to be subsiding. *I can only hope.*

Going into the second week of treatments, I haven't had to sleep as much during the day. If I have something planned in the evening I force myself to rest for an hour or so, which allows me to make it through whatever the evening entails. I can definitely tell, though, when I'm pushing it because my arm starts hurting, imploring me to slow down. But by then it's too late because the ache quickly turns into throbbing.

Also around the second week of radiation, on occasion, I've begun feeling a slight burning inside my left breast, like the mildest of sunburns. Sometimes I also feel an ever so slight burning on my lung, and I mean ever so *slight*, which is normally accompanied with a dry yet liquid feeling in my throat that I attempt to clear to no avail. Always I'm thirsty after treatments, not to the point of dying of thirst, but more so the feeling of *hmmm . . . I'd love a tall glass of ice water with lemon.*

And just as they said—yes, obviously, two weeks of radiation is a pivotal time period—I definitely have one brown nipple and one *(ahem)* not so brown nipple. I told Ken he needs to take me to the French Rivera so I can even out the colors! And that's when I noticed a swath of dark brown skin under the crease of my left breast. It doesn't hurt or itch, and after consulting with Ken, I decided there's no urgency and I'd bring it up the next time I see the Radiation Man.

The most bothersome issues are my left shoulder and arm. They *really* hurt at times. Primarily it's a deep dull ache that sometimes makes me very irritable—*sorry, Ken*. A muscle from my bicep down to the palm of my hand acts, at times, as if it's never been used in my life. When I attempt to extend my arm and lift it over my head it feels as if it's going to snap. Other days, it's just my normal arm—*go figure*. My left shoulder blade has the deep dull ache too, but that seems to go away when Ken massages the area.

I'm happy to report my left breast seems to be doing well, although my nipple is *extremely* sensitive. Sometimes I feel a blast of sharp pain in the area Jorge vacated, but that's fleeting. And since the swelling has gone down, when I lean forward, a crevasse can be seen in my breast. Nothing that can't be fixed by our Shape Shifter of course!

Yes, I'm a bit lopsided, but it's nothing anyone would notice other than Ken and me. I did try a bra on, albeit I'm too sore to wear one, but it doesn't matter because one cup fits and the other doesn't. And since my breasts are two different sizes I decided to find a bra that would accommodate them both without having to bother with a prosthetic. And that's when I came across lace bras sized in small, medium and large. Since they're not based on cup size, the stretchy lace molds to the size of both breasts, offering all the support I require. I actually find them to be more comfortable than my *pre-Jorge* bras.

Truthfully, I wasn't expecting the scar where the Lymph-Along-Kid was to look this, shall we say . . . *mean*. I've been assured over and over in time it will fade. I hope it does before summer; I enjoy wearing tank tops.

At the Radiation Man's office, everyone's delightful. They make this type of visit all the more palatable. I know this is going to sound strange, but I actually enjoy coming here! The only disappointment I've experienced so far is that they rotate the technicians occasionally.

Attempting not to sound nosy, "Is Thomas on vacation? I haven't seen him in a couple of days."

"No. He's been transferred to another location. We techs are contracted employees and rotate in and out of various facilities."

"Oh ... I'm so sad to hear that." I truly was disheartened. I had come to trust Thomas and then one day he's simply gone? Not to belittle the older woman who took his place, but I didn't have much faith in her abilities. First, she couldn't see my tattoos to align the equipment—*heck, I can barely see them*—and it took her a while to get the rhythm of things. She ended up working out fine.

Nonetheless, when it comes to healthcare, as I've said before, you build trust in people. When they suddenly vanish, their absence leaves you kind of cold, as if you're just another piece of equipment or something. You aren't even given the chance to say goodbye. I guess I'm one of those people who gets attached to those in whom I've entrusted my life, and I don't like change in this area.

Speaking of change, I'm not looking forward to my next appointment with the Mad Scientist. I understand now why our Shape Shifter mentioned that we should not only like the doctor but his office too. I literally took it as meaning the physical surroundings and didn't consider the staff. Knowing now what I didn't know then, I probably would have looked into other oncologists. But everything happens for a reason. If I hadn't gone to him I wouldn't have met this group of people.

As for the Mad Scientist, unless he convinces us 100 percent I need to be on one of the drugs he's recommending, I'm definitely foregoing this portion of the treatment. In all honesty, the thought of his office nauseates me. I guess it's time to start searching for a new oncologist.

I cancelled the appointment with the Mad Scientist. When I called to do so, the operator asked if I planned on rescheduling.

That's an odd question I thought to myself and simply replied, "I don't know."

The whole debacle had been too much for me and I still can't stomach the thought of riding that elevator up to the fourth floor. Instead, I've decided to focus my energies on my current treatments. And, quite frankly, I don't feel like visiting vampires either. As for the pills he's proposing, there'll be time enough to discuss that at a later date. After all, he said I wouldn't start them until after the radiation treatments were over.

Now to more pertinent matters . . . it's the third week of radiation treatments and my breast feels as if it has a slight sunburn. I decided since we have an aloe plant I'd use some of its gel to relieve my symptoms. To say the least, I found the whole ordeal to be incredibly messy and I kept sticking myself with its thorns, although the gel did provide temporary relief.

In the past an esthetician who, after noticing I'd had a little too much sun, suggested I try a cucumber gel mask that contained aloe vera. The gel was amazing and soothed my sun-drenched skin. Remembering this, I checked online and to my amazement found it was still being sold. Purchasing a few jars, I was thrilled to find it worked *wonders* for me, exactly as it did when I was younger! Now, at night before I go to bed, I put it on my breast for a period of 10 minutes and wash it off with cool water. It seems to alleviate any irritability I have in this area. Afterwards I place aloe lip balm on my scars. This has become my nightly ritual.

Since the start of these treatments, every Tuesday the Radiation Man examines me just to make sure everything is going as planned. He always ends these appointments by asking if I have any questions. I took this opportunity to inform him about the swath of brown skin that had appeared under the crease of my left breast, and the fact that my bicep and middle forearm muscles were still incredibly sore. He recommended I contact the Medicine Woman; he hadn't seen anything like the deep brown color and, as for my arm, he wasn't sure about that either.

Feeling a bit like a hypochondriac I phone Mabel and, after relaying my concern to the Medicine Woman, she suggested I come in that afternoon. They all agreed I shouldn't be feeling this much pain in my arm.

Reflecting back to my early 20s, I had popped my left shoulder out of place while water skiing, although it did immediately go back into place. Ever since then my shoulder has been a bit problematic, although nothing to write home about. I wonder if this could be contributing to the pain since she had to pull my pectoral muscles apart during surgery. It seems to have affected all of the muscles in this area, including my shoulder blade, which is still completely numb.

Another crazy thing I've noticed when standing in front of the mirror, if I hold my arms out horizontally, my left triceps seems to be flabby and far less firm compared to my right arm that has muscle tone. And strangely my left upper arm looks larger than my right. Up until my surgery I did Pilates three times a week and weight training with a personal trainer twice a week. I want to start up again, but have been waiting for my left arm to feel better, and let's not forget my stamina. I feel so . . . *old*—*I wasn't going to say it and instead just leave the sentence hanging, but I didn't want to freak anyone out! If your imagination is anything like mine . . . well, I'll let you finish that thought.*

Now back to my visit with the Medicine Woman . . . looking me over, she says, "Everything appears to be doing *really* well. I recommend you see your dermatologist about the browning. I haven't seen that before, but since there's no itching or burning in that area I'm going to say it's nothing serious."

"Okay, but what about my left arm, it's just killing me."

"Have you been doing your exercises?" she inquired.

"If you mean raising my hands over my head twice a day, yes, I'm actually doing it three to four times a day, but it seems to make no difference. Plus, look at my left triceps . . ." I make a muscle with my left arm while simultaneously wiggling the triceps with my right hand. "See? It looks all loosey-goosey! Is this normal?"

The Medicine Woman, looking stupefied, stares at me. She then closed her eyes, I think appearing to hold back laughter, but her personality is so dry it could have been for any reason. When she opened her eyes again she said, "Apryl, your body just needs time to heal. It will return to its normal self in approximately eight months from your surgery date . . . just give it time."

"Okay, but what about the soreness?"

"Mabel has a handout with a few additional exercises which should help out."

The next day I made an appointment with my dermatologist for October 28th, and for the remainder of the week I faithfully did the additional two exercises, which did absolutely *nothing* for my arm. I couldn't attain the stretch my arm so desperately required. Then it dawned on me that I should contact my personal trainer, who is amazing at sports stretches. He has you lay on top of a massage table while working studiously on your body, stretching it every which way until, sadly it seems, the final stretch comes all too soon. But once you're standing on your own two feet again you feel as if you're five inches taller! After ringing my trainer and telling him about my problematic arm, he scheduled me for a stretch on Wednesday, October 30th.

I'm getting tired of my daily routine and decided to do something *other* than what has become my norm of doctors' appointments. I arranged to have a manicure and pedicure this morning. While relishing the foot massage, my phone chimed indicating I had a voicemail; it didn't even ring. I opted to listen to it later . . . I was too into the massage, it felt fantastic!

After my relaxing spa treatment, I went to my sunshine appointment and returned home for lunch. After appeasing my hunger pangs, I sat down on the living room sofa to play a game on my iPad when I remembered I hadn't listened to the voicemail I had received earlier.

After punching a series of buttons on my phone I hear the quizzical voice of my dermatologist's receptionist. "Apryl, we have you scheduled this morning for a 9:30 appointment and are wondering if you'll be in?" She had phoned at 9:45; I had completely forgotten about the appointment.

What's wrong with me? I never do this. Laying on our living room sofa I stare off into space. I felt as if I were a million miles away from reality and felt horrible about missing the appointment, primarily because the doctor had gone out of her way to fit me in. I continue to lie here despondently, sinking deeper into the sofa. I couldn't bring myself to phone and apologize, let alone *reschedule*. Instead I fell fast asleep, all the while thinking, *I'll call them tomorrow.*

I never did reschedule the appointment, primarily because the brown swath of skin had faded and was completely gone within a couple of days. I figured if my doctors weren't concerned, then why should I be?

Thankfully I remembered the appointment with my trainer for a stretch—it did wonders for me! Thereafter, like clockwork, I scheduled a stretch with my trainer two to three times every week, wherein he focused solely on my arm. And my arm, with his help, began returning to its former self!

Remember how I said I've been wearing my mom's dog tag from WWII since this all began? Well, I've noticed, around this three and a half weeks of radiation, the tag is feeling kind of funky against my skin. It's as if the dog tag itself is *hot* from being in the sun and I'm inside! It actually feels as if it's burning my skin where it touches me. I mention this to the Radiation Man and he suggested I stop wearing it during this treatment period. Sadly, I took it off when Ken and I returned home.

Ken could see the heartbreak in my eyes after doing so because it has brought me an inordinate amount of courage and strength during these past months. "Apryl, give it to me," and I watch as he places it tenderly around his neck. He then kisses it and says, "I'll keep it safe until you're able to wear it again." *See what I mean? Who thinks of stuff like this? That's right—Mr. Wonderful! Maybe I should be thanking his mother; oh yeah, I have!!!*

A few days after the removal of the dog tag, I noticed a few white pimples had appeared on my chest close to my left breast. I haven't been able to exfoliate this area due to the sunburn feeling and therefore attempted to pop the nasty little white-headed pimples. *Yikes* . . . they're not pimples, they're blisters. There weren't that many and, quite frankly I was the only one who noticed them, so I decided to just let them run their course. Thankfully they went away about two weeks after the treatments ended.

This last week and a half of radiation treatments are taking their toll on me. I've completely stopped sending e-mails to The Inquisitive Minds. I'm simply too tired and my head seems to be in a foggy place, continuously spinning round and round and up and down. As I had mentioned previously, I find myself forgetting scheduled appointments and either miss them completely or run *extremely* late.

On Monday I had a dream that one of the techs came to me and told me I no longer require these treatments and am *free* to go. Honestly, I think my body's telling me I no longer need them; Jorge has left, never to return. During tomorrow's appointment with the Radiation Man, I'm going to tell him I no longer need the treatments and walk out the door. I long for my former life.

When I arrive on Tuesday, I sign in and am told by the beautiful smile, "The Radiation Man is not here today. However, if you have any questions or concerns, you're welcome to meet with Mimi, his nurse practitioner." Okay, everything happens for a reason and I'll dispassionately continue with the treatments. I'm beginning to resent my daily routine and long for my former life . . . *am I repeating myself?*

Finally . . . the last three treatments are ahead of me. I'm told on Monday instead of the machine turning, the bed will now be joining in on the fun; together they'll be performing a new kind of dance. Listlessly I lie on the bed as it jerks back and forth to the intended positions the Radiation Man has dictated, all the while mechanical arms expertly move up and down in all directions. I've succumbed to its every whim and helplessly watch as the beast moves wildly around me. *I'm getting tired . . . really tired of this dance and desperately want it to end.* Then it's over.

That evening Ken and I watch the final 100th episode of *Fringe*. Funny . . . we began the series when all of this craziness started. Honestly, it helped lessen the burden of what I'm going through because it's about doctors, science and technology. Whenever I'd get scared around some of the machines, I'd secretly pretend I was in one of the episodes. I'll miss watching it, but am glad it's over.

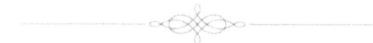

My head feels foggy and I'm frantically attempting to pick up the pieces from my former *life* — my former *self*. However, I find this endeavor to be far too cumbersome; quite frankly, I'm spent. I attempt to divert my attention to something simpler, *something* that has the ability to take me away from *everything*. I begin playing the mind-numbing game *Spider* on my iPad.

Every day from morning until night, any chance I have, I'm playing it. It's mesmerizing, intoxicating, challenging and takes me away to the foggy land my mind so desperately wishes to drift to. I can't get enough; I *hate* it when I'm interrupted. And because I have it on my iPhone, I'm able to take it *everywhere* with me. Ken despises it, but allows me to continue because it seems to pacify whatever it is I'm attempting to escape from. *Please excuse me now while I get back to my Spider and the tangled web we're weaving . . .*

20

Tangled
Maroon 5

The web the *Spider* and I have spun is quite intricate, captivating me with its complexity. It's never-ending and I find myself being comforted by its ability to hold me in its lifeless realm, a kingdom in and of itself. I lie here tangled helplessly, yet shielded, hidden away from the realities of life. No one expects anything from me and frankly, I'm not interested in offering anything in return.

I begin pondering the metaphorical glass pitcher of water . . . I can feel it in my hands, holding it, peering through it. The water is neither cold nor hot. Testing its contents, I tip the container and watch as the first droplets begin to fall. It splashes down around my feet, upon the parched earth waiting to drink it in.

As the water continues to drain from this pitcher I notice it reflects a world within—*my world!* It's unstoppable and continues to fall to the ground *soundlessly*. No one hears it or sees it—but I can *see* it and I can *feel* it splashing down around my feet. The water seems to be never-ending. I have no control over it and I can't keep myself from pouring it.

I then realize the water is just about gone, but when will the last drops fall to the ground below? Eventually there will be no sign it ever was except for the marks it made upon the earth. Ultimately those too will disappear.

Can this be life? I feel it's been mine ever since I was made aware of Jorge's presence. Even though he's gone I know he was here, or was he? Is this a nightmare? Will there ever be an end? Eventually there's no more water and the pitcher I hold within my hands is *empty*.

I take refuge in our living room to escape once again within the *Spider*'s web. Ken's in the kitchen doing something and, quite frankly, I don't concern myself much with what he does anymore. There's going to be a full moon tonight but nothing seems to be of interest to me other than my *Spider*. Suddenly Ken appears standing before me, interrupting my reverie, my refuge.

As I pry my eyes from my seductive paramour, I lock eyes with Ken. Daggers of jealousy, anger and concern are hurling in my direction over the fact I've given in completely to this illicit lover. Within his unkempt rage a thunderous cry erupts deep within, "Get up off your *fat* ass and do something—*anything!*"

I am so enraged with his unexpected fury I take the iPad and run for the shelter of our bedroom and slam the door shut. I melt into a torrent of tears and sob uncontrollably. I await his penance begging me for forgiveness—*fat ass? But he loves my ass!* He never comes to apologize. I wait an hour for him to open the door and offer solace. Still it does not come. Anger begins to well up inside and my blood begins to boil. Once again the Comanche Warrior rears its mighty head and I'm on the warpath.

I fling the bedroom door open and storm down the hallway towards our media room. I stand in its entryway and scream at him. We go on like this for I don't know how long, with neither one of us winning. *But I want to win.* I'm tired of not having a voice. I'm tired of not being heard and having to be the one paying the price for whatever this unknown atrocity is that has brought on a scourge for a second time in my life. I'm *angry* about *everything.* Life has stolen precious moments from me and I'm expected to just be okay with it? I look for something to throw at him to end this tirade of screaming.

And that's when I lock eyes on three things I know are inexpensive and, quite frankly, I could care less if they break. There they sit to my left on their beautiful iron candelabras—*candles.* Each one hefty enough to cause damage to the one I love. Without giving it anymore thought, I grab the first candle from its cradle. Its weight is about three pounds and I fling it towards my target—Ken!

With wide disbelieving eyes he escapes the first flying candle of anger with ease. I then grasp the next candle and throw it, this time with all my might. He blocks it with athletic grace using his arm as a shield. I hear the candle as it makes contact and then Ken lets out a painful shriek. I accomplished what I set out to do—wreaking havoc on the one I love and once again I find myself running for the shelter of our bedroom, sobbing.

Shortly Ken comes in holding his arm in pain and takes to mending his wound.

"Apryl, I think you may have broken my arm." Reality sets in.

"Oh Ken . . ." The one thing in my life that has been unbending and I have finally succeeded in breaking it. "I am so very sorry. I don't know what got into me."

Not knowing what else to do I fling myself into his arms. "I am so sorry . . . I didn't mean to hurt you." I vowed I'd *never* do so again. I felt horrible, like a wretched troll who unleashed the anger and sorrows of his world on an innocent bystander. Not only an innocent bystander, but one who's attempting to protect me from *everything*, not caring what I look like nor the fact that I had an ill-gotten disease.

This is what it took to break me free from the web *I had chosen* to create . . . the foggy world where I didn't have to face the consequences of reality. Ken had freed me from the chains that bound me from my life and my future. We gave one another what we both were so desperately seeking at that moment . . . *love*.

Thankfully his arm was not broken—instead badly bruised. I am so disgusted with myself—yet he still *loves* me. And I love him more than I ever knew possible.

After breaking the chains of my downward spiral, it was time to face the music and schedule the appointment I've been attempting to avoid at all costs—the replacement of the Mad Scientist. Since *El Tango*, I find myself wondering whether I'm strong enough to attempt another go at it.

An acquaintance—happily now a friend—made some phone calls on my behalf when I was first diagnosed with Jorge. She went out of her way for me on so many levels, and hardly knowing me at the time. After doing so, she gave me the name of the head oncologist at a local cancer facility whose specialty is *Breast Cancer*. As he came highly recommended, and after completing research on the now all too familiar medical websites, I found he was considered a *five-star* doctor.

Picking up the phone, I dial his number; I'm literally shaking. I'm transferred to his scheduler, and she begins the normal deluge of questions. It's at this moment I lose my breath and burst into tears. I can barely speak and have to ask her to hold while I attempt, with every fiber of my being, to gain control of my emotions. I don't quite understand why I'm so emotional. I mean, I've already received the news of Jorge and finished the radiation treatments . . . it's smooth sailing from here—right?

But here I sit with the receiver in my hand covering it so this new scheduler wouldn't hear my despair. The emotional angst is still so raw, and it takes everything within me to realign myself. My voice cracks as I attempt to continue the conversation. "I apologize. This has been a difficult period for me. The Mad Scientist I had previously was not the best experience."

The scheduler was so kind to me, showing deep compassion for what I had just been through; she talked with me a bit on a personal level prior to continuing the inquisition. Once all her questions were satisfied, and being that I dropped the name of my friend in hopes of obtaining a not-too-distant appointment, she gave me a date much sooner than I had anticipated—on Christmas Eve.

Phoning Ken, he chuckled at the date and exclaimed, "What a great way to start Christmas!"

Later that day, I received a strange bill in the mail. It was for an out-of-network surgical assistant. Placing it aside I opted to discuss it with the Medicine Woman at our next appointment. There's just too many items requiring my attention.

The days of December seemed to pass in the twinkling of an eye. All too soon it was Christmas Eve and we had closed our office for the remainder of the year. That morning Ken and I readied ourselves for the fateful appointment. When we arrived we were directed to check in and approached the desk with a bit of apprehension.

Pleasantly a jolly man greeted us. "I'm sorry, who did you say you were here to see?" I repeated the oncologist's name and watched as a light of recognition and huge smile enveloped his face. "Oh—you're here to see *The King*! You're just going to love him!" he exclaimed. *I hope so* I thought to myself. And that's how my second oncologist received his name.

He then inquires of my paperwork and, after looking them over, asks that I complete a couple more pages. No sooner was I seated and put pen to paper than a check-in clerk appeared and asked that we follow her. Again a joyous attitude and, as if she were one of Santa's elves, she begins with her merriment, "You can finish your paperwork upstairs," she cheerfully offered. What a pleasant change from the Mad Scientist's office, or could it be I'm simply on the receiving end of holiday cheer?

After reviewing my initial telephone intake information, she hands me the few sheets of paper I'm expected to sign and collects my co-pay. She then ushers Ken and I out of her glass office, back through the small waiting area and points to a bank of elevators. "You'll take that elevator to see The King." Extending to us holiday greetings, she leaves us to face the steel gray doors alone.

The elevator is quite large inside. Silently we ride it to the intended floor, then the doors slide open revealing a beautiful spacious glass building. There's a glass handrail in front of us that overlooks the floors below. Turning right, we head toward the next in-take desk. Floor-to-ceiling glass windows are on our left. Tables with various games and puzzles silently promising to amuse and titillate are everywhere and I wonder, *have I entered the North Pole?*

Checking in with the third desk, we're asked to have a seat. "Someone will be with you shortly."

I quickly fill in the blank lines on the paperwork I was previously given, and return it to the check-in clerk when my name's called by a nurse. "Wow, there's no waiting here," I say to Ken.

A pleasant young man greets us at two swinging doors. Stepping through one of them, he holds it open, allowing both Ken and I to enter. We follow him around a corner and into a huge hallway that continued to heaven only knows where, but we stop at what appears to be a nurse's station at the beginning of it.

"Please have a seat." He points to a small row of chairs up against a wall. I look around and see all the normal gadgets required for my vitals, as the young man begins with the familiar procedures—clip on finger, blood pressure taken from my right arm; of course, I remind myself to uncross my ankles. He then takes my temperature using a gun-type thermometer and ends with weighing me. *I've got to do something about that number.*

After the young man satisfies his *I want to know your most intimate details*, he then asks us to follow him down another hall and into an examining room. "The King will be with you shortly," he informs us. "Please change into this gown with the opening in the front," and he leaves us to comply with his wishes.

No sooner have I closed the gown around me and am making my way to the examining table than a slight rap is heard on the door and my heart skips a beat as the doorknob turns. The handsome King enters my chamber offering cordialities. Unexpectedly my eyes fill with tears. I look at him and shudder, "You scare me!"

While holding a chart I know contains my utmost personal details in one hand, he responds to my fear with a wonderful full of life expression only Latin men have the ability to project. With a huge gesture, he flings both arms out to his sides. "Why? You don't even know me yet!" *God, does he have to have the sexy accent too?*

"Because you're going to ask me to put poison in my body." Tears begin to fall.

To lighten the moment he says, "You're too *young* to be here. How old are you?" he inquires as he opens to the page containing my particulars.

"I'm 65," I reply knowing full-well I'd catch him off-guard and hoping to put the smile back on my own face.

"No, you're not!" he replies with the anticipated response I've grown accustomed to, from people who feel it's okay to ask the age of a younger woman dating an older man.

Holding a piece of my hair in front of my face, "Yes, I am; I dye my hair and know a great plastic surgeon!"

He absolutely does not know what to think of me and looks to Ken for a more truthful response. Ken of course laughs. "No, she's not. She's only 46!" We're all tickled with laughter. Thankfully, the tears have stopped falling and I wipe the remaining droplets with the back of my hand.

We then began discussing Jorge and his darkest secrets. The King then examines the areas that Jorge and the Lymph-Along-Kid have vacated. "Are you aware there's a new procedure that allows surgeons to check your lymph nodes for cancer while you're in surgery, negating the need to take a scoopful of them out?" *Was he serious? Oh why didn't I meet with The King before I decided on the Medicine Woman?*

"Really? Did I make a mistake?" *God, how did I not find this in my research?*

Realizing I was silently berating myself, he says, "Apryl, I didn't mean to cause you to question the procedure you had done. You accomplished what was needed and that was ridding your body of Jorge." I think in an attempt to lighten the exam he then asked, "You do know you're lopsided?" but it felt as if he intended to inform me of something new.

"Yes, we know. We decided to wait on the reconstructive surgery until my body has had time to heal. That's what our friend the Shape Shifter recommended."

"And you know when it comes time your insurance will cover the surgery?"

"Yes, but I don't plan on having it for a year or so," I said, scanning his face for any concern over this decision. Thankfully none was to be seen.

He then perused more of my intimate details as I began asking questions previously posed to all my doctors. Thankfully, he offered similar responses to what I'd already received. Of course The King took this opportunity to say, "You've done all the hard parts, and I agree with your former Mad Scientist; the next protocol is Tamoxifen."

"I know and I don't want to take it—I do terrible on prescription medications." And I went through all the reasons why I shouldn't be on the drug.

"But Apryl, you're so *young!* It could prolong your life and help you avoid any reoccurrence in the future." I shot back with the percentages of how much this drug could offer me.

For several moments he stares at me deep in thought. I don't know if his mesmerizing brown eyes were attempting to figure out what it would take to get someone like me on this drug. Or was he attempting to instill confidence and at minimum get me to try it? If it was the latter, I began to cave.

"Dang, why do you have to be Latin?" I inquired. "Latin men are my weakness," meaning it in the best sense, of course!

Aghast at my remark, "Your husband's standing right here!" he exclaimed, nodding his head towards Ken.

"I know, but he knows I have a thing for Latin men!" We snicker at my naughtiness. Taking a breath and glancing at Ken, my heart gushed, *and we love and trust each other implicitly!*

A Tango with Cancer

He then got serious again, "Listen, I have a patient who's about your age and she has the same aversion to prescription medications. Instead of taking one 20-milligrams pill daily, I proposed she split the dosage and take 10 milligrams in the morning and 10 at night. It seems to be working very well for her. And the pills come in that dosage so you won't have to mess with cutting them."

All I could do at that moment was tell him I would *consider* taking it. I don't know what I was expecting. I think he knew at this point he wasn't going to get a definitive answer from me and offered, "I'll have the prescription called in. I'd really like you to seriously consider taking it." I like The King—*I like him a lot!* He was beginning to instill within me some vague form of trust within this crazy healthcare system.

On the ride home Ken said, "You know Apryl, if it were me, I'd at least try it." He totally caught me off-guard.

"But you said you'd support my decision? I didn't realize you felt I should be taking it." Why are these choices so complicated and confusing?

"Honey, whatever your ultimate decision is, I'm with you 100 percent. I just feel I should let you know what I'd do." Then, as an afterthought, "Let's leave this decision for January. You've had enough this year." I watched as The King's castle vanished from our view. Then, with a smile, I decided it was time to enjoy Christmas—Merry, Merry!

The ache in my back had become more pronounced during radiation treatments, to the point the techs had to assist me when attempting to right myself. Albeit, it didn't help that the treatment bed I was laying on, in actuality, was a *hard plastic table*. It had become my mission to determine the cause for this unrelenting pain. In November, Mimi had mentioned it could be a cyst on an ovary which she had spotted on my PET/CT Scan. Therefore, it was only logical I enlist the help of Dr. Gyno.

I won't even begin to delve into the circus tricks it took to have two MRIs and a very intrusive, not to mention embarrassing, ultrasound completed. Can you believe it took two months to get the approvals for them? And the procedures themselves were literally nightmares! With that behind me, the results were sent to both Dr. Gyno and Dr. KnowItAll in mid-December. It was smooth sailing from here and a welcome change to focus on something other than Jorge.

Like clockwork my gynecologist phones the next day to inform me he's received and read the results from the ultrasound and MRIs. "Apryl, there's no sign of cancer and everything as far as the cyst goes looks completely healthy. But because I'm not an expert as far as your lower back goes, there's really nothing more I can tell you than that."

"That's fine," I reply, "I primarily wanted to rule out it was a problem caused by the cyst. I'll contact Dr. KnowItAll; he'll know what to do." And we end our call extending holiday wishes.

I phone Ken to let him know of the findings. "It's odd that Dr. KnowItAll hasn't called; he usually does the next morning after he's received results. I'll call him and see if by chance he's available." Ken agreed; he too thought it was strange we hadn't heard from him.

Dr. KnowItAll will know what to do, I thought to myself as I dialed his number. Ruford answered the phone and I informed him about my MRIs and the fact that Dr. Gyno ruled out my back problem being from the cyst.

"I'll pass your message on to the doctor, but he doesn't have time to call you back today, it will have to be tomorrow."

"No problem. My main concern was getting the MRIs completed prior to year-end since I've met this year's deductible. It can wait until tomorrow."

Tomorrow came and went, along with year-end finance meetings at the office, our company holiday party, and my first meeting with The King on Christmas Eve—to say the least, my attention was diverted. It wasn't until Christmas Day I realized Dr. KnowItAll never phoned back.

"Wow, that's really strange, Ken."

"I agree . . . that's not like him." We both assumed there must have been a mix-up with my message.

On Thursday morning the thought occurred I should call his office. *Really? What are the chances his office will be open today? It's probably closed until after the New Year.* To my astonishment the phone was answered.

"Hi, this is Apryl Allen calling. I had results faxed over from Imaging Center #1 a couple of weeks ago and I'd like to speak with Dr. KnowItAll regarding the results."

"In order to speak with Dr. KnowItAll you're required to schedule an appointment." *Really? Another doctor's appointment? Can't he take pity on me with everything that's happened over these last six months and speak to me on the phone? I'd gladly pay him if that's what he wants.*

"Okay..." I say with a lilt of disappointment.

"Can you come in today at 10:30?" *Wow... that's less than an hour from now and I haven't showered.*

"No we can't... we have an appointment at 12:30." Ken and I had purchased movie tickets online. Since we gave our staff the week off, why not take some much needed time for ourselves too?!

"Okay, what about 11:30; we can have you in and out in no time."

Rats, why didn't I call his office first prior to purchasing the tickets? "Sorry no, that doesn't work either. Do you have anything later in the afternoon?"

Her tone then took on an incredulous inflection, as if to say, *"Really? You do realize you're asking to schedule an appointment with God — and you don't have the time?"* Okay, this was a bit annoying but I figured she wasn't so happy due to the fact she was working the day after Christmas. "No, nothing this afternoon..." *long pause.* "Can you be here tomorrow at 2:30?"

"That works fine; look forward to seeing you then." I hang up the phone and apologize profusely to Ken because I've now scheduled yet another doctor's appointment during the only week we have off from the office. This is the last thing either of us wants to be doing during the holidays.

"Honey, it's not a problem at all," Ken replies. He has literally been a prince through this entire... well cRaZiNeSs! So it was confirmed, and I was that much closer to having this behind me. I truly am doing my best not to complain about my surgery, my back or the great fear I have lulling deep inside.

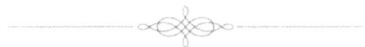

We're about five minutes late for the appointment — Dr. KnowItAll is *always* on time. Signing in, I'm greeted by his receptionist and see Ruford sitting in the reception area too.

"Hi, Ruford," I say enthusiastically.

He gives me a half-hearted smile and a strange "Hello" in response. *That's odd; he seems to be indifferent to me. Hmmm . . . probably just my imagination or maybe I'm just being overly sensitive.*

Since we're the only people in the waiting room we take the chairs closest to the table with the latest tabloid gossip readily displayed. In less than five minutes my name is called. I turn to Ken, "You are coming with me, right?"

"If you want me to . . ." The question didn't require a response; my face said it all.

Yuck! As normal, they ask me to step on the scale prior to entering their examining room. *Really?! Can't they forgo this just once?* Looking at the metal slider indicating my weight I question, *why is it always this number?*

His receptionist shows us into an examining room and thankfully does not ask me to change into the infamous frock. I take my usual place at the end of the examining table. As we wait, we notice the temperature in this room is particularly *HOT!*

Being thirsty, Ken informs me as he opens the door, "I'm going to get some water; do you want any?"

"No, I'm fine. But mention to the receptionist how warm it is in here."

"I was planning on doing exactly that." Leaving the room, he left the door ajar so cooler air could enter. Returning, he mentions how warm it is to the receptionist whose desk is across the hall.

Surprisingly, she answers Ken as if we're complete strangers to them. "This is the temperature doctor prefers for those patients needing to change into gowns." *Really? We've never experienced it being this hot before—and we've been coming here for years!*

We continue to wait. It's really odd to me we're waiting so long; Dr. KnowItAll is always punctual. Well, he does get upset if you're even the slightest bit late so maybe this is his way of punishing me. We hear his comings and goings with other patients. Ken is literally melting in the office and decides to get more water. He returns, this time leaving the door open. I again reiterate to Ruford and the receptionist who are nearby, "It is *REALLY* hot in here."

"Doctor prefers the office warm for those having physicals," she replied again, using a smug tone. *Seriously? It feels like summertime in Phoenix in this room.*

Before I go on, I'd like to tell you of my experience with Dr. KnowItAll over the years. I find he gets a bit exacerbated because I question everything, and when he prescribes medication, I usually don't take it. You see, I'm the type of person if I'm sick, don't ask me why, I listen to my heart.

After my hysterectomy in 2003 I had bouts with nausea. After seeing Dr. KnowItAll, he told me it was acid reflux and prescribed Nexium. (I know what you're thinking, why go to him and not your gynecologist? I was between gynecologists at the time—don't ask, that's another story.) In my heart I knew it wasn't acid reflux, and even though I purchased the prescribed medication, I didn't take it. Instead I found if I worked out it dissipated, so I stopped complaining.

Again I found myself questioning another diagnosis in 2006 when I hurt my right knee; I had attempted to pick up a moving box while wearing high heels. Dr. KnowItAll's prognosis was arthritis and quickly dismissed it; of course he prescribed medication for the pain, which I declined. I found it hard to believe that the symptoms of arthritis simply appear overnight. Needless to say, I continued my pursuit for the cause and found I had actually torn my meniscus. When I informed him of my findings it pretty much pissed him off.

On the other hand, if I come down with the flu I've always taken whatever he prescribes. If you recall I mentioned previously my bout with mono in 2011—again, another misdiagnosis, but you know how that ended. After this experience is when I told Ken I wanted him in the room with me during doctors' appointments.

Dr. KnowItAll was wearing me down; he'd listen to my symptoms, but was quick to dismiss anything I wanted to discuss in more depth. He made me feel as if I was a hypochondriac, complaining much about naught.

In June of 2012, when we had our annual exams, Dr. KnowItAll asked I bring the blood work we had completed by our naturopath. I could tell he wasn't too happy we were seeing her. I, of course, in his mind, was the one to blame for this decision, not Ken. He didn't appear to be pleased that she had diagnosed me with mono either and completely dismissed the fact I felt better after taking her prescribed vitamins.

Then came my favorite part of the physical. *"Is there anything out of the ordinary you want to address?"* Why . . . so you can tell me it's all in my head?

"Actually, I've noticed this little red blotch in the crease of my left breast. It's about the size of a quarter."

"That's just from the suction cup on the EKG machine," was his response. And we finished discussing whatever else it was he wanted to dismiss. I realized, after the fact, that I was lying on the examining table the entire time. So how exactly did he figure I saw the little red blotch? Big breath, deep sigh. *Now back to the calamity and eventual implosion of Dr. KnowItAll . . .*

Just prior to Dr. KnowItAll walking into his *hot* jail cell I said to Ken, "You didn't realize you were marrying such a disaster, did you?"

His fun-loving response, "No . . . I didn't. But our years together have been pretty spectacular!" We were laughing aloud when Dr. KnowItAll walked in and inquired of our gaiety.

I reiterated our conversation after greeting one another. "How long have you two been married?" he inquired.

"Thirteen years!" Ken and I chimed together.

"Well, it only gets better from here," Dr. KnowItAll added and we all laughed, although I'm not quite sure why.

Dr. KnowItAll is into everything—biking, hiking, swimming, and deep sea diving—the man appears to be in fantastic shape. But something was off today. I'm getting the same strange vibe I use to feel when I'd meet with him by myself. It's odd, he doesn't make me feel this way during my annual physicals, only if I have a health concern.

"So tell me about your lower back pain, is it on the right or left side?" He stands ready with my medical file and pen in hand.

"Left side," I reply.

"How bad is the pain?"

"Some days pretty intolerable, but mostly just a constant annoyance."

"For how long has this been bothering you? I know you've mentioned it to me in the past, but for how long *exactly*?"

"I'd say about two years."

"Are you currently having chemo, radiation or taking any medication? Specifically, Tamoxifen?"

"No, nothing and I was wanting to speak with you about . . ." Abruptly, Dr. KnowItAll cuts me off. "Okay, undo your pants so I may examine your lower back." Feeling around, he pushes here and there.

When he got to my left hip, "*Ouch! That's painful!*"

"Okay, just as I suspected. I recommend you go on the following medications—a muscle relaxant, pain pills . . ." *and blah, blah, blah.*

Because his attention is solely on my chart I lean over and attempt to see what he's writing and unknowingly crinkle my nose.

"Yeah, I know . . . you don't like taking medications," he slaps my medical chart closed. "I'll tell you what, when you're ready to have your back fixed give me a call." His *sort of* pleasant manner changes radically and his nose begins to turn a deep crimson.

Ken and I simultaneously ask the same question, only each using our own words. "We'd at least like to hear what you'd recommend?"

His nose continues to betray his attempt at a calm demeanor as its color continues to deepen. "I recommend for a period of 90 days you do no physical activity whatsoever—no dishes, no laundry, no driving a car, no picking up your pets. Lay in a fetal position while sleeping with a pillow between your legs . . ."

"But for the past four months I've basically done that due to my surgery and it's only gotten worse . . . *and* I'd prefer not to take pills. Wouldn't it be better to go to a physical therapist and . . ."

Again Dr. KnowItAll rudely interjects. "Yeah, I know you don't like taking medications. And, quite frankly too many cooks in the kitchen spoil the food." *When did I become pasta primavera?* "If you want to go see a physical therapist, a naturopath, a chiropractor or an acupuncturist, *be my guest*. When you're *ready* to fix your back, come and see me at that time."

"Well, could you at least tell me what the results were from my MRIs?" I asked in a proactive way.

"I have an extreme dislike for Imaging Center #1. I'm friends with the owner, but after sending my daughter there for a mammogram and spending 45 minutes on hold waiting for him to decipher her results—to no avail—I have chosen to no longer use their services. The last thing I'm going to do is spend my time reading reports for *you*; I *refuse* to do so!" He angrily said this all the while waving the reports in my face. *Wow! I can't believe he's so enraged!*

"So what you're saying is the two months I spent attempting to schedule the MRI's, and the days it took to have them completed, was for nothing?"

"Listen, I've personally had numerous MRIs, along with surgery, and know *exactly* how to fix your back. None of these so-called experts know how. So when you're READY to have it fixed give me a call. I don't mean to upset you . . ." and he looks to Ken as if to say *your wife is wacked.*

"You're not upsetting me," I said, using an expressionless tenor. I might have been *stunned,* but definitely not upset.

Ken then attempted to weigh in. "Dr. KnowItAll, Apryl has been through so much these past few months with doctors and . . ."

Dr. KnowItAll haughtily cuts him off and looks back at me. "Like I said, when you're ready to *fix* your back, give me a call. Until then go and do whatever you feel you need to do." He then placed my chart under his arm and, while avoiding eye contact, extended his hand for me to shake, which of course I stupidly did. While shaking it he utters a not so meaningful "Have a good day . . . goodbye."

Okay . . . that went well! This was the last thing I thought would happen today. Ken and I sat shell-shocked briefly. I then did my pants up and we left Dr. KnowItAll's jail cell. Prior to leaving we actually paid our co-pay and after signing the receipt his receptionist squawked, "Have a Happy New Year!"

Despondently I reply, "Yeah, you too."

Numbly we walk to our car. Climbing into the vehicle we sit in silence from the shock and distress of the appointment. Eventually I find my voice. "This is why I've been having you come to my appointments. He seemed to get angrier each time I saw him."

"I know you said it—not that I didn't believe you—but I didn't think it was like that." Ken was completely aghast.

"He's never been this irate; something must have happened to him personally." Was I actually making excuses for him?

"Apryl, he didn't even ask how you were doing, nor how your Tango or treatments were going. It's as if he didn't care."

"I don't understand . . . how can people be so angry?" I wanted to cry but didn't have it within me to do so. Not anymore.

"Honey, what he did was unconscionable. You said it a few years ago, and now I understand; it's time we find a new family physician. Until we find this person, just in case we need something in the interim from Dr. KnowItAll, we won't ask for our records."

Dejectedly we drove out of the parking lot, wondering if the New Year would bring a happier and healthier future.

21

Tightrope
Stevie Ray Vaughan

Fate lingers in the air, never revealing exactly what is to be. Instead, it teases relentlessly with the possibilities of *"what-if."* The last week of December was sheer torment; I was incredibly stressed. It felt as if my world was crumbling. I *wanted* to trust in someone but there simply wasn't anyone there. I *wanted* to believe in our healthcare system, but ultimately I was running out of faith in its providers.

Over our morning coffee I questioned Ken, "I don't understand . . . I don't understand why people act the way they do in this world." Reading the papers was depressing; too many people on this planet are choosing to create chaos—*on all fronts*. It's no different within the healthcare system; there's a lot of angry people out there.

"Honey, as I said before, there's no black and white—no definitive answer."

"But I want to know *truth*. I want to *feel* it!" At that moment *truth* was out of reach, and I was willing to grasp at *anything*. "I want to *believe* Tamoxifen is the next step for me, but I'm terrified of what it will do to my body. There hasn't been one doctor who has convinced me otherwise."

Ken pondered for several moments. He wanted to offer a solution and help me find the peace of mind I was so desperately seeking. And then it happened . . . a light went off. Or was it divine inspiration he claims he's not privy to?

"Apryl . . . *choose* what you want to *believe*. Find it within your heart and believe in it. I've seen you do it before." For someone not particularly religious, Ken is incredibly insightful.

I took a deep breath and let go of all my anxiety, every ounce of stress I was holding on to and I *simply* let it all go. He was right, I had done it before. But what was it that I did precisely? Then I realized, Ken had said exactly how I did it. Truth is what we believe in our hearts. Ultimately I will know *truth* when I feel peace. And thus I began searching . . . for *peace*.

Over the next couple of weeks I did feel a little better, although I think my stress manifested itself in other ways. The last week of December, after the calamity with Dr. KnowItAll, it reared its ugly face as a sty in my eye, requiring me to make yet another doctor's appointment, with our ophthalmologist. No sooner was I relieved of that annoyance than it reappeared under the guise of a cold sore on my lip the first week of January.

Then the unexpected happened: my lower back completely went out on me. I couldn't stand, sit, walk or lie down. I was completely immobilized and disheartened. Everything I have been through and now I was being punished again? Why is it that some people who are unkind, mean and vindictive often walk free of any illness or disease? Why do they get to live long lives untethered by the plagues of this world? Again the words of my mother echoed, *"How can life be so cruel?"*

With everything going on, I felt as if I were walking a tightrope. But I had a choice. I could choose to be *happy* or choose to be *defeated* and I chose happiness. No matter what life throws at me, I won't let it knock me down. Even though at this moment I feel I'm flailing at the bottom, there's only one direction left—*UP!*

In an effort to lift my spirits I decided to change tracks; I had to find something worthy on which to focus. Since Ken and I are in desperate need of a break, because we never really had a reprieve through the holiday season, I chose to focus my energies on a couple upcoming excursions. The first, a trip to San Francisco in February. Second, a two-week vacation in Mexico for my birthday. Everything else in my life I'd treat as if it were a business. In between planning our trips, I continued dealing with the bills that were piling up, and a few upcoming doctors' appointments. But infuriatingly, I'm now forced to figure out my aching back.

Instead of wreaking havoc on two business days for Ken, I opted to schedule my two follow-up Jorge appointments the same afternoon; the first was with the Radiation Man and the second with the Medicine Woman. They were both on Friday, January 10th. My visit to the Radiation Man was uneventful. After a quick examination, he asked if anything was out of the ordinary or bothersome.

"Only my back at this point but I plan on enlisting the help of my former physical therapist," I informed him.

"I think that's a good idea," he agreed. "What have you decided about Tamoxifen? Do you plan on taking it?" he inquired.

"With all the research I've done, and the fact that it can only offer me an additional 3 percent security, I'm opting not to take it." In truth I was beginning to wonder if I was actually attempting to convince *myself* of my decision.

The Radiation Man didn't really concern himself with the fact I had chosen not to take the drug. He wrote a few notes down in my file. "I'd like to see you again in six months for a follow-up. You can schedule that on your way out," and he bid us goodbye.

As directed, I stopped at the front desk and asked if Malaika, the young woman with the beautiful smile, was available to schedule an appointment for me. "I hope we didn't miss her. Is she still at lunch?"

"I'm sorry Apryl, but Malaika no longer works here."

"What?!" The smile is gone?

"Yes, she was let go the afternoon of your last treatment here."

I couldn't believe what I was hearing. How could she be dismissed while the Imp-Worm was allowed to continue with her employment? Something is really wrong with this treatment center. Of course the doctors, not wanting to sully their hands in the matter, turn a blind eye and deaf ear to the situation. How sad.

It's not often you meet a special individual with such a generous soul. When faced with a life-altering event such as Jorge you begin to tumble and sometimes crumble. She listened to my fear of the unknown and then selflessly went out of her way to find the answers to my questions. She didn't have to do that; she actually cared and made me feel as if I were a *person* and not a patient. And now I'm being told she is simply gone.

I was disheartened and wasn't the only patient that felt this way. Malaika was the one person at this center who boosted everyone's confidence. I know because we patients discussed it while waiting for our appointments. *Everyone* despised upstairs. With the exception of this floor, the administrative staff at this facility are an angry group of people.

There was nothing that could be done. The powers above on the fourth floor had made their decision. I can only imagine the type of person who runs a facility like this, hiring and firing people on a whim, disposing of the compassionate and instead employing unhappy souls who have no reason to be working at this type of treatment center. *Let it go, Apryl . . .* I know in my heart wherever she goes, Malaika will find her way. And the company that hires her will be that much more successful—because of her!

On to the next appointment of the day—the Medicine Woman. We sign in, waiting no more than 10 minutes and then we're called back by Mabel. She takes us into one of the three examining rooms. I change into the frock with the opening in the front, taking a seat on the examining table while Ken takes the chair next to it.

After a couple of minutes the Medicine Woman lightly raps on the door and enters, wheeling her computer in tow. Taking a seat, she begins recounting and questioning all my personal information, procedures and therapies to date. *This is really beginning to irritate me.*

"I show I did a lumpectomy and lymph node dissection on your left breast back on August 26th—correct?" She peers at me over her glasses. *Seriously, can she write some tickler notes down to make me feel as if she remembers me?*

"Yes, that's correct."

"And I'm showing you have completed your radiation treatments and did not require chemotherapy—correct?"

This is ridiculous. "Yes, that is correct."

"What medications are you currently on?"

"Nothing."

"You're not taking anything?" *I know what she wants me to say.*

"No, I'm not taking anything." *Isn't that what I just said?*

"So you're not taking Tamoxifen?" she asks, a bit perplexed.

"That's correct. At this point, I've decided *not* to take Tamoxifen."

"Why?" I now have her full and undivided attention.

I began reiterating how I came to this decision. "As it states on the pathology report, I'm at low risk, meaning a less than 10 percent chance of the cancer reoccurring if I did *nothing at all.*"

"No, it doesn't say that on the report." The Medicine Woman was adamant I didn't know what I was talking about. (At the time, I didn't realize my pathology and the genomic profile from Agendia were different reports.)

Using my most polite voice, so as not to upset her or cause difficulties in our relationship, "Yes it does. It says so in italics under the section that reads *'Low Risk.'* Because I was diagnosed with early stage breast cancer I have an excellent prognosis for survival without any form of therapy." I quickly scanned her, looking for any signs that I was going to be browbeaten again. *Lord knows I've had enough of that during this past year.* She appeared to be calm, so I continued, "And the probability of reoccurrence is less than 10 percent." Once again I did the math out loud and finished with, "Mostly I'm concerned about its side effects."

She sat for a brief moment digesting everything I had just thrown at her. Then blatantly she struck back, "Suck it up and take the pill."

Wow . . . *"Suck it up."* Now, I know she didn't mean it the way it came out, but *really*, *"Suck it up?"* If she was attempting to convince me to take the pill, those were not the words that were going to change my mind.

Eventually she continued, "If it were me I'd take it—I really don't want you back in here due to another Tango, and 3 percent is a huge factor when you look at the statistics."

"I haven't decided 100 percent I won't take it, but I'm leaning that direction," was how we ended the debate.

She then continued on with more questions, all the while typing my answers into her computer. "We're finished with the questions. Let's examine you." Leaning back on the table she began probing my right breast, nipple and underarm. "Have you noticed any changes in your right breast?"

"No—none." She then began examining my left breast. When she got to my left nipple she squeezed it so hard I thought surely she had drawn blood. "OUCH!" I flailed, shocked she squeezed it so mercilessly.

"Oh, sorry. It still must be tender from the radiation treatments. When did you say you finished them?" *Seriously, does she not remember anything?*

"On November 20th."

"It'll be tender for a few months longer," she informed me while probing my left underarm.

"No discharge in either of your nipples?"

"No," *although you may have caused some with that last tweak!*

"Everything looks good. But you need to seriously rethink your decision on Tamoxifen."

"I'll do that. I do have one other question—I received a strange invoice in the mail last month. The company said it was for a surgical assistant contracted for my surgery. Apparently, I'm responsible for the invoice since she was out-of-network. Can this be correct?" I feel like I'm questioning an authority I have no right to question.

"I have no idea; you'll need to get with Mabel on that." Without giving it another thought, "I'd like to see you again in three months—which will be . . ." she counted the months off in her head, "April."

Thrilled I received an A-Okay check-up twice in one day, I happily booked my next appointment. I didn't bother with the out-of-network surgical assistant; I'd deal with that another time. I think this is called avoidance.

At last, I can now take a much needed break from Jorge. But I still need to figure out what to do about my aching back. I decided, while looking into that, I'd simultaneously attempt to find us a new physician. June would be here before I knew it, and that's the month we schedule our annual exams. Plus, I wanted to stay ahead of any unforeseen and unexpected events, in particular the flu. I *refuse* to ask for help from Dr. KnowItAll.

During these past few months, Ken and I narrowed our search for a new internist down to two doctors, one female and one male physician. After googling each doctor I was incredibly pleased with what I found. The female internist has a rating of four and a half stars, while the male internist has a five-star rating. Perusing the patient comments about the male internist, I see they match exactly what I want in a primary care physician. He listened, took his time and is compassionate.

But can you believe of all the people we've contacted and all the doctors we've been referred to, who would guess we'd narrow it down to two doctors working at the same office? I was disappointed to learn they were both aligned with a local hospital and did not have a private practice. *Apryl, let it go—you've been told this is where the medical world is going.* It's either this or one of those concierge doctors, and who needs that additional expense in this roller coaster economy?

Scheduling a consultation appointment with each of these physicians was a work of futile effort—there is no such thing. Instead, we're required to schedule "New Patient" appointments. Worse, prior to meeting with a potential doctor, it's mandatory we give them *all* of our personal information, even though in the end the doctor may not be our physician. To add insult to injury, we're required to pay for the privilege of meeting the doctors in person and allow them to take our vitals!

Furthering my disdain for our healthcare system, scheduling the actual appointments proved almost impossible. It took several phone calls to people I'll refer to as Admin Junkies, all clamoring, *"That's against our rules!"*

In the end I was able to obtain a "New Patient" appointment with the *female* internist in mid-April *for me*. And after an *unbelievable* amount of torment, the *male* internist is eventually scheduled at the end of April—*for Ken*. We weren't allowed to schedule "New Patient" appointments for both of us with each doctor; because they're in the same office and are only allowed to bill once for the appointment. It was up to me to get creative, scheduling one appointment separately with each doctor that we'd both attend. It shouldn't be this difficult when it comes to one's health.

Thankfully, due to my knee surgery, it only took one phone call to my former physical therapist to schedule an appointment with a back doctor. Since January 22nd I've been working studiously on a fix for my aching back. But, miserably, because of my back, we had to cancel our trip to San Francisco, along with a few local excursions Ken and I had planned here in town. I feel horrible, too, because I know how much Ken was looking forward to them. It's now getting awfully close to our Mexico trip on March 30th.

Feeling like a sitting duck in a pond on the opening day of hunting season, I decided it was time to figure out exactly what The King was going to do for me. I mean, was there any real purpose to have a doctor like this in my life if all he's there for is to dispense poison?

Knowing his facility was easy to schedule appointments with, I dialed the number on The King's business card. Thankfully, within less than three minutes, I had an appointment scheduled for May 1st. I made the decision at that time to hold off on scheduling my mammogram until I met with The King.

22

Money
Pink Floyd

Dancing a Tango is a full-time job. Biopsies, researching doctors, consultations, tests, aligning schedules, the actual surgery itself, the therapies that follow, prescription drugs, insurance—everything is exhausting. And none of this takes into account time for healing or physical therapy; that is, if you're lucky enough to have a doctor suggest you do it.

And now, as much as I detest the thought of it, it's time to face the mounting medical bills. The one I'm attempting to avoid in particular is a bill for a surgical assistant. The date of the invoice is December 10th, almost four months after my surgery. It states in bold black letters NOW DUE: $300. If I don't pay it within a 90-day period the amount will jump to $1,345.99. And, because the surgical assistant does not take ACME Insurance, the responsibility is mine. Reluctantly I pick up the phone and dial the billing department for this surgical assistant.

I got right to the point. "Who authorized this out-of-network assistant?"

"Your Medicine Woman did."

"But I told her my insurance was with ACME."

"I understand, but the Medicine Woman specifically requested this type of assistant. You should have clarified it with her prior to your surgery."

"I don't understand; how would I have known she required one? Besides, I told the Medicine Woman my insurance was through ACME when I engaged her services. Shouldn't this invoice be her responsibility?"

"No, it's yours. This often happens when doctors choose a surgical assistant. And prior to your surgery they can't very well ask for your approval when you're under the effects of anesthesia."

"So basically I'm over a barrel. The Medicine Woman has given you all my personal information, so unless I succumb and pay the invoice you'll send me to collections, correct?"

"Well, there's always the option of contacting your insurance company to appeal; they may cover it. We've submitted the invoice ourselves but since the surgical assistant is out of your network, they have declined to pay."

"You're telling me it's my responsibility to get the insurer to pay your $300? As far as I'm concerned this isn't my responsibility. I'll take it up with the Medicine Woman myself." I ended the call with a not-so-pleasant demeanor.

How could the Medicine Woman have done this? I did all the right things and now it's my responsibility? I'll deal with this at another time; I simply don't have the energy, and I toss the invoice to the side.

Over the next couple of weeks, I continue faithfully with physical therapy. During this same period I thought it prudent to schedule a visit with my Shape Shifter. I wanted him to look at my surgery areas and confirm all is normal. I'm also interested in knowing when he thinks a good time would be to do my reconstructive surgery. After speaking with Brianna, we scheduled an appointment for February 27th.

"Everything looks fantastic! How did all your treatments go?" he inquired with heartfelt concern. Minus *El Tango*, I filled him in on the past six months, ending with the Big T debate.

"Apryl, you know I care for you like my own sister. *Please* . . . go on Tamoxifen. It could potentially save your life."

"But I don't do well . . ." reiterating my sentiments for prescription drugs. "Plus I spoke with eight women across the country—all of whom within a period of two weeks to two years went off the drug due to its side effects. I can't do that to Ken or myself."

"But I'm sure Ken would much rather deal with side effects than the alternative. It's science, Apryl. I'd hate to hear that you're one of the 3 percent who has to dance another Tango. And I'm speaking from personal experience . . . my sister-in-law opted to forego chemo because she couldn't stand the thought of losing her hair. She wouldn't listen to my knowledge of medical treatments and died, leaving two precious kids behind. Please don't make the same mistake."

God, I know my Shape Shifter is speaking from the heart, but does he realize what he's asking? I'm already marked for life by this unwanted Tango and now he wants me to go on this horrid drug? "Apryl, if you won't do it for yourself, then do it for Ken. We love you and want to see you live a long and healthy life."

What exactly do you say to someone who has your best interests at heart, especially when he's throwing in heart-wrenching pleas like these? *What to do—I feel so confused!* "Okay—I'll have a prescription called in."

"And please keep in touch; I want to know how you're doing. As far as the surgery goes, I think you need a break from everything. Let's not consider it for another year or so. Only you and Ken will notice your difference in size."

He was right, but it really wasn't my different sized breasts I was concerned about. I didn't want to go on that damn pill. We left his office with me promising to take the hideous drug, but by the time I got home I had convinced myself otherwise. There were more pertinent matters to attend to—like my aching back!

Exasperating, pesky and irksome ... medical bills are like a perpetually incessant old aunt who nags you all the time simply because she can. I'm still reeling from the aforementioned invoice for the surgical assistant who's *not* in network. I know it's only $300, but it's the *principle* of the matter. I've yet to question Mabel on how or why this happened. Frankly, I don't want to be disappointed again in life by someone I trust, especially someone I have trusted to safeguard my life.

Returning to the previous medical bills accounting project, I attempt to organize and match bills to EOBs for a second time. However, after sorting through the paperwork, I find the majority of them still to be EOBs. That's when I realized, since my surgeries 10 years ago the medical world has changed. Doctors, facilities, laboratories and Lord only knows who else they've enlisted (i.e., surgical assistants) appear to no longer send patients invoices.

Exactly how am I supposed to know what services I'm being charged for? I've received only a few actual bills. I felt sick to my stomach. What if more bills like that for the surgical assistant start coming in? Then what do I do? I sat back staring at the paperwork.

Pondering my dilemma, I reflected on past surgeries, recalling how I enlisted the help of our insurance agent. There's an individual at their office who speaks and understands this language. She could help me sort through all the craziness of this Tango. With high hopes I dial her number.

"Hi, Olivia, it's Apryl Allen calling. Unfortunately, I think I'm going to require your assistance in deciphering a pile of medical bills I inherited from my recent Tango. Would you by chance be willing to help with them? I'll buy you lunch!"

"You don't have to buy me lunch," she giggled. "Yes, I'd be more than happy to help with your bills. What I'll need is everything you've received to date."

"Fantastic, I'll get them organized. Is there any specific way you want them?"

"You don't need to organize them; I can do that for you." I don't think she realizes what she's offering. After all, this surgery was for Jorge, not an everyday illness or surgery.

"I can't bring them to you like this; I haven't even opened half the envelopes. They're literally sitting on my desk in a disorganized pile. Would it help if I sorted them by doctor and then date?"

"Yes, that would be most helpful. I'll take it from there."

"I should mention, back in November I entered what invoices and EOBs I had received into an excel spreadsheet, to determine whether payments were applied correctly to my deductible—which I believe they were. However, I only received a handful of actual invoices, and had to primarily go off the EOBs, which, quite frankly, are another language. Eventually I gave up, thinking I'd receive invoices at a later date but haven't."

"The doctors and facilities didn't provide invoices?"

"No. The only time they did is if it wasn't covered by my insurance. In total I've received maybe five invoices; it's really quite confusing."

"You'll need to contact your doctors and ask them to send over their invoices. You're right, without them, there's no way to determine what's been billed." Obviously she didn't realize what she was asking of me. I've received *maybe* four or five bills and the EOBs are verging on 100 pages.

Taking a deep breath, I let out a, *this just got more complicated* sigh. "Okay, this may take a while to do, at least a month," I informed her.

Discouraged, I hung up the phone. Might as well start with the bill that claims I owe money for the surgical assistant. I called the number on the statement and was put through to the billing clerk.

"Sorry, that's not how healthcare works anymore. To receive invoices you're required to contact ACME Insurance and request that a copy be sent to you; it's due to all the privacy acts put in place."

"Are you kidding me?"

"No, I'm not. Otherwise, if you want *us* to send an invoice directly, you'll have to fax or mail us your request in writing before we can do so." I literally felt myself sinking to the bottom of the insipid barrel.

I called Olivia back. "You're not going to believe what I was just told . . ." repeating the conversation to her.

"That's ridiculous! Well, rather than have you go through all that red tape, I'll contact ACME insurance and request they send them over." *How can she sound so nonchalant about this?* "When can you drop off the paperwork?" she inquired.

Looking at my schedule, "I'm available on March 5th . . ."

"That works for me. Would it be possible to meet at our office?" She could have asked me to meet her in Pompeii!

"Absolutely. Then we'll go to lunch!" She didn't have a choice.

When I hung up the phone, I began organizing every piece of paper I'd received on Jorge since the beginning of our Tango. In an effort to help clarify charges, I made notes on the paperwork itself, at least on those I could decipher after cross-referencing the dates with my calendar. It literally took a week of my time to rummage through the carnage.

Every morning I'd start first thing and wouldn't stop until Ken got home at night. I felt like I was on a merry-go-round, although this one wasn't so merry and I wanted off. The task eventually took over our dining room table and a few chairs. It was excruciating. I was reliving the last year while sorting through the unwanted Tango now relegated to paper. To be perfectly honest, I even broke down a few times—no wonder I was avoiding this.

Finally, the intricate puzzle created specifically for me was now ready for Olivia's desperately needed help and expertise. The jumbled mess had turned into a stack of organized pages and folders a foot in height.

When I arrived at Olivia's office and pulled them from my briefcase she couldn't believe her eyes.

"I didn't realize how much paperwork you had," she exclaimed, fingering through the folders. "I'm so glad you organized them. And it appears you have all the paperwork too. Most people bring only a small portion of what they've received."

"Frankly it would have been too difficult for you to organize. And since this is my tango, I kind of had a heads-up on what was what."

While Olivia rummaged through each file, I pulled up the excel spreadsheet on my laptop. "That's fantastic! Can you make me a copy so I can enter the remaining EOBs?"

"You mean the majority that I haven't entered?" We both laugh. "Sure!"

She then came to the surgical assistant's invoice. "This makes me so upset; doctors don't require surgical assistants. Basically, they're similar to a student intern and you're paying for their education."

"Are you kidding me? I don't want to be paying for someone's education I don't know. Not to mention I don't particularly like the thought of my body as a textbook." My stomach churned at the thought of a stranger learning the dos and don'ts during my surgery. "What exactly do they do during surgery—take notes?"

"No, basically they take over the nurse's job, such as scanning instruments, handing them to the doctor and whatever else the doctor deems appropriate." She continued to sift through the last year of my life. "The first thing I recommend we do is appeal this invoice. We'll need to write a letter to ACME's claims department. I notice here it stipulates if you pay the invoice now you'll only be responsible for $300, versus the $1,300 they claim is the normal rate for this type of procedure. To avoid the excessive fee, you may want to pay the $300 now and let ACME Insurance reimburse you later."

"When I spoke with the billing clerk, she said as long as I keep in contact with her she'll continue to put a hold on my account. I know it's only $300, but I feel this surgical center is taking advantage of the situation and I refuse to give in to their dodgy ways of doing business."

"As long as you're sure. I'd hate to hear you're responsible for the full fee." Unease reflected within her eyes.

"Thanks, Olivia, but I believe the billing clerk will treat me fairly. Plus, I take meticulous notes during each phone call. I'll call her this afternoon and inform her of the appeal."

"There's only one other bill I'm concerned about, but I only see an EOB for it. Did you receive an invoice from this company called Agendia? The service date was on August 22nd; do you know what it's for?" *Now she's heightened my concern too.*

"Agendia . . . I believe that was the entity that determined Jorge's risk factor and the type of therapy I'd require. And no, I haven't received an invoice from them. That was completed so long ago I just assumed it was taken care of."

She pointed to a total line on the paper. "It says here on the EOB the amount you owe is $1,177. 50 and this EOB was processed on January 2nd. Are you sure you didn't receive an invoice from them?"

"No, I'm positive; any medical bills I received were all placed in the same pile on my desk." *Great—another headache to deal with.*

"I suggest you call them and inquire about your account balance. Don't tell them your EOB reflects a balance due. That's a can of worms you definitely want to leave unopened." *I love people who think a step ahead of the game.*

"Okay, I'll call them this afternoon. Is there anything else you're concerned about?" *Please say no; I truly can't take one more thing on my plate!*

"Nope—these are just the two I've noticed off the top. Everything else looks in order but you never know. By chance did you bring your quarterly statements from ACME?"

"No, I didn't realize they were needed." *I'd been shoving them in a "to be filed" box at home with Ken's.*

"Yeah, I like to cross-reference them; you'll know immediately if an EOB is missing." *This girl is on top of her game.*

"All right, I'll e-mail them to you this afternoon as well," silently hoping the list of to-do's wouldn't get any longer. It was then a thought caught in my throat. "Olivia . . . how do people, who don't have someone like you to help, make sense of their medical bills?" The thought was nauseating as I reflected back on the sweet little old man and his wife who preceded me during my radiation treatments.

"They either just pay the bills—hopefully they can afford them—or if not, they end up with a negative on their credit report and it's turned over to collections."

"That's a hideous thought." I couldn't imagine facing this beast on my own. Dealing with the actual Tango of Jorge was devastating enough, and now I have to deal with medical bills. It's overwhelming, and I have a great support system!

Then another thought occurred to me: what about a single mother having to go through this alone? The notion was repugnant as other scenarios began flashing before my eyes. *I need to stop; this will make me crazy!*

Somehow I redirected my attention and set Jorge aside. It was time to revel in life and hear the tales of Olivia's new family. We happily left for lunch together, and I was all too thrilled to be leaving the burden of decoding my tango in the hands of an expert.

That afternoon I worked on my to-do list, contacting Agendia first. And as Olivia stipulated, "I'm inquiring as to the balance of my account."

The polite girl on the other end of the phone responded, "May I please have your account number?" Reading the numbers to her, "Oh . . . you're one of my accounts. Hold on, let me see." Thankfully, she didn't place me on hold and within a matter of 10 seconds, "Your account balance is zero. Is there anything else I can help you with?"

Thrilled with her answer, I replied, "Nope, that's all I needed to know. I appreciate your help." And I happily ended my two-minute phone call.

Next on the list is to write an appeal letter. I quickly compose it based on my discussion with Olivia, sign and scan the letter, both for my records and to e-mail Olivia for her to review and submit on my behalf.

Ringing the billing clerk for the surgical assistant, I informed her of my appeal. She in turn reminded me I would still need to phone her each month upon receiving the statement, "Otherwise your account will be taken off hold and you'll be responsible for the full amount."

Now for the last item on my to-do list—scan my quarterly statements and e-mail them to Olivia along with the appeal letter. When I clicked the send button I felt the dance of this Tango actually beginning to slow—*the end was near.*

Closing my eyes, I took in a deep soulful breath that completely filled my lungs. As I let the air slowly escape my lips, I envisioned myself holding the pile of medical bills and EOBs, all of those many, many pages grasped within my hands. Using all my might, I flung them as high as I possibly could into the air. With much pleasure I watched as a gust of wind took over and scattered them, vanquishing them from sight and mind.

23
Windmills of Your Mind
Sting

The day before we left for Mexico, we took our beloved babies to our dog trainer for boarding; loco Hugo desperately needed help with his manners. Truthfully, it's Ken and I who are in need of training, but we'll attempt that feat upon our return. It was during this time that a strange happenstance occurred . . .

It was a beautiful spring day with not a cloud in the sky. Feeling energized from the warmth of the sun, we happily toured this doggie halfway-house. While discussing our naughty little boy, I turned around to face the trainer and was blinded by the sun.

With no warning whatsoever the sun suddenly aimed all of its rays directly at my left breast, as if attempting to ignite it on fire. It was so painful! I couldn't bear to stay within its wicked grasp and quickly sought shelter from nearby shade. I found myself wishing I had one of those lavender scented ice-water washcloths some hotels keep in soaking dishes throughout their spa. It would have dampened the burning sensation and brought welcomed relief!

It was such a strange feeling, similar yet very different from having a really, *really* bad sunburn; we all know what it's like to stand in the sun with one of those. Luckily we weren't there long, but now I'm concerned about Mexico.

So why didn't any of my many doctors warn me about this? Or why wasn't it listed as one of the potential side effects? Didn't I mention to a couple of the doctors I planned on having Ken take me to the French Rivera to even out my tan?

Well . . . it's neither here nor there now. I'm one of those who slather myself in sunscreen when I know I'll be in the sun. Hopefully that will help deter any future pyro attempts while in Mexico. If it becomes too problematic, I'll just stay completely in the shade, or at least as best I can.

Worst case, I'll make my own version of ice-water soaked washcloths . . . keeping them within arm's reach, of course!

Our nonstop flight arrived in Mexico City that afternoon and I was exhausted. After we had a quick bite to eat, I decided to lie down for a bit. Well, that intended short slumber turned into 12 straight hours; I couldn't believe it was the next morning when I woke up. I was both disappointed and concerned because I didn't want this to be another trip where all I did was stay in the room and stare at . . . *whatever*.

Ken assured me it was just the stress of travel. "Honey, your body's still recovering from surgery and radiation; give yourself a break. I'm here and you're with me—that's all that matters." He was right. This trip is for the two of us and I won't let anything take that away.

The remainder of our trip was invigorating. We spent a few days in Mexico City, then drove to San Miguel de Allende to visit friends and enjoy the treasures of the old majestic colonial village. Its enchanting cobblestone streets are lined with colorful stone walls and doors that open into arched flowering courtyards containing shops and galleries.

While stumbling in and out of storefronts, we weren't looking to buy anything, but weren't opposed to it either. Entering through one of the many wrought iron gates, we were lured to an antique armoire with glass doors containing heirloom jewelry. One item in particular caught our fancy—an ivory bracelet with animals carved on it.

After closer examination of the carving its story came to life—an elephant and lion were battling over an antelope. Each side of the bracelet depicted two very different endings to the same story—one the elephant as the victor, the other the lion. The bracelet was very old and had a slightly bent metal pin that, when slid within its intended holes, locked the bracelet securely closed. I had never seen anything like it.

The saleswoman was more than happy to help me try it on. It was a *perfect* fit and I felt shivers down my spine when she locked it in place. I looked to Ken and conveyed in a glance, *I love it but I'm sure the price is astronomical.*

Admiring it long enough, I prepared to remove it when Ken announced, "We'll take it!"

"What?! Honey . . . we can't." Yes, I *wanted* it, but I didn't *need* it.

"After what you've been through this year . . . you deserve it! Happy Birthday, honey!"

I opened my mouth to debate the purchase but the saleswoman found her voice first. "Don't ever argue with a handsome man wanting to buy you something!" She was right—who am I to argue?!

Besides, there was *something* about this bracelet . . . neither I nor Ken could quite put a finger on it. Yes, it was lovely, but it was more than that. It felt as if it had been a part of me—a part of *us* before. We left the store with the bracelet safely wrapped within my purse. I was so excited; I couldn't wait to wear it!

When we returned to the hotel later that afternoon we carefully pulled the bracelet from its silken satchel to look at it again. It was a stunning piece of art that was obviously well-cared for over the years.

The next day we met dear friends for dinner. Wearing the bracelet, all four of us relished its splendor. Later that evening, retiring to our hotel room, Ken helped me take it off, protectively returning it to its satchel; I placed it deep inside the safe within our room. While readying ourselves for bed I began brushing my teeth. That's when Ken reached into the safe for his jewelry box. *Thunk!*

Gurgling through a mouthful of toothpaste, "Oh no, Ken, tell me you didn't drop your watch?" I felt sick to my stomach for him.

His watch took a fateful spill last year at a Ritz Carlton on the marble floor. It landed on its crown, bending the stem to the point it could no longer be wound. After months of idly sitting in his jewelry drawer, I had it repaired and gave it to him as a gift—for the second time—over the holidays.

Ken said nothing, yet I could feel how upset he was. I rinsed my mouth and began patting it dry while watching him in the mirror. He was examining it over his sink under the light. But he wasn't holding his watch; instead it was the satchel that held my bracelet.

"Oh no, Ken, don't tell me it was the bracelet that fell. I only wore it once!" I blamed myself for not taking more care while placing it within the safe.

Of course Ken was blaming himself and just stood there with blinking eyes peering into the satchel. He then did the inevitable and pulled it from the bag. The beautiful bracelet was now a broken circle. The side depicting the lion as the victor had fallen from grace, separating its champion from his world. Its continuous sphere changed in a heartbeat, relegated to simply three chunks of ivory.

I felt like a child looking at a beloved toy that had been taken away—because it really wasn't mine to play with in the first place. I buried my eyes into the crook of my arm. I couldn't bear to look anymore and sobbed, "Oh, honey . . ." It was a one-of-a-kind piece—at least to us—and now it was *broken*.

Heart wrenchingly Ken implored, "I'll find a way to fix this."

"Oh, Ken . . . there's no way it'll ever look the same." We stood staring at the broken bracelet, then into each other's eyes and back to the bracelet again. We attempted to fit the pieces together, but had neither the knowledge nor ability to return it to its former luster.

"Apryl, don't ask me how, but I'm going to find someone who can restore it." I knew the chances were against us. Quite frankly, I believed the broken bracelet would lie within my jewelry drawer ruined forever. At least I got to enjoy its beauty for one night.

Lying in bed, neither of us could sleep. "Ken, you do know I don't blame you for it breaking."

"I know . . . but I do!" It broke my heart to hear him mentally berate himself.

"Honey, look inside the safe, all my jewelry has been thrown haphazardly in there. I should have taken more care when putting it away."

Unexpectedly using a force of strength, Ken grabbed and pulled me towards him. Crying aloud, our tears stained both our faces and the sheets. I've never known us to weep with such anguish—*together*.

Unsure of our grief, I questioned whether our heartbreak was for an exquisite piece of art, or what it represented—a broken body, a broken world or broken hearts. Only those of us who've encountered the shock of a life-altering event could possibly understand. When it fell, life came to a standstill. On so many levels Ken and I clung to one another. It was then I knew it was not because a material object had broken.

We cried ourselves to sleep that night, awakening the next morning with hearts that appeared to have mended during our hours of rest. Ken didn't allow me to see the bag, nor its broken contents, for the remainder of our trip.

It wasn't until we returned home, not knowing which bag he pulled it from, Ken stood holding the silken satchel. I watched as his serene expression changed to angst. Feebly attempting to deflect our heartaches, "Honey, let me put it in my jewelry drawer." Silently thinking to myself, *out of sight out of mind.* He tenderly handed me the soft gray bag with purple lining and watched as I carefully placed it in the drawer.

The next day, returning home from work, Ken asked I switch on our computer. Taking over the controls, he expertly navigated to a website for a Master Craftsman who restored fine art, paintings and *ivory!* "I'm not sure this is the person, but I did a lot of research and believe this is who can repair your bracelet. I'll send him an e-mail tomorrow."

Copying me on the e-mail, we received a response from the Craftsman requesting we send pictures. Elated, I took photos and forwarded them to Ken. Another e-mail was sent and within an hour we received an unexpected response:

> *From:*   *Pedro*
> *Sent:*   *Thursday, April 17, 2014 1:10 PM*
> *To:*   *Ken*
> *Subject:*   *Ivory Bracelet Repair*
>
> *Dear Ken,*
>
> *Interesting, my wife has an almost identical bracelet she inherited. She had a similar problem due to her dropping the piece. Yes, I can repair it back to its original state—I have also restored countless bracelets during the last 30 years of restoring ivory, many with similar problems due to the grain of the tusk.*
>
> *I can definitely work on your wife's piece. I have, however, a 2- to 3-week backlog. Would that be a problem for you? I could work on it right away if it is an urgent situation for you.*
>
> *Kind Regards,*
>
> *Pedro*

The time frame was insignificant as long as the bracelet was in good hands. And the next morning we FedEx'd it to the Craftsman; I had to force myself not to dwell on it.

Next on our never-ending list of doctor engagements was our "New Patient" appointments. First up, the *female* practitioner. (Sigh.) After a round of *"that's against our rules,"* we're allowed in. We reviewed with her in detail our medical history, needs, and the reason why we're in the market for a new internist. We liked her a lot, but weren't thrilled with her staff.

While inflating the cuff to take my blood pressure, she took the opportunity to voice a worry. "My only concern for you, Apryl, regarding your Tango with Jorge, is the choice you've made regarding Tamoxifen. *If* in 10 years from now he returns, you won't berate yourself over the decision you've made, will you?" This was a question no one had asked before and it genuinely seemed to come from her heart.

"No, the decision is mine and mine alone. Should he return for a second Tango, at that time, I'll opt for a Double M." *But he won't be returning*, I add silently.

"Okay, I just want you to know there is a very serious possibility he could return, and you should be aware of the potential fallout from your decision." I like her; she has a kind way with words and she knew I hadn't come by this decision without serious contemplation.

At the beginning of our "New Patient" appointment with the *male* practitioner some unexpected acrobatics were required when we initially arrive, due to these same Admin Junkies. Eventually we're seated in his examining room; this time Ken is on the table. No more than five minutes pass when there's a polite rap on the door and in walks the physician. I like him immediately! Don't ask me why; there's just something about the way he carries himself, his thoughtful introduction and his calming demeanor.

After greetings, I ask, "I'm interested in knowing why you're a five-star doctor?" I get right to the details at hand.

"You know ... I think it's because I take pride in treating my patients as I would my own family," and thus we began discussing at length our reason for being here.

He was thoughtful while listening to our needs and concerns and we didn't feel rushed in the slightest. Nor did he seem overly spent or stressed, which you'd expect at 4:30 in the afternoon when he's seeing his last patent. I knew it when he first walked in the door, but now I was certain, we just met with our new internist. At long last we feel confident in the doctors we have.

Pedro, the Master Craftsman, comes from a family of architects. His grandfather was the personal architect to Emperor Maximillian and traveled with him from Austria to Mexico. Both Pedro's father and uncle followed in their father's footsteps, as did Pedro's brother. Yes, Pedro is well acquainted with architecture and those who create it.

During their initial e-mails, Ken mentioned to Pedro that our bracelet had a very special meaning. *"Circumstances that preceded the purchase was one of the reasons we had acquired it."* Shortly thereafter Ken received a phone call from Pedro; he was curious about its unique significance. Without going into grave detail, Ken told him of my tango with Jorge.

Pedro, taken aback by the meaning of Ken's gift—more so what the bracelet represented—in turn conveyed the importance of his wife's bracelet. It happened to be an almost identical twin to mine and appeared to have been made by the same artisan. But what made the significance of these two bracelets so profound is how Aliza, Pedro's wife, came into possession of hers.

A family friend was the original caretaker of Aliza's bracelet, which she had inherited from her mother. Ironically, this friend was a Tango survivor herself, and years later the family friend handed down her bracelet to Aliza as a token of admiration and kinship.

Genuine compassion could be felt as Pedro continued, "Within the first two years of our marriage we were told Aliza had an ill-fated Tango; she was in her late 20s and doctors gave her two years to live. Thankfully, she surpassed the two-year mark. But sadly, during this period, her mother began a Tango very different from hers and was tragically taken from our family."

Pedro ended his tale with great enthusiasm. "Aliza and I will be celebrating our 19th wedding anniversary in May!!!" Ken was in disbelief.

Phoning me, he recounted the meaning of my bracelet's twin. I found myself overtaken by emotion.

This bracelet ... it wasn't a mere *bracelet*. It had meaning that obviously went beyond our comprehension. Its purpose, yet to be discovered, had brought our worlds together. *Fate*—alluring and intoxicating—continued to linger in my world.

Reflecting back to when I first slipped the bracelet on, I contemplated whether there are such things as past lives. Could by chance this beautiful piece of work have possibly adorned one's soul before? Or, maybe, within its circle it had brought together two very different stories—as depicted on the bracelet itself. Two worlds and lives set apart from everything, and one misfortune—this one turn of *fate* was meant to bring us together?

With remarkable skill, Pedro repaired the bracelet and returned it to us within a week of receiving it. Ken sent an e-mail thanking him for the unanticipated quick repair. Within minutes Pedro responded:

> *From:*   Pedro
> *Sent:*   *Tuesday, May 06, 2014 3:17 PM*
> *To:*   *Ken*
> *Subject:*   *Very Brave Ladies*
>
> *Dearest Ken,*
>
> *You and I share the unfortunate journey of being caretakers of very brave ladies. I've had the privilege to do so for 16 years now! Our latest scare was over the weekend due to pain and the possibility of an implant breaking. In fact, we just came from the radiologist—thank God all is well.*
>
> *The fear of Jorge returning never goes away. For years to come, you will be your wife's source of strength and support as a partner ... always holding onto one's belief of hope, that in turn keeps our loved ones alive. Why do I tell you this? Maybe because I'm 15 years ahead of you with the situation! I'm here anytime for anything you*

need from paintings, woodworks and ivory to friendship and support.

Thank you for appreciating my ability to restore fine arts. I am blessed with the opportunity to do what I love—and I get paid for it! To me, it's not a job, it brings me great joy and fun! We found some cool original frescos in the cathedral restoration that I undertook last week—the original date is 1867!

I'm so happy to know your wife is pleased with the restoration. Stay well and feel free to contact me anytime.

Pedro

I was in awe of Pedro's craftsmanship when I received our bracelet. He had restored it back to its original beauty. You would never have imagined this bracelet had fallen from a protective haven and lay broken on a cold stone floor. But the words still echoed within my mind—*broken body, broken world, broken hearts*. It truly is remarkable—two worlds and lives set apart—and a *broken* bracelet was to bring us together? But why? I had to thank him for the repair, but more so for sharing their story with us.

From:	*Apryl*
Sent:	*Tuesday, May 06, 2014 5:58 PM*
To:	*Pedro*
Subject:	*Thank You . . .*

Dearest Pedro~

We received our beautiful bracelet on Friday. To say we were stunned with your workmanship is an understatement—Pedro, you are incredibly talented! As Ken had mentioned to you in previous e-mails, we were heartbroken when it fell from the safe onto the stone floor of our hotel room. At the time I had only worn it once.

One can't help but wonder, could this be fate? The shivering of my spine when it was placed on my wrist. The thoughtfulness of purchasing it as a gift. The falling and breaking into many pieces. The search for a Master Craftsman to put it back together—this time with the strength to endure many years to come. How many more worlds will this bracelet touch? The delicacy of life is something we all too often take for granted.

Thank you for restoring our piece. I know the story of this bracelet will not end here. It's obvious to Ken and I it was meant we were to make one another's acquaintance. Although I went through only an inkling of what your wife had to endure, the shock of catastrophic news such as this reverberates throughout a lifetime. Leaving you always wondering when, if, and ultimately thank God it's over—but is it ever really over?

Again, thank you . . . you have our deepest appreciation for the return of a gift that will forever—on so many levels—be dear to my heart.

With kindest wishes and loving appreciation,

Apryl.

Driving to see The King the next morning, my phone notified me I had received an e-mail—it was from Pedro.

From:	*Pedro*
Sent:	*Tuesday, May 08, 2014 9:26 AM*
To:	*Apryl*
Subject:	*You're Welcome . . .*

Dearest Apryl,

I don't know how to thank you for your sweet incredible e-mail—it has brought tears to my eyes. I completely understand what it means to go through a life-changing circumstance such as this. Maybe being an artist allows me to feel the world in a different way, and I in turn allow myself to let go and have tears. Thank you for giving us the opportunity to restore the pieces of your bracelet—to make it whole once again—and for choosing to add the necessary strength to the original piece. Strength for a long lasting repair . . . one that can be handed down over years to come! My hope is that the restoration of your bracelet translates to a restoration of your health and well-being! When you have a moment my wife wishes to tell you herself of the very similar stories your bracelets share.

Kind regards,

Pedro

On so many levels I wanted to speak with his wife, and quickly sent a response to his e-mail.

From:	*Apryl*
Sent:	*Tuesday, May 08, 2014 9:46 AM*
To:	*Pedro*
Subject:	*Love to speak with Aliza!*

We're headed to an oncologist appointment as I type this. Yes . . . I'd love to speak with Aliza sometime in the future!

Kindly,

Apryl

Stepping on the elevator, we ascend to The King's floor. Cordially greeted, we respond to the usual compulsory questions and pay my co-pay, after which we're asked to complete two pages of paperwork. But no sooner did I start filling in the blank lines then my name was called.

Before I could respond, the check-in clerk, hearing my name, answered on my behalf, "Apryl will be with you in a moment." Looking to me she directed, "Finish the paperwork . . . it won't take long; the nurse will wait." *Wow, that's a change; the nurse will wait.*

Scribbling as fast as I could, I returned the completed form to the check-in clerk. A little nervously, I plod towards the swinging doors with the nurse patiently awaiting my arrival. Greeting us with a smile, he leads us down the short hallway and takes my vitals. "Hmmm . . . your blood pressure seems to be a bit elevated. You'll need to keep an eye on that." *Okay . . . I thought to myself, but I think I know what's causing it.*

Following him into The King's chamber, he directs me to change into the gown neatly folded on the examining table and excused himself. I slipped it on and then The King himself lightly rapped on the door. He entered with the same charisma I remembered him having at our first meeting. After brief cordialities, he recounted our last appointment, remembering practically every detail; *he must use tickler notes.*

His eyes then flooded with concern and a raised eyebrow. "When I last saw you I prescribed Tamoxifen, but you're not taking it. Why?"

Shrugging my shoulders, "I'm worried about my mental well-being, not to mention the other side effects it causes."

"I understand, Apryl . . . but this is your *life* we're talking about," he stresses.

This has been a heart-wrenching decision and I thought I'd made it. "So you feel that strongly I should be taking it . . . even though it will only give me an additional 3 percent of added protection—and with no guarantee?" The King could see my anguish.

"As I mentioned during our last appointment, I have another patient about your age on it and she has the same aversion to prescription drugs. We've divided her dosage in two; she takes it twice a day and appears to be doing just fine."

"I don't know . . . this is all so scary to me." I was truly at a stalemate and finding it difficult to commit to this drug.

"Apryl . . . it's time you make a decision; otherwise it will be too late. You've only got a short time frame now before the opportunity is gone." He could see my anxiety as he looked deep into my eyes. "How about this . . . just commit to it for one month. It takes about three weeks for the drug to completely enter your system. If after a month it's absolutely horrific and you can't handle it, then go off it."

It sounded reasonable. "Okay, I can commit to *one* month." I was willing to place the wretched pill in my mouth. Now I just need the persuasion to swallow it.

Changing the subject, I ask, "So why do I need an oncologist and why should I continue the follow-up appointments with the Medicine Woman and Radiation Man?"

"I'll be watching you for the next couple of years. I know what to look for and will immediately know if Jorge decides to make another appearance. As for your Medicine Woman, honestly, there's no reason to see her more than once or twice *after* your surgery. It's really up to you at this point. As for your Radiation Man, he'll want to keep an eye on the aftereffects of his treatment. You'll probably only need to see him one or two more times at most." The King was being ever so diplomatic.

"The Medicine Woman has given me an order for another mammogram. I was considering going back to Imaging Center #1, but wanted to get your opinion."

"It would be more beneficial for you at this time if you came to our facility. That way the reports and mammograms are easily accessible to me and, should anything cause me concern, I know exactly who to speak with."

"Fine . . . I'll come here." It made perfect sense and I feel confident in The King.

Somehow I got it in my head it wasn't the best idea to have surgery on radiated tissue; maybe it was because THE Shape Shifter had made such a fuss over it. *My* Shape Shifter said not to concern myself with it, but of course I am. I thought who better to ask than The King!

"Is it problematic to have reconstructive surgery on tissue that's been radiated? I mean, have you heard of any problems when doing so?" *God, let this not be problematic.*

"As long as you've given your body time to heal it's not an issue. I know some really great Shape Shifters, so when you're ready let me know and I'll get you their names." *Whew . . . check that worry off the list!*

"I have one final question. Over the past couple of years I've noticed a red blotch that comes and goes in the crease of my left breast. No one seems to know what it is and during radiation the entire crease under my breast turned brown. Is this something I should be concerned about?"

"No, I've seen it before. Some women get yeast in their breasts. Similar to a yeast infection with relatively no side effects other than the red blotches and yes . . . it would turn brown after radiation. It's nothing you need to worry about."

Finally . . . someone confident in an answer. "Now that you said it, I vaguely recall showing the red blotches to my dermatologist years ago. I believe that's what she said it was, too." *Yippee . . . I can officially cross another worry off my list!*

Exhibiting no signs of feeling rushed, The King *listened* to my every concern and was thoughtful in his responses to questions. With heartfelt care, he circumnavigated my indecisiveness about Tamoxifen. Ultimately, he left us to schedule my annual mammogram—which we did for May 14th. And then—what I've been dreading most—his assistant again phoned in a prescription for Tamoxifen.

His last request was an easy one. "I'd like to see you again in September." Ken and I left feeling more on track than we have since this whole convoluted Tango began.

During our meeting with The King, Pedro had gone to my website and purchased both of my albums. Immediately I sent him an e-mail:

From:	*Apryl*
Sent:	*Tuesday, May 08, 2014 11:18 AM*
To:	*Pedro*
Subject:	*They were supposed to be a gift!*

Pedro!!!

I was going to send my CDs as a thank you — a gift! I can't believe you did that . . .

Apryl.

From: Pedro
Sent: Tuesday, May 08, 2014 1:12 PM
To: Apryl
Subject: They are a gift!

Apryl!!!!

Thanks so much for thinking about sending them as a gift, but I believe in supporting fellow artists! Besides, they are a gift . . . our anniversary is coming up! Can you overnight them? I'll reimburse you. I hope all went well with your oncologist today.

I better run as I'm writing from the cathedral and my carpenter has questions. Have a great day and let's stay in touch!

Pedro

From: Apryl
Sent: Tuesday, May 08, 2014 3:35 PM
To: Pedro
Subject: The gift has been shipped!

Pedro~

The CDs are being sent overnight and should arrive to you by 10:30 tomorrow morning. And please, you do not need to reimburse me for the shipping . . . Happy Anniversary!

The King's appointment went well. He wants me to go on Tamoxifen. I've finally given in and told him I'd try it for 1 month—I don't do well on medication. Do you know if Aliza is or has taken this drug? I'm interested in talking to her about this as it's been a heart-wrenching decision for me.

With that being said, I will definitely call her! Is there a particular time that's best to reach her? I may not be able to phone until the early part of next week. I'll try to get an e-mail off to her though . . .

Apryl.

From:	Pedro
Sent:	Tuesday, May 08, 2014 3:51 PM
To:	Apryl
Subject:	Call Aliza

That's great news!

Please talk to Aliza, she has been on it for well over a decade and feels it's been an important factor for her being alive—she swears by it!

She's had so much exposure and experience on the subject—of course, that's added to all her medical research since she's a nurse. Text or call her right now if you want.

Pedro

It seemed Pedro knew I was attempting to postpone the call—or maybe my mother intervened sending him her urgent little nudges. Whatever the explanation, within minutes I received another e-mail.

From: *Pedro*
Sent: *Tuesday, May 08, 2014 3:55 PM*
To: *Apryl*
Subject: *Call Now . . .*

I told Aliza you'll be calling . . . she is so excited. She has her mobile with her at this moment, so by all means call her.

Pedro

Rats . . . I was hoping to have this conversation another day. But since I'm now at the office waiting for Ken to finish with a meeting, I might as well call her.

"Hi, Aliza, it's Apryl Allen!" Of course we immediately hit it off. She has quite the enthusiastic personality! But what I loved most was how passionate she was about her Tango. She's a year older than me and has been Tangoing for nearly *20 years*; of course she's passionate!

She spoke candidly about her Tango and how aggressive it was, unlike mine. She went on to explain, "I did the math of percentages too; however I went in the opposite direction. I kept asking myself, '*What can I do to raise my percentages of survival?*'" Interestingly she added, "I don't know if you're aware, but if ever Jorge returns, no matter what form he takes, he'll be considered *metastatic breast cancer*."

"No . . . I didn't know that."

Aliza continued discussing her Tango. "I did everything you did, including five rounds of chemotherapy, meaning five different types, each requiring its own protocol." I felt a lump form in my throat and tears filled my eyes; *Apryl, this could have been so much worse*. She then explained, "As a preventative measure, I even went as far as having a stem cell transplant in efforts to eliminate Jorge completely." I couldn't believe what I was hearing. *What this poor girl has gone through!* "So when Tamoxifen came along I couldn't get it fast enough; I truly believe this drug has kept me alive!"

"What about the side effects?"

"The only thing I can remember were the hot flashes, but I didn't care; they just weren't that bothersome to me. Maybe because of how desperate I was to live. During this period I had decided to finish my nursing degree; I loved going to class because they kept the rooms cold. But like I said, this drug was saving my life so I was willing to put up with *anything!*" While listening to her Tango tale, I contemplated mine and realized, *but I'm at low risk—and not in as desperate a situation as she was.*

As if working on the final pieces of a puzzle, the meaning of the *broken bracelet* began to fit together when she told me about her family friend whose Tango was very similar to *mine*. She had been in her late 40s when she met Jorge and did *exactly* what I did—surgery, radiation and, thankfully, she too did not require chemo. Now she's 80-years-old and sadly her Tango has returned, only this time it has taken one of her lungs.

I sat in disbelief. And, just to dispel *any* potential uncertainties, Aliza said, "Apryl, after Pedro forwarded your e-mail I wanted to respond immediately . . . but nothing came to me. This might sound strange to you, but if ever I need inspiration or want to speak with my mother I go outside and look to clouds for answers . . ." Okay, Aliza now has my complete and undivided attention. ". . . She's always there for me. However, this time there was nothing. Instead, all I could hear was her voice repeating what she constantly said to me when she was alive, *'there are no coincidences.'*"

I couldn't believe what I was hearing. I imagine my mother is standing next to me whispering, *"I'm here Apryl—follow your heart and you'll be fine!"* "Aliza, I know the reason for the bracelet . . . all of this has happened so I could learn of your and your friend's Tangos. I understand now, even though I'm faced with a terrifying disease, I still have choices. It's ultimately up to me to decide what is best. More importantly, I have a choice when it comes to Tamoxifen . . . and because you did so well on it, I'll at least give it a try."

After ending the call, I filled Ken in on every detail of our conversation while driving directly to the pharmacy to pick up my very own bottle of Tamoxifen! This phone call took place on Thursday, May 8th. For whatever reason, when I begin a new routine I have a tendency to start it on Sundays. This also gave me a little more time to contemplate whether I would take the pills.

Mulling decisions within the windmills of your mind is probably not the optimal way to come to a conclusion. I stare at the bottle. I open it and peer inside at the little white pills. I even smell them to see if they have a particular odor . . . *nothing*.

Friday and Saturday came and went. On Sunday I greet Ken with our usual morning hug. Sitting down at our kitchen counter I reach for the bottle of Tamoxifen and take my first pill, not realizing on this particular Sunday, May 11th, it's *Mother's Day!* Amused, I laugh inwardly. *Aliza . . . your mother's right, there are no coincidences!*

24

Velvet Voice

Apryl Allen, Julio Fernandez & Richie Cannata

It's the morning of my annual mammogram ... I'm nervous. I have literally come full circle. I know in my heart of hearts my tango is over—but all the emotions, angst, fear and heartache are still very real and very raw. Opening my closet door, I contemplate wearing one of my long skirts because they're comfortable and easy to maneuver in.

Searching through the hangers I come across the beautiful tranquil blue and purple skirt, my favorite. Suddenly a flash of lightning from last year's mammogram strikes and I realize I was wearing this exact skirt at the time. Hanging it back in its place, I make a mental note to wear *another* skirt.

I finish drying my hair and Ken asks how much longer I'll be. "It's going to take us 30 minutes to get there and that's 10 minutes from now." Feeling a bit rushed I quickly finish and we drive to what is now my inescapable appointment.

Once seated in the waiting room, I look down at my hands nervously folded on my lap and can't believe my eyes; I'm wearing the blue and purple skirt, the one I *wasn't* going to wear. I inhale deeply—*everything is going to be just fine!*

Soon after this realization, my name is called. I follow the young woman down a few short halls to what looks like a locker room. Peering down a very long hallway, one side is lined with doors to dressing rooms and the other are the treatment rooms. I was taken to one of the changing rooms and step inside. It's only large enough for one person to maneuver within. The locker is tall and thin with a bench next to it that's a little on the high side; meaning, if you sat on it, your feet would dangle below, not touching the ground.

"There's a gown in the locker; please change into it from the waist up with the opening in the front." I didn't have the heart to tell the young woman I knew the routine all too well. She left me to follow her instructions and I slipped off my blouse; however, when I opened the locker, someone's clothes were already in it. I could hear a tech in the hall finishing up with another woman and I just knew these were her clothes. I quickly placed my top back on and exited the small dressing room.

Sure enough it was a much older woman's clothes. She had to be in her 80s and looked extremely tired. The tech ushered her into the changing room and closed the door. Turning to me, "Can I help you? Is something wrong?" She could see the concerned look on my face.

I quickly explained the situation. "Yeah—the older women always forget to lock their doors." *Then why don't you double-check the lockers when you come to get them? Is nobody thoughtful? It's life and sometimes we all could use a helpful hand!* With no thought at all she escorted me into another nearby room.

Once changed, I open the door and sit on the bench to wait. I assume that's what I'm supposed to do—leave the door open so the tech sees me when she comes back. Sure enough she arrives and takes me into a corner treatment room.

"I just love your skirt! Where did you get it?" And would you believe we have almost the exact conversation as I had a year ago with the other mammo tech?! Life really is cyclical!!!

"Please drop your right arm out of your gown and place it on this bar. While I position your breast you may feel a bit of a pinch ... I hope I don't hurt you." She then smashed my right breast to the height of a pancake using the mammo machine. After several poses, we performed the same ones on my left breast, adding a few more, for good measure I guess.

I did shed a few tears. I didn't expect to, but I guess it's due to the emotional roller coaster I've just gotten off of. Finally, it's over. "Please have a seat back in your changing room; *our* Breast Investigator will be out to go over your results shortly. Also, don't change into your clothing until he meets with you, just in case he needs a couple of more pictures." *God, please let this Breast Investigator be happy with what he sees.*

I waited for maybe 10 minutes when a young thin man came walking down the hall. Peering into my changing room he inquired, "Apryl Allen?"

"Yes . . ." This time I was calm and knew in my heart *everything was perfectly fine!*

"I reviewed your mammogram and everything looks good. We'd like to see you back in November, simply due to your Tango."

Thanking this young Breast Investigator, I changed as quickly as I could back into my clothes. Then, as fast as I could walk I raced to the door I knew Ken was waiting behind—attempting not to break into a run. Opening the door, I turn the corner . . . *and there he was.* All the emotions from this past year came flooding back as tears began streaking my face.

"Honey . . . is everything okay?" I could only nod my head yes. "Oh, honey . . . come on, let's go have lunch."

During lunch Ken asked again, "Are you okay?"

"I just want to go home and cry," I said, attempting to hold the tears at bay.

"Finish your lunch, sweetheart." I watch as his fingers moved fervently over the letters on his phone.

When we return home he followed me inside. "Ken . . . I'm really okay."

"I'm not leaving you alone; we're spending the afternoon *together!*" His velvet voice was calm and tender.

A couple of weeks later, after collecting our mail, I received the response from ACME Insurance regarding the surgical assistant. ACME had received the appeal on April 9th and responded on May 23rd:

> "We approved network benefits because the service was rendered at a network hospital and you had no control over which surgical assistant the physician would use. Therefore, the claim was reprocessed at the network level of benefits to allow 10 percent of the MAF. An Explanation of Benefits is forthcoming indicating ACME paid $78.17. ACME does not consider the unpaid portion to be your responsibility; however, non-network providers may bill you for any amount not paid by ACME."

This was maddening! Basically I saved myself $80 — taking hours out of my day to appeal the unpaid charges, and now I'm responsible for the remaining $220. I love how ACME notated it *"does not consider the unpaid portion to be my responsibility"* — how exactly does that help me? Try telling that to the surgical facility which has all of my personal information, freely given to them *without my authorization!*

Of course I can choose not to pay the bill, and would be within my rights to do so. However, this out-of-network surgical assistant can legally send any unpaid portion of her bill to collections. All the pains my husband and I have meticulously taken over the years to insure we have *perfect* credit, in one push of a button, would end.

We've worked diligently cultivating and caring for the credit we have today and now this surgical facility is holding our perfect score for ransom — $221.83, to be exact. She's getting paid more than three times the normal fee. What a *great system.*

Reluctantly I phone the Medicine Woman's office to discuss why an out-of-network surgical assistant was engaged, fully expecting Mabel to answer the phone. To my surprise, the Medicine Woman herself answers. Therefore, I opted to start with a more innocuous subject, with a question I had regarding the specimen date on the Agendia report.

"I noticed that the specimen sent in for the Agendia report had a collection date of July 9th — when the Breast Investigator did the initial biopsy of Jorge. Can this be correct?" *This answer ought to be interesting.*

"Yes; we as surgeons have the choice to send in the biopsy or a portion of the tumor from the surgery. I prefer to send in the biopsy."

Holy Crap!!!!! IF they had sent my biopsy in when it was initially done, I would have known I was at low risk from the get-go. Having the knowledge there was no urgency to my surgery, I would have done things so differently. Instead, under duress, I had to make decisions about my future and life. Not to mention all the bullshit "what-ifs!" And *El Tango* would never have happened.

My breath caught and all I could muster was a feeble "Okay." I had to change the subject.

Explaining I had appealed the invoice for the surgical assistant and ACME's decision to pay the $80, I questioned, "I don't understand why services for an out-of-network surgical assistant were engaged?"

Well, the Medicine Woman was all talk today. "If the surgery is over an hour I engage the services of a surgical assistant, primarily because it's far too cumbersome and alleviates some of the physical duress my body takes on during surgeries such as this." *Okay, shouldn't she have informed me one would be required?* "And, no, I didn't verify whether the surgical assistant was in your network. That's who was available at the time we booked your surgery."

Ultimately the conversation ended with her blaming the healthcare system and how unfair it is to those in need. "You should contact the surgical assistant's billing office and discuss it with them. Maybe since your insurance company will be paying the $80, it will be willing to drop the other charges." *Yeah, right, and I have some oceanfront property I'd like to sell you down the street.* "I know they'll take payments if that's the difficulty here."

"No, we can afford to pay it. It's the principle of the matter I have the issue with. I have perfectly good insurance that would have covered these charges had someone been chosen in-network. It's especially annoying since we're already paying astronomical rates for insurance."

Again, the same response. "I recommend you contact the billing department for the surgical assistant; it may very well drop the charges."

"I can't imagine it would do that; the billing department is going to insist I pay the remaining balance. They basically have me over a barrel."

"Yeah, that's how insurance is." *But it's the inflated rate of the out-of-network surgical assistant I'm upset about. Obviously there's nothing that can be done.*

"Okay . . . well, I'm also calling to schedule my next appointment with you . . ."

"Hold on. I'll get Mabel," and I'm placed on hold.

When the receiver is again picked up, Mabel greets me. "Hi, Apryl! Let's get your next appointment scheduled . . ." I could hear her plucking away at the keys on her computer.

"Exactly how long will I be needing these follow-up appointments?"

"Forever . . ."

"Really?" That totally contradicted what The King said to me.

"Yes, for the next two years you will have appointments with the Medicine Woman every four months. Then the two years that follow, you will see her every six months. The fifth year is considered your 'cure year' and you'll only need to see her annually from that point forward."

"Seriously? I had no idea . . ."

"Yes, the Medicine Woman is an expert when it comes to breasts. For instance, she caught the fact a Tango had returned four years later on another patient—and that patient had just been to her oncologist who didn't catch it."

"Wow . . . okay." Honestly, I was in more disbelief I'm now a lifetime patient of the Medicine Woman, at least until she decides to retire.

And then, having overheard my conversation with the Medicine Woman, "Consider yourself lucky your insurance is covering anything at all towards the surgical assistant. We're finding patients who've not been diagnosed with breast cancer, yet have tested positive for the BRCA genes, are being denied coverage for mastectomies." *How horrible, but that's a completely different battle,* I thought to myself. We ended the call after scheduling my next appointment in August.

Note to self: In the future, if ever I find myself or a loved one facing some sort of Tango, whomever we have chosen as our specialist will be given a letter stipulating he or she is only allowed to engage the services of those who are within our network.

Now I understand there's that rare possibility an out-of-network service provider is required and the entity wanting to be engaged is someone whom the doctor prefers and trusts—but at least give me the courtesy of knowing. This way I can plan accordingly, with no surprises, nor added stress to an already stressful situation. I can then do my due diligence and find out what my financial obligation will be, thus leaving me, the individual attempting to heal, with peace of mind and the ability to actually *heal.*

It's June 16th and I have yet to receive a statement from the surgical assistant's facility. Rather than waiting for the invoice, I decide to inquire about my balance. Prior to doing so I enlist the help of Olivia, to decipher the meaning of *"10 Percent of MAF"*—ACME referred to it regarding the decision on my appeal.

It means *Maximum Allowable Fee*. Basically, it's the maximum amount ACME will pay a provider for a procedure. How it works is ACME contracts with providers, wherein a provider agrees to take a percentage of their fee as payment. Ergo, had the surgical assistant been contracted with ACME, she would have been required to accept the $78.17 as payment in full. Instead she's billing for more than three times the amount. *How is this legal?*

Armed with all the information I think I'll need, I phone the billing clerk and get right to the matter at hand. "It appears my appeal has been resolved and ACME Insurance has agreed to pay 10 percent of the MAF, which is $78.17." Butterflies in my stomach begin fluttering, but I decide to go for it. "I've spoken with both the Medicine Woman and our insurance agent and they're both in agreement with ACME Insurance. The overage is technically not my responsibility."

"I understand, but it's up to the surgical assistant to decide whether she'll take it as payment in full. I can e-mail her, but I can't guarantee anything."

I have to admit the billing clerk has a calm demeanor and doesn't let my anxiety-driven frustration fluster her in the slightest. "What I'm *really* perplexed about is *why*, when the Medicine Woman requested a surgical assistant, neither the doctor nor your facility went the extra mile to ensure that person was in my network." For heaven's sake, they had weeks before my surgery to figure this out.

Calmly she replied, "That's not how it works. The hospital requests the first assistant and we're the company with which it contracts. So basically it's whoever's on duty the day of your surgery."

My head was doing somersaults attempting to digest her explanation. "Let me get this straight: A first assistant and surgical assistant are the same thing, correct?"

"Yes, that is correct."

"And the Medicine Woman didn't have a choice; she just informed the hospital that she required a surgical assistant on that particular day for my surgery." As I said this the Medicine Woman's response reverberated within my head: *"That's who was available at the time we booked your surgery."*

"Yes, that's correct. There was no way for her to know whether the surgical assistant was in or out of your net-work. She just happened to be the individual on duty that day."

My head was reeling. *If the company the surgical assistant is employed with is contracted with an in-network hospital, doesn't it make sense the surgical assistant should be required to take the negotiated rate as payment in full?* I knew she couldn't answer this question and didn't waste my breath asking it.

Prior to ending the call, the billing clerk assured me, "I'll send an e-mail to the surgical assistant and ask if she'll accept the $78.17 from ACME as payment in full. But like I said, at minimum her normal fee for something like this is $300. I'll call you when I receive her response." Well, at least she didn't say *no, make the payment in full.*

It seems everything has just about come full circle. Would you believe when Ken brought the mail in, I received a check from the Mad Scientist's office for that $45 *"El Tango"* credit. It appears it was never applied to any of my bills and the office finally got around to refunding it, *nine months later!*

On June 26th it will be one year exactly since I was made aware of Jorge. I feel it befitting to have all the loose ends of my tango tied up prior to this day. Therefore, on Monday I contacted the surgical assistant's billing clerk regarding another statement we received on Saturday. This time it reflects the payment from ACME Insurance, with a remaining balance of $221.83.

"I haven't received her response yet. It usually takes a few days due to her hectic schedule." *Yeah . . . well, I'd like to get back to my former self and she's keeping me from doing so.*

"All I can do is send another e-mail." *What's wrong with calling her?* I thought. *Does anyone even use the phone anymore?* The billing clerk continued, "There's always the possibility she's out-of-town on vacation. I'll let you know as soon as I hear anything."

Five days after that phone call I received another statement in the mail. The balance due reflected $71.83. Highlighted on the bottom left corner of the page was the following note from the billing clerk:

> "The surgical assistant has agreed to accept $150 minus the amount the insurance paid of $78.17. The total

> *amount due by you is $71.83 and that will make your account paid in full. Thank you"*

I guess the billing clerk couldn't bother herself to make a phone call. Of course I immediately wrote the check for $71.83 and put it in the mail.

Being curious, I phoned both Mabel and Iris to better understand why the specimen from my biopsy, taken on July 9th, wasn't sent into Agendia at that time by the Imaging Center. Both women wanted to look at my records to assure me they followed procedures correctly, which they did—but I wasn't questioning that. They both seemed perplexed by my query. Their reasoning . . . that's what the surgeon does and I hadn't chosen mine at the time.

The period that lapsed during this time alarms me for two reasons. First, how do I know my specimen wasn't mixed up with another person's? I mean, it was shelved from July 9th until August 22nd and lesser things have been known to happen. And second, you're telling me, we as patients are expected to *wait* to hear about every detail pertaining to our future health? I truly don't understand how our healthcare system is allowed to do this.

Seriously . . . doesn't it make sense that it should be your internist's responsibility to send it in? Imagine how confident you'd feel to have your personal physician, whom presumably you trust, help you understand Jorge and assist in putting a game plan together for your Tango. They're the ones with all the medical knowledge and know intimately our personal health issues. Can you imagine the amount of stress this would eliminate?

I guess I'm just expected to be happy my tango with Jorge is over. I pray, should you ever find yourself in my shoes, you're able to tango better than me. Now I have a whole new perspective when I hear another individual say he or she is celebrating their umpteenth anniversary of a tango. Thank you to all of the entities and individuals attempting to find the cure—stay your course! Your efforts have prolonged my life!

I can't believe it's been a year since I was made aware of Jorge. It feels as if it were a lifetime ago. Shockingly, I find the most trying moments to have been the endless waiting periods, and having to deal with those individuals who appear to have no compassion for the patients. The treatments, at least for me, were relatively easy.

As for Tamoxifen, I've officially been on it for 46 days. I'm happy to report I feel relatively normal. It's funny because when Ken and I have a little tiff, I find I start scanning myself and question, *"Am I upset because it's a normal argument OR is it the pill causing me to overreact emotionally?"* Always I come back to the same conclusion: *"It's just a little argument . . . nothing more"* and Ken always backs me up on this belief. I do find, however, I shed a tear a little more than usual, nothing over the top, thank goodness.

Around the three-week time frame I began feeling bloated and sometimes find I have a tingling sensation in my fingers, hands, calves and feet. It feels as if I've eaten a meal high in sodium. I've also noticed that occasionally I feel dizzy. For instance, if I bend down and stand back up too quickly I feel light-headed. At night, while sleeping, my legs will occasionally cramp and strangely, my calves feel tight and have hardened. Working out doesn't appear to lessen the tightness nor does a good stretch.

Around the fourth week I felt kind of woozy down below, sort of like I use to feel before my period would start when I was younger. However, this was more pronounced and lasted for a week, maybe a week and a half; as of today I no longer feel it. Also, I seem to switch from being a bit on the warm side to being a little chilly. Again, nothing horrible either way.

As for how my body is recovering from surgery, my arm occasionally has a dull achy feeling, but as long as I keep up with my workouts and stretches it appears to alleviate it. Mysteriously, the muscle from my bicep to the palm of my hand some days feels as if it's never been used and could snap; other days I feel nothing at all. It doesn't appear to be associated with stretches or workouts.

My left breast still has the tan, although it has lightened up quite a bit. It's strange; you can see how the beams went across my breast, forming the corner of a square starting at the bottom of my left underarm. As for my scars, where Jorge was, it's still a thin, three-inch, gray line and I definitely am concaved in that area. And where the Lymph-Along-Kid was, that scar looks the best and is quickly fading to just a thin line; you probably wouldn't even notice it was there. Where the drain was, that is still a round red scar about the size of a dime, but it too is fading.

How do I feel? I feel happy! My body feels strong and healthy and I simply adore my life! How do I feel about my future with Tamoxifen? To be honest . . . I'm not sure. If Ms. Hyde decides to rear her ugly head, it will be at that time Ken and I get to make a decision. Basically I'm going take one day at a time . . . because that's what I have, *time*!

25

Million Years Ago
Adele

The King is *dead* . . . yes, you read correctly. On Saturday, July 5th, I received a letter dated June 30th from the *Management Team* at the cancer center where The King resides. It stated, *"As of July 4th, The King will no longer be practicing at our facility."* Offering, *"During this transition, it is our goal to continue to provide you with excellent and uninterrupted care"* and listed names of *other* oncologists at their facility.

I know I've said it before, but trust in doctors is hard to find. It seems any confidence I've had for our healthcare system is being stripped away! How can a doctor who seemed to genuinely care about his patients simply up and leave? I don't even get a personal letter, only a dreary unsigned black and white *copy*. I feel empty . . . completely blank. I don't have it in me to search for another doctor. And now I'm on Tamoxifen with no one to monitor me? What about the side effects I've begun to have? Who will address those?

The week following this news, I receive a bill dated July 4th for my annual mammogram in the amount of $402. 86. This can't be right, and I contact the facility to inquire of the invoice. The woman I speak with offers to look into it on my behalf and said she'd get back with me.

Having received no return call from Woman #1, on August 6th I try again; of course she isn't available and I start over with a different person. Woman #2 claims there is no error and tells me I need to pay the invoice in full. I in turn ask to speak with her manager.

After being transferred to Woman #3, she informs me the procedure was coded as a mammogram with a history of breast cancer. Further research finds the code on the doctor's form has caused ACME to request medical records to verify there was indeed a prior history of breast cancer. *Duh . . . can't ACME find it in their records?* Since the records have been sent to ACME, I am to phone back in two weeks regarding its status. Another hour from my life . . . *gone.*

It's now been two weeks since my last call and, prior to speaking with The King's facility, I decide to contact ACME Insurance first with hopes they can shed some light on it. ACME informs me because my mammogram was performed at a hospital, it was billed at a higher rate. It's also considered an outpatient procedure, which of course goes towards my annual $2,000 deductible. And since I haven't met my deductible for 2014, I'm required to pay for the mammogram. Had The King coded it as a preventative mammo, I wouldn't have owed anything. *Are you kidding me?*

"You can ask the facility to recode and resubmit the bill if you think it will do that."

Now I have a mission and dial The King's facility once again. Of course the previous three women are unavailable to speak with and I'm told by Woman #4, "In order to have a procedure considered for recoding, you'll need to write a letter to Management for their review." *No freaking way!* And I ask to speak with yet *another* manager.

Once again I find myself repeating the conversations I had with Women #1 through #4 *and* I include my recent call with ACME Insurance to Woman #5. At first, she's slightly heated that I'm not willing to write the letter. She then offers to call ACME and discuss my findings with them and places me on hold. Returning to my call she tells me whomever I spoke with at ACME incorrectly informed me about the hospital rates being higher than an independent imaging center. And I'm having to pay for my mammogram due to the fact it was coded as a *diagnostic* versus *preventative.*

"What about the fact I was told ACME had requested my medical records from your facility?"

"I have no idea how Woman #3 came to that conclusion. It says nothing about it in our notes."

"So you're telling me, since I've been diagnosed with Jorge I will no longer receive preventative mammograms? And unless my deductible has been met I will be required to pay for them? I've been told I'm supposed to have these *twice* a year plus ultrasounds, and I'm not allowed *one* as a preventative?"

Woman #5 could hear my distress. "Yes . . . that's what it sounds like." She then added, "I feel like you're being punished for having had Jorge." *Just terrific.* Feeling pity for me, she offers to recode it but can't promise anything, plus she needs to obtain approval to do so. Prior to hanging up I ask for her phone number, simply because I don't want to go through another mind-numbing explanation with a potential Woman #6. Thankfully, she gave her number to me.

A few days later she phoned back with the approval to recode and resubmit it to ACME. The code she changed it to basically means, *"Yes I had breast cancer, but this is my annual exam I'm having."* After changing the code, my account returned to a zero balance and we're now awaiting the response from ACME . . . which could take a couple of months.

During this same period, unbeknownst to me, a claim had been processed for my anesthesiologist, almost an entire year *after* my surgery. How can that be possible? Thankfully he was in-network and the bill was covered 100 percent.

It's September 30th and tomorrow is the start of my favorite time of year—autumn with the holidays soon to follow. However, *drum roll please* . . . in the mail today we receive a form letter from our newly found internist. On the hospital letterhead he's aligned with, in black and white, it reads, *"I wanted to inform you that effective November 13th, 2014, I will no longer be practicing internal medicine at this hospital. I have decided to change my career path and practice another type of medicine."* This letter too is an unsigned copy.

Wow! I don't even know what to think. I haven't found it in me to search for a new oncologist. The thought of researching, scheduling doctor appointments, and flashing my lovelies at even more strangers is stomach-turning. And now, after all the angst we went through to find this new internist, out of the blue he's leaving? He could have simply said he's no longer taking patients, which would have been the admirable thing to do.

Losing two doctors in a period of three months is devastating. Where do we turn? Who do we see in the interim? This is healthcare in the United State of America? The best advice I can offer . . . *Don't get sick!*

Almost as if a reminder I'm due for another mammogram, I receive the response from ACME Insurance regarding the recoding of my May 14th mammo—*nada!* It reflects the same amount towards my deductible which, having not been met, I'm required to pay—*lovely*. Unfortunately, it also reminds me it's time to find an oncologist, primarily because I want this individual overseeing my next mammogram. Ironically, our ophthalmologist and a specialist Ken sees recommended the same oncologist. Separately, they both said this is who they would use or recommend if they or a family member were diagnosed with a Tango. So . . . the week before Thanksgiving I phoned to schedule an appointment—can you believe he had an opening on Tuesday, November 25th? *Go figure.*

My first impression of this Oncologist Man—he's Dr. Cool! He's casual in conversation, funny and banters humorously with my teasing personality. We discuss everything, including the current status of my left arm. I showed him my range of motion, which is 100 percent lifting it over my head but reaching backwards, I'm around 95. He informed me I may not get that range back, but to keep up with my workouts. I could try physical therapy, but truthfully having done so much already, he feels if it does return it will be due to my own sheer will.

We then discuss my current side effects with Tamoxifen. I start with the first week of September, when I had what I consider the worst cramps in my life. It physically hurt to sit down, but ibuprofen quickly put an end to it. That's the only time I've experienced cramps like that since I've started the drug. As one woman wrote online who's taking the Big T, "My ovaries are screaming!" That's exactly what it felt like.

Of course I still get cramps in my extremities which occur in the strangest of places—my forearms, hips, the outside of my calves and feet, even the left side of my chest and left shoulder blade. At night they'll occasionally sneak up on me, but I'm able to work them out. Of course during Pilates, my feet and calves contort and I grit my teeth flexing them, attempting to put an end to those. I've also noticed my joints, especially my ankles and hips, seem to snap, crackle and pop. Truthfully, it's nothing I can't tolerate.

Sadly, my left breast has encapsulated completely from radiation. And just today I've noticed a muscle that looks like a vertical line. It runs for a couple inches starting under the crease of my breast, and even though it can't be seen, I can feel it all the way down over my rib cage, ending at my stomach. We all agree this is due to the encapsulation and once I have my reconstructive surgery it will be a thing of the past.

The most recent nuisance is my left knee has begun to hurt. It feels as if I've hyperextended it. Dr. Cool's only concern is it could be a blood clot and wants me to have an ultrasound. I mentioned the Mad Scientist had performed the test for deep vein thrombosis and that it came back negative. Dr. Cool said that test only lets us know if there is a *tendency* for them, and just to alleviate any concerns, he'd like me to have it checked out.

Continuing on, I inform him my face occasionally flushes, leaving my cheeks a rosy pink. Some days it looks like rosacea and at other times it appears as if I have acne. I've never had issues with either of these; I wonder if this is the onset of hot flashes? Although, I consider myself lucky because I've been told the women in our family only have a slight warming of the body with no sweats. *Thank goodness!*

The last annoyance I've noticed is . . . dang . . . what was it . . . oh yeah, I forget things. It's so frustrating, verging on embarrassing at times. I'll be in the middle of a conversation and completely forget what I'm talking about. Or I can't remember an expression or word and have to play a game of charades or guess what I'm thinking.

I was elated to hear each time I go in for mammograms Dr. Cool will be requesting a diagnostic mammogram *and* sonogram which will be performed on *both* breasts. Of course I informed him about my last mammo. "It's not considered preventative and I'll be required to meet my deductible before insurance kicks in."

His response was simply, "Insurance companies are all different and there's no way to guarantee what will be covered." *I'm learning that.*

Ending our exchange about Tamoxifen, I told him I've recently been toying with the idea of going off of it, simply because I don't want any more side effects. However, Dr. Cool countered, "Most side effects occur within the first 30 days of taking a new drug." Therefore, I shouldn't worry about Ms. Hyde because she would have already reared her hostile head— thank goodness she hasn't!

Dr. Cool further concurred with both The King and the Mad Scientist, I absolutely *should* be taking Tamoxifen. He was adamant I continue with the drug primarily due to my one lymph node involvement. Okay, he has me there and I agree to continue taking it provided the side effects go away once I stop taking it, *and* so long as I don't encounter any *horrendous* side effects.

He assures me once I discontinue the pill, all side effects will cease. We then discussed how long he feels I should be on the drug—five or 10 years. He said he'd like to see how I'm doing at the five-year mark. If I feel as I do today, he'd like me to continue on; if not, I can stop.

I then ask whether I should continue seeing the Medicine Woman and Radiation Man. Unlike The King, Dr. Cool suggests I continue with the Medicine Woman, primarily because her focus is solely on breasts and she's able to catch things others wouldn't. He also commended me for choosing a surgeon whose sole focus is exactly that—breasts! As for the Radiation Man, he's only looking for fallout from treatments. Once he's confident there's no serious side effects he'll more than likely conclude his services.

So there you have it . . . from this point forward, monitoring only. I'm to see Dr. Cool again in six months. As for the mammogram, sonogram and ultrasound, since my deductible has not been met this year, I opted to wait until January to have them. I plan on having my reconstructive surgery in 2015 and would rather not spend the additional $400 it would cost me in 2014. Actually, it'll probably be more since he's added the additional tests.

My mammogram, sonogram and ultrasound were scheduled for January 12th, which ended up being a two-hour appointment, minus the ultrasound for my knee. In my ineptness, I left the order sitting on my desk at home. Without the order, the imaging center couldn't obtain the authorization to have it done.

It appeared this mammo, unlike The King's, seemed to be much more extensive. The tech smashed my breasts every which way, asking me to hold my breath, then not to hold it, all the while scanning away. While the tech was reviewing the mammogram, I decided to take a gander too. That's when I noticed several horizontal white lines in the area where the Lymph-Along-Kid was, around nine in total.

After asking what they were I was told—*are you ready for this?*— "They're staples. It's normal to have them after a lymph node dissection." *What?!* Why on earth wouldn't I have been told that I'd be *stapled* back together?

After speaking to the Medicine Woman about the "staples" she informed me they are titanium clips used to seal the lymphatic channels after my dissection. And no, they won't disappear, they're there for the rest of my life. No wonder my arm hurts like the dickens! But happily, because of them, I have a life!

As for the sonogram—it's the same as an ultrasound, although no one's been able to tell me why the two different names—this one took forever. My right breast is so lumpy bumpy the tech was capturing so many of them I thought for sure I'd require another biopsy, *or two—God forbid*.

Both of these procedures were a bit on the painful side. I didn't realize it, but I bit my bottom lip so hard during the sonogram it turned black and blue. I also became extremely lethargic during the procedure, due to all the stress, I'm sure. Oh the joys of getting older . . . even though it has been a bumpy ride, at least I can say I am!!!

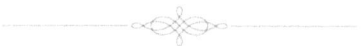

On April 30th I'm given the all clear from the Radiation Man; I no longer require follow-up appointments with him. It's also coming up on my one-year anniversary of being on Tamoxifen. I'm sad to report the side effects have worsened. My calves are unbelievably tight and hard and my joint pain is starting to become intolerable. Everything—wrist, fingers, toes, hips, and knees—hurts. And my tailbone seems to be taking on a deep dull ache while seated. All of my extremities have occasional bouts with cramps, and strangely sometimes my chest, stomach and shoulder blades join in. Worse, a couple have occurred simultaneously—just to the right of where Jorge was located and to the right of my left shoulder blade—leaving me unable to breath!

My fingernails are weak, brittle and peel, and I'm having serious bouts with dizziness. My face at times will flush bright red from my neck up and my upper lip occasionally sweats. I'm also noticing a few pimples, and while attempting to extract them, I'm seeing facial hairs I've never had before. And where I've paid to have hair removed in the past, it's now growing back. And, I can officially add I'm becoming a *sappy* woman— while speaking to a couple of girlfriends, I began discussing an article I had read in the newspaper. I got so choked up, you'd have thought it had happened to me.

To make matters worse, I'll be in the middle of a major project and realize I need something in another room. However, when I get there, I have no recollection whatsoever of the project I'm working on and I start a new one. The other project remains on an indefinite hold until I wander back into that room and find it in limbo land. I also find it difficult to cook because I often forget I have something on the stove top. One of the scarier side effects is when I'm driving; my brain becomes foggy and I feel discombobulated. I'm unsure of where I am or where I'm going. I'll recognize the intersection or street, but have to search deep within to recall why I'm driving there.

On top of all this I've noticed a molar feels funky and have mentioned it to my dentist, who's asked I see an endodontist. This specialist can't find anything wrong with the tooth and feels the culprit may be another tooth that will show itself in six months. In the meantime, I've noticed a stain on my bottom front tooth which I attempt to remove with my electric toothbrush to no avail. A week later I feel as if I'm losing my mind because several of my teeth start to have this funky feeling. Then suddenly *all* of my teeth become sensitive, as if I've just had them whitened and left the product on too long. I start cutting out acidic foods from my diet but the symptoms persist.

Picking up the phone I start dialing my endodontist, but decide to google the symptoms first. Upon doing so I find several chat rooms with women claiming they too have these same symptoms; some go on to say they've been taking Tamoxifen for one year. The response they're given is these side effects are caused by chemo. But since I didn't require chemo I can attest it's a side effect from Tamoxifen.

Delving further into the topic a few women actually have been told their teeth are decaying; even worse, some are having issues with breaking teeth, while others require teeth to be pulled. One individual mentioned her dentist noticed her sinuses were inflamed and suggested that could be the culprit of the decay. While reviewing my X-ray with my endodontist, he too had mentioned my sinuses were inflamed and asked if I had sinus problems. I've *never* had problems with my sinuses.

Shortly after this finding, the joint of my second toe, on both the top and ball of my left foot, have completely swelled up and I'm unable to walk on it for a couple of days. I have no recollection of hurting my foot whatsoever. After a trip to the podiatrist, I'm told its considered pre-dislocation syndrome and, after googling it, I find stiff calves contribute to it.

This is when I shriek *"Mercy!"* All of these aggravating and painful symptoms for an added 3 percent security that Jorge will not return? And there's no guarantee! The side effects are not worth it to me and on May 2nd I discontinue Tamoxifen.

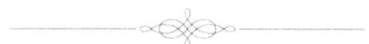

On May 15th I had my biannual appointment with Dr. Cool and on May 21st I had my quarterly meeting with the Medicine Woman. During these appointments I told them about my decision to go off Tamoxifen. None of the doctors were aware of teeth issues while being on the big T; yet, I was able to report after being off the drug for two weeks, the sensitivity has dissipated and the funky feeling of the one molar is now gone.

On May 22nd we met with our Shape Shifter to schedule my first phase of reconstructive surgery. It was initially scheduled for Wednesday, June 17th, but ultimately it had to be changed to Wednesday, June 24th. (You'll know why momentarily.)

Prior to reconstructive surgery, I'm required to have a pre-surgery clearance appointment that includes blood work, a chest X-ray and EKG of my heart. Since Imaging Center #1 would be completing the X-ray, I included the ultrasound on my leg that never happened. However, I'm asked to obtain a new order from Dr. Cool since the other was from November. In doing so, because both of my knees are now bothering me, Dr. Cool has requested both legs be done. Thankfully all was normal and I'm free to go.

On Monday, June 8th I feel unbelievably nauseous and on Tuesday I have major stomach cramps. They were so bad I was curled up in a ball on our couch, eventually causing me to vomit. After doing so I feel much better and it appears everything in my system is back to normal, with the exception I still have the waves of nausea.

Strangely, one week later, exactly on Tuesday morning, I awake to the stomach cramps again. This time I'm in agony for the entire day. I throw up, but it doesn't alleviate the symptoms and I continue on in this manner until I have the dry heaves. During this period, several attempts are made with an Admin Junkie to leave a message for our female internist (we opted for her as our primary practitioner). But, because it's her day off and it's against their rules to contact her, I'm only allowed to leave a message for her nurse, who ultimately poo-pooed my symptoms and suggests I take Pepto-Bismol for my *"upset tummy."* Of course that came right back up and the cramps have worsened.

A few more rounds with the Admin Junkie, who threatens to sic her higher power on me (I'm elated at this suggestion) and, after doing so, I'm told they'll attempt to contact my physician. Ringing me at home, our internist suggests I take a Valium to see if it will alleviate the cramps (luckily I still have 40 of the 50 prescribed by the Mad Scientist). After taking it, I'm able to keep it down for 15 minutes and, even though it came back up, mercifully the cramps somewhat subsided.

I then force myself to take five spoonfuls of chicken broth (strangely, it tastes as if an entire shaker of salt has been dumped in it) and am able to keep it down. My body takes two days to recover from this episode. None of my doctors can figure out the cause. For the remainder of the week I have waves of nausea, headaches and dizzy spells. I'm downing water, Gatorade and anything salty like crazy. I hope the nausea subsides prior to my surgery on the 24th.

During one of the waves of nausea, I'm reminded of the bouts I had after my hysterectomy. I realize Tamoxifen is hormonal therapy and has tricked my body into thinking I'm menopausal. But now that I've gone off of it, my body is confused and has obviously begun producing estrogen and progestogen again. And because of my missing parts, my body doesn't know what to do with it, thus causing the nausea. To add insult to injury I feel like I'm having PMS, not mood swings, but I feel extremely bloated and my ovaries feel as if their getting ready to scream.

I'm now concerned because it's Monday and my surgery is scheduled for Wednesday. God, I hope the stomach cramps don't occur again. I'm coming up on two months of being off the drug and my foot still hurts, as do my joints. I'm in disbelief of the side effects from going off of Tamoxifen; I was expecting this going on the drug, not coming off of it. I pray these side effects go away; I'll be disheartened if I've wreaked lifetime damage to my body.

Thankfully I had no more stomach cramps and was able to have my surgery the morning of June 24th. It was a relatively easy surgery; my Shape Shifter removed my implants and cleaned up the encapsulation and scar tissue. The surgery took a total of 30 minutes. My main concern was my left arm; I didn't want it to become problematic once again. Our Shape Shifter took note and made sure my arm was in a comfortable position prior to surgery.

I remember closing my eyes, and after opening them I wondered when they were going to start the surgery—not realizing it was over. I went home afterwards and was completely fine, extremely ravenous, though, and had no problem eating.

The next morning we went in for my post-op appointment with the Shape Shifter. After greeting us he informs me, when I initially woke from surgery—are you ready for this—I began singing. *I'm so embarrassed!* He said they were all impressed because I stayed on key during my impromptu performance. During my phase two surgery I'm going to request he tape my mouth shut!

We then took a look at his work. Everything looked great, other than the fact I appear to have 80-year-old breasts—officially they're sagging. After pinching them this way and that, our Shape Shifter feels all I need is a breast lift as I have ample breast tissue. And yes he can fix the crevasse where Jorge once was.

Phase two is planned for October. I'm still unsure whether I'll have implants put back in. If I do, they will definitely be on the small side. Ultimately it depends on how I feel about my breasts.

After surgery I've still been craving sodium. The nausea did lessen for a few days, but eventually came back. I think because I'm taking Tylenol with codeine all my aches and pains have subsided. I hope they've gone away, and the drug isn't just masking the issues. I do take a Valium at night before I go to bed, simply due to the fact I can't physically take another bout of stomach cramps. In doing so, my calf muscles seem to be softening. And I'm not having any issues with cramps in my extremities.

I had my annual with Dr. Gyno on June 30th. He said the nausea is definitely hormonal and should eventually subside. He does, however, want to see me again in six months, just to make sure there are no lingering side effects from the Big T.

I have to admit, I was terrified of this surgery. I kept having nightmares that our Shape Shifter, after opening me, informed us Jorge had come back and was throughout my entire body. I think it's due to my upcoming two-year anniversary of being Jorge-free. You see, that's when my mom was informed her Tango had come back and was given six months to live.

Thank God this is over. (Big sigh.) I look forward to returning to my former self!

Looking back to when my *Tango* began, the most shocking truth about healthcare ... it's broken. I don't know if it can or will be fixed during my lifetime—there are simply far too many fingers in the pie neglecting its fundamentals.

Recently, I found myself revisiting the Hippocratic Oath and realized the vision from our past has been lost. The reality of today's medical world? It's completely engrossed with infrastructure and business models hence neglecting the one thing it was put into place for: healing living, feeling human beings.

I then contemplated what changes would have made a difference for me as a patient. Here is the short list:

1. Preventative Healthcare. It's time to refocus our priorities. The Hippocratic Oath even favors it: "prevention is preferable to cure."
2. Personalized Healthcare. Healthcare is cutting edge when it comes to Personalized Medicine (think genetic and microbial signatures). Now it's time to transform the role of the Primary Care Physician— *individualizing the patient*. Your Internist *should* know you, your personality, your lifestyle, your family and most importantly your medical history.
3. Compassionate Healthcare. Providing compassion during a period of the unknown is essential for the healing process. To accomplish this, three things must happen:

a) Health professionals, their staff and patients need a stable and stress-free work environment.
b) Doctors should determine the patient load that enables them to provide accurate and empathetic care.
c) Every individual who works in healthcare (from professionals to their administrative staff) should be educated in understanding the human aspects of an illness—anxiety, fear, and pain.
4. Biopsies. When a biopsy is initially taken a genomic test (if available) should be completed first; the results should then be given to your primary care physician *(see #2 above)*. Knowing the severity of a health misfortune from the get-go will enable the individual and their internist to determine what specialists and protocol best suits you. In turn it will alleviate unwarranted stress, allowing the individual to focus on *healing*.
5. In-Network Facilities. The fees for health professionals, who are contracted by a hospital or medical facility, should fall under the umbrella of that facilities negotiated in-network insurance rates.
6. Prescription Drugs. *Seriously?!* These companies are supposed to be in the business to help *heal* and in some instances *save lives*, not inflict financial ruin.

I've been astonished to learn how many people have similar health misfortunes. Maybe it's because technology has progressed to the point it's catching things before they turn catastrophic. Nonetheless, when you least expect it, you'll encounter others who are or have Tangoed. It's quite stunning how we support one another, sharing our fears, concerns and ultimately our expectations and hopes for our future.

Lastly, I'd be remiss if I didn't discuss the sexual aspect of what one experiences. What I can tell you is I feel broken as a woman. Maybe this is due to my breast being misshapen, or the fact I've lost a portion of my breast. And even though Ken assures me it's now his *favorite* breast, I have to admit I feel uneasy when he kisses me there. It's a sad reminder life will never be the same.

During an intimate moment, Ken happened to glance up and noticed I had my eyes squeezed tightly shut. Immediately he was concerned he was hurting me. I assured him, "No, I just hate this is what I am now."

"Apryl . . . *THIS* does not define you—you beat it!!! And I especially love this scar because it means I have you that much longer!" as he traced its thin gray line with his finger.

It was shortly after this period when Ken and I were on a date sipping martinis after a concert. We were seated next to a woman, her son and her sister, all visiting from out of town. At some point during our conversation, the subject of Tangos came up; she too had danced. Having exchanged contact information, she later sent a beautiful unsolicited note, and described the sentiments I currently feel about my body.

> *From:* Emma
> *Sent:* Monday, March 02, 2015 4:02 PM
> *To:* Apryl
> *Subject:* Life after Breast Cancer
>
> *Apryl,*
>
> *It was a pleasure to meet you and Ken last week. You are truly a delight! My sister, son, and I enjoyed the rest of our stay in your sunny state and were not excited to return to our less than balmy temperatures.*
>
> *I was thinking about our conversation and our experiences with breast cancer, and I am always amazed at how sharing a similar event can instantly create a bond between women. It was easy to feel the support you have from Ken, and I truly believe that is special.*

This disease is such a sensual deflator for us as women, since it is our bodies that get physically altered, but I know there is light at the end of the tunnel to regain that sexy feeling. Stay with the reconstruction program and focus your sights on the new body you and Ken will get to share. I will be waiting for your book to be published. The world needs to know there is life after breast cancer!

Wishing you all the best!

Emma

    Throughout this Tango you can and will find loving support. Actually, I highly recommend *prior* to starting your Tango, recruit help from loved ones—a spouse, sibling, son, daughter, extended family and friends. Yes, you will require more than one person during this Tango. It can become extremely challenging for family and caretakers—often one and the same—since they too will be required to put their lives on hold. Their normal day-to-day activities will become burdensome and in some instances overwhelming.

    Another reason I suggest you enlist the help of more than one person during this time is because a Tango takes a toll on everyone, not only mentally, but physically too. I know this because Ken, in August of 2014, experienced his own health issue due to all the stress he was experiencing. It's imperative these individuals take care of their health too—keeping up with exercise and the simple things in life that bring comfort and relaxation. Simply put, having additional loved ones around to take turns during hospital stays, doctors' appointments, and even everyday chores around the home is the best support you can offer a caregiver.

    Remember, others before you have taken this beaten path, and I can attest it truly is not the end. Instead, look at it as an awakening of who you are, where you are going and appreciate the fragility of life. The best thing you can do during this time . . . surround yourself with loved ones.

    And yes, you do have a choice when it comes to life. You can either see its drudgeries or you can choose to see the splendor life has to offer! Eventually all of this will seem as if it happened a million years ago.

A Final Note

When I was first diagnosed with Jorge I was desperate to read about what I could expect. I wanted to learn as much as I could about this *Tango* from treatments, feelings, what I would be experiencing, the types of doctors I required. I wanted to know *EVERYTHING*! And honestly I didn't feel like one of those extraordinary people seen occasionally in the media embracing the illness with open arms.

After researching books on the subject, I found they could be divided into several categories: "My *Spiritual* Journey," "My Journal," "Survival Guides," "Memoirs of *Someone Famous*" (we're not privy to their preferential treatments or makeup artists), along with a plethora of doctors writing about "Diets for Breast Cancer" and worse, stone cold medical books. None of which addressed what I was *feeling* as a living being, nor what it was going to be like to face this alternate world. During this same period, I spoke with several women who had breast cancer but none could recall in detail what their treatments were like.

My hopes were further shattered by the images we're bombarded with by the media. The illusion that a little breast cancer fairy would swoop me up and fly me away to her ethereal world, all the while sprinkling me with pink healing fairy dust. It wasn't until I was midway through my *Tango* that I realized, no one knew really anything more than I did. Thus my *Tango with Cancer* began.

I'd like to make something very clear: this is not nor will it ever be a *vanity* project. Back in January 2014, before I started writing, I actually began to feel the *"Spiritual"* phase we often hear people speak of. All the craziness began seeping from my mind and I actually started to forget many of the horrific sordid details. I felt a sort of lightening of my soul as if I had just crossed the Sahara Desert with an eight-ounce bottle of water, and lived to tell about it!

It was around that time my phone started ringing. My Inquisitive Minds were asking if I would be willing to forward my e-mails to a friend of theirs who had had just been diagnosed with a *Tango*. Like me, others weren't interested in the retelling of a "journey," but instead were desperate to hear what they were going to be up against from someone who had experienced it firsthand. It was then I realized there was a need for this type of book and I began compiling my e-mails. I was shocked at how much I had already begun to forget but reading them brought it back to life.

The time it has taken me to write this book has been one of the most excruciating periods in my life and one I never care to revisit. Every chapter I have written has caused me to relive this experience in its entirety. At one point I thought *forget it, it's not worth it*—thinking it wasn't doing me, nor would it do *anyone* any good. But I persevered . . . primarily for those who find themselves at the beginning of their own *Tango*. I wish someone had chronicled their experience in detail, in this fashion, for me. I would have done many things differently if I had a book like this as a resource.

I feel this book goes beyond my type of *Tango*; you can apply my experience to any unexpected health misfortune. The most important factor I have taken away from this encounter is how much *compassion* plays a role in healing. And speaking of healing, now it's time for me! I'm ready to put this Tango in the past and focus on my family, myself and my life . . . there will *not* be a sequel to this book!

Acknowledgements

Ken, I can't imagine where I'd be without you. You have been my rock, my will, and at times the only hope I had. Thank you for your constant prodding of *'You can and will'* during this unfortunate twist of fate—a terrifying period peppered with uncertainties and torment. All too often you magnanimously gave of your inner-strength for me to cling to when I had none. And through it all, you've held steadfast to the promise you made my mother—her dying wish for me—and for that I'm in awe. As for this book, where do I start? The constant reminder and reliving of what was, has been as difficult on you as it has been for me. Thank you once again for your belief in a talent I never knew I had—I love you.

Kimberly, Cionne, Judy, Ed, Pat, Stanley, Cindy, Esperanza, Anne, Becca, Beth, Linda and Danny, thank you for supporting me during a time when it was hard to find my smile. And to all my friends who found the time to brighten my day . . . thank you.

Ken, Pat, Catherine, Billie Jo, Scott, Dino and a couple others who were willing to take time out of your busy schedules to review this not so pleasant reality-of-life book—thank you for the extraordinary encouragement, advice and feedback!

My dear friend and mentor Catherine . . . you have left me speechless! You have freely and selflessly offered guidance and support. The many, many phone calls answering the mundane. Helping me navigate this other world known as publishing. *(Yikes!)*

A special thank you to Craig for your knowledge of the programs required to create the cover art—you are an amazingly talented individual!

Lastly, I'd like to thank those doctors, technicians and administrative staff who know how to care with compassion—specifically: Marc, Joseph, Clare, Jimmy, Carol, Dohna, Brittney and TC. You listened from the heart and did your best to guide me through the unknown—I'll be forever grateful for your kindness.

About the Author

APRYL ALLEN has written and recorded two award-winning albums, *Morningstar* and *Shape Shifter*. As a member of the Comanche Nation she is actively involved to preserve her tribe's dying language and stories handed down. Her current project, *Shape Shifter (Na ~~Unu~~ Nahai)*, takes these narratives and weaves them into a fictional Native American trilogy based on historical fantasy. The Comanche Nation has acknowledged her efforts by proclamation on November 7, 2008 naming it "Apryl Allen Day." As a survivor of breast cancer and child abuse, Apryl views life as sacred—a gift we should all cherish. Her dream, as a survivor and member of a dying culture, is to be a voice that echoes throughout time. *Nasutam̶,̶ nasutam̶*.̶ . . (Remember, remember . . .) She lives in Phoenix, Arizona.

Albums

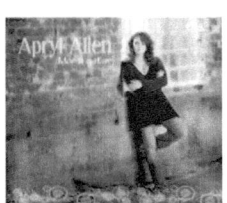 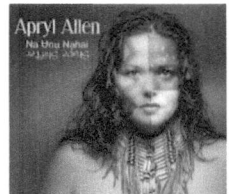

Coming soon to a Bookshelf or eBook near you

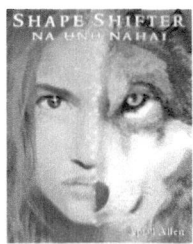

Visit
www.AprylAllen.com